Twin Block Functional Therapy

Second Edition

To Sheila, Fiona and Alastair for their love, support and understanding over the years during the development of the Twin Block technique. This book is based principally on the treatment of children, and I make a special dedication to our grandchildren:

With love
To Rebecca, Cameron, Alastair, Joanna and Ellie

Commissioning Editor: Michael Parkinson
Project Development Manager: Lynn Watt
Project Manager: Frances Affleck
Designer: Judith Wright, George Ajayi

Twin Block Functional Therapy
Applications in Dentofacial Orthopaedics
Second Edition

William J Clark BDS DDO

Orthodontist, Fife, UK

With contributions from

Gary G Baker DDM, Orthodontist, Vancouver, Canada

A Gordon Kluzak DDS LDS (M)RCDC, Paedodontist, Calgary, Canada

Forbes Leishman BDS DDOrth MscO, Orthodontist, Auckland, New Zealand

Christine Mills DDS MS, Assistant Clinical Professor, University of British Columbia, Vancouver, Canada

G D Singh DDSc PhD BDS, Associate Professor, San Juan, Puerto Rico

Mel Taskey BSc, DDS, MSc, Prosthodontist, Edmonton, Canada

Foreword by
Professor T Graber Clinical Professor of Orthodontics, University of Illinois, Chicago, USA

Illustrated by Frank Dingwall

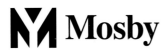

EDINBURGH LONDON NEW YORK PHILADELPHIA ST LOUIS SYDNEY TORONTO 2002

MOSBY
An imprint of Elsevier Science Limited

First edition 1995
Second edition 2002

ISBN 0723 43170 1

British Library Cataloguing in Publication Data
A catalogue record for this book is available from the British Library

Library of Congress Cataloging in Publication Data
A catalog record for this book is available from the Library of Congress

Note
Medical knowledge is constantly changing. As new information
becomes available, changes in treatment, procedures, equipment and
the use of drugs become necessary. The authors and the publishers
have taken care to ensure that the information given in this text is accurate and up to date. However, readers are strongly advised to confirm
that the information, especially with regard to drug usage, complies
with the latest legislation and standards of practice.

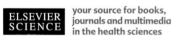
**ELSEVIER
SCIENCE**
your source for books,
journals and multimedia
in the health sciences
www.elsevierhealth.com

The
publisher's
policy is to use
**paper manufactured
from sustainable forests**

Typeset by Palimpsest Book Production Limited,
Polmont, Stirlingshire, UK
Printed in Spain

Foreword

It is never too late to give up on your prejudices
Henry David Thoreau

As we enter the new millennium, it is only fitting and proper to ask, 'What is new?' Of course, what is new is not always the best. As a long time student of orthodontic history, I had the rare opportunity to associate with the movers and shakers of orthodontics, since I first met Benno E. Lischer, orthodontic pioneer and Dean in 1935, when I entered Washington University. I was fortunate to have Edmund Wuerpel, the great artist associate of Edward H. Angle, as a teacher of art appreciation after I entered the university. Facial form was my religion. I think my time-tested perspective should be objective. I have seen many approaches, touted as 'the latest and best', disappear in the dust of time, even as some early orthodontic philosophies have waxed and waned, only to appear brighter and stronger than ever, as evidence-based treatment confirmed the claims made. Never was this more true than in dentofacial ortho-paedics and growth guidance of the craniofacial complex. Truly, the test of time is the one to apply.

It is now abundantly clear in our field that the most important consideration is not the tool, but why you use it, how you use it, when you use it, for how long you use it and do the therapeutic results stand the test of time years later?

Early pioneers were mechanically oriented. Particularly in North America, under the influence of Edward H. Angle, the movement of teeth was the overwhelming consideration and American mechanical ingenuity was not lacking when it came to efficient tooth moving appliances. But if we know anything now, it is that orthodontists must be applied biol-ogists. The interrelationships of morphogenetic pattern, of teeth, bone and neuromuscular components, determine to a large degree what we can or cannot do. Basal jaw mal-relationships in three planes of space comprise a significant percentage of orthodontic practices. Space age materials in brackets, bands, wires and plastics make the Procrustean bed of mechanotherapy more efficient. But we cannot ignore the biologic continuum. A sober look at adults who had orthodontic treatment earlier, with subsequent relaps-ing malocclusion characteristics, begs the question, 'Was it all worth it?'

Medicine and dentistry are under an increasingly critical assessment of our professions. Prince Charles said in 1998, 'Medicine remains too often one sided in its approach' and, again 'Science has tried to assume a monopoly, even a tyranny over our understanding.'

The vaunted legal profession has cast a jaundiced eye on our efforts, looking for iatrogenic responses to our ministra-tions and making off with an increasing number of lottery type awards, of which they get one third. What a breath of fresh air of objectivity Dr Clark has provided in this book, while still presenting the technical details in lucid prose, with case reports to demonstrate specific problems and solutions.

This new edition by William Clark is the culmination of a lifetime of dedication to answering the biologic chal-lenges, as well as the mechanotherapy demands. I was fortu-nate to do the Foreword for the previous edition of this superb book and thought it was surely the latest and best, but the exhaustive and exhausting revision, incorporating the latest research from world class clinicians and researchers not only makes the appliance details easier to understand and use, but provides a *raison d'être* and biologi-cally balanced perspective for long-term assessment of treat-ment results. As an author of books myself, I can well appreciate the many thousands of hours devoted to the new edition, the consummate detail in the hundreds of cephalo-metric tracings done by him personally, the fine tuning of myriad details. Read, learn, enjoy and let your patients benefit!

A brief résumé of the chapter contents gives an overview of the extensive coverage of diagnostic and therapeutic aspects, quoting pertinent research to validate the concepts.

Chapter 1 on the art of orthodontics discusses the philo-sophical challenge, in that art and science are of equal proportions in our field. He stresses that this was recognised by Angle at the turn of the last century:

The study of orthodontia is indissolubly connected with that of art as related to the human face.

Edmund Wuerpel, the artist, played an important role in the courses taught by Angle.

An important distinction is made between orthodontics and dentofacial orthopaedics. We cannot serve our patients' needs with tooth movement alone.

In Chapter 2, design and construction are described and profusely illustrated with excellent drawings, making it easy to understand, even for the neophyte. Ample case reports demonstrate appliance use and results. The clever merging of profile views of patients, before, during and after, shows the significant facial changes produced. Dr Clark recognises the limitations of the superimposing of lateral cephalograms on the anterior cranial base, which ignores the spheno-occipital synchondrosis and growth changes that can occur during treatment. He ascribes to the approach of Eugene Coben and Robert Ricketts on the use of nasion–basion as the cranial base plane. I strongly recommend this approach for both research and clinical studies! It is high time that we get out of the nasion–basion rut of the last century. Current radiographic techniques make visualisation of basion, the posterior base plane terminus, easy to pick up.

Chapter 3 on form and function again emphasises the need for a broader diagnostic perspective than provided by two-dimensional lateral headfilms. Topics covered are the role of extraction therapy, therapeutic limitations of the genetic paradigm, bone remodelling response to functional appliances, development of the temporomandibular joint, evolution and limitations of functional appliances, objectives, bite registration, activation, and control of all sagittal and vertical dimensions. The acronym is WYSIWYG.

Chapter 4 is current and choice research, and clinical analysis, of growth studies in experimental animals. The landmark research of McNamara, Harvold and others has been validated by more sophisticated armamentaria and methodology. A long neglected aspect is the influence of functional appliances on the glenoid fossa. We have concentrated on the mandible, ignoring the membranous temporal bone. The recent (2000) visco-elastic hypothesis of Voudouris supports changes noted, and is much easier to understand than ascribing changes to muscle attachments alone.

Chapter 5 on diagnosis and treatment planning is a magnificent exercise that is bound to help the reader, regardless of the appliance used. We are dealing with a three-dimensional problem and the author stresses control of all three dimensions in proper sequence.

Chapter 6 carries the diagnostic discipline a step forward as the Clark Cephalometric Analysis, based on the research and clinical experiences of Broadbent, Coben, Ricketts, Bimler, McNamara and others. This chapter alone justifies the book, as the implications transcend functional appliances.

Chapter 7 is devoted to appliance design and construction and is well illustrated to prevent any misunderstanding.

Chapter 8 discusses treatment of Class II, Division 1 deep overbite problems. The Twin Block design and use are beautifully adapted to handling multi-dimension malocclusion challenges. It is clear that we are not a generation of profiles, as Sam Weinstein once critically noted, with our obsession on anteroposterior correction.

Chapter 9 elaborates on treatment in the mixed dentition. This is one of the most rapidly growing aspects of skeletal malocclusion correction, as current research clearly shows the beneficial effects. Long term records show the justification of properly chosen and managed skeletal and neuromuscular problems.

Chapter 10 on Combination therapy—fixed and functional treatment—was important in the previous edition (it is not 'either' or!) It has been updated, again with evidence-based research and choice case reports.

Chapter 11 on the Twin Block traction technique shows a neat way of employing extraoral force to withhold maxillary downward and forward movement with the Concorde facebow, developed by Dr Clark. Does it work? Look at the accompanying case reports and decide for yourself!

Chapter 12 addresses the open bite and vertical problems. The Achilles heel of most functional appliances is control of the maxilla. With time-tested and proven orthopaedic results from headgear, it just makes good sense to control vertical and horizontal maxillary development, with its beneficial effects on open bite cases, excessive vertical dimension etc.

A plethora of beautiful, meticulously drawn cephalometric tracings of treated cases demonstrates the potential of vertical control. A short section on rare earth magnetic augmentation, à la Dellinger, shows that this is, indeed, a most adaptive approach. This is covered more extensively in Chapter 19.

Chapter 13 is devoted to Class II, Division 2 treatment. My own experience with this category of malocclusion demonstrates that predominance of the morphogenetic pattern lasts throughout life. (My wife had this treated three times and the lateral incisors came out, the central incisors moved lingually without wearing a Hawley biteplane. Of course, a modified Twin Block appliance can perform the same function. I am sure Charles Tweed was thinking about Class II, Division 2 malocclusion when he said, 'Retention is forever!')

Chapter 14 covers Class III malocclusion treatment with the reverse Twin Block appliances. Perhaps here, more than any other category, the limitations of removable appliances is apparent. However, with extraoral force, with early growth guidance, with elimination of 'convenience bites', Twin Blocks can be used successfully in mild to moderate Class III cases. The consummate clinical skill of Dr Clark is apparent in the accompanying case reports.

Chapter 15 is a broader discussion of differential diagnosis, as the clinician explores the orthodontic, orthopaedic or surgical approaches. With exponentially decreasing insurance coverage for orthognathic surgery these days, the last alternative is less likely. Being innovative with a combination of fixed and removable appliance can produce surprisingly good results.

Chapter 16 addresses the problem of correction of crowding. Combination fixed/functional therapy can be the way to go, given a proper diagnosis.

The use of extraction therapy, explicitly with Twin Blocks is explored in Chapter 17. Obviously it ties in with the previous two chapters!

Occasionally, we are confronted with facial asymmetry, along with a dental malocclusion. Can Twin Blocks be used to correct unilateral problems? Ample case reports in Chapter 18 show the diversity of Twin Blocks in successful treatment.

Chapter 19 explores the use of rare earth magnets in more detail, as they are incorporated with Twin Blocks. They can assist in correction in all three planes of space and there is some evidence of enhancement of tissue response. This is surely true in de-impaction of lingually malposed maxillary canines, as our own research shows!

Chapter 20 on adult treatment shows specific problems that are amenable to Twin Block appliances usually in combination with fixed mechanics.

Chapter 21 takes advantage of a well known mechanism for controlling and correcting TMJ problems—forward posturing of the mandible is amazingly easy with Twin Blocks, and vertical control is also feasible. The case reports supplied by Dr Mel Taskey support the concept that it is not only the tool but also how you use it.

Chapter 22 , a projection into the future, is a fascinating brainstorming voyage by Dr Clark on problems of arch development, innovative fixed lingual appliances with unique attachments like his Trombone appliance, the Transforce maxillary lingual appliance, which is exceedingly stable and efficient in maxillary arch expansion, and fixed Twin Blocks, cemented for specific problems. The fascinating pre-fabricated occlusal inclined planes must be seen in the illustrations to appreciate their potential. Studying the case reports in this chapter, as all others, is time spent exceedingly well.

Chapter 23 is a joy to behold, as well as read. The title alone would attract you, 'The flat earth concept of facial growth.' What a devastatingly correct appraisal of our archaic concepts, prejudices and dogma—all orthodontic residents should have this alone as required reading! Three dimensional diagnosis for the present, with much of the material based on Jim Moss's three-dimensional facial reconstructions is no longer an option, but a necessity.

Chapter 24 is entitled 'Growth response to Twin Block treatment,' but it is a potpourri of related subjects. The Twin Block traction technique research is reported. Evaluation of the value of mean growth changes in treating individual patients, the relationship with fixed appliances, reference to contributions to this book by Mills and Kluzak of Canada and Leishman of New Zealand, a comparison of the Bass, bionator and Twin Blocks, related to control; comparison with the FR-2 and controls, treatment effects and post treatment stability make this a valuable prelude for the conclusion section. With tongue in cheek, with all the ways of harnessing growth, Bill Clark finishes with a quote from an Epistle to a young friend, by Robert Burns.

To catch Dame Fortune's golden smile
Assiduous wait upon her,
And gather gear by every wile,
That's justified by honour.

Epistle to a Young Friend,
Robert Burns, 1759–1796

T.M. GRABER

Preface to the second edition

I am too much of a sceptic to deny the possibility of anything.
Thomas Henry Huxley 1825–1895

It is surprising that after a century of investigation of functional orthopaedic techniques, opinions still vary regarding the effectiveness of orthopaedic techniques in promoting or modifying dentofacial growth and development. Limitations, based on past experience, continue to restrict the teaching and practice of orthopaedics.

During the twentieth century two areas of orthodontic philosophy consistently failed to be resolved, in spite of all efforts to clarify the underlying principles by clinical and academic research.

The first was the question 'To extract or not to extract ?' The pendulum swung from Angle's non-extraction philosophy at the beginning of the century through the Tweed and Begg extraction philosophies in mid century, until during the last two decades, a non-extraction approach gained further popularity in clinical practice.

Secondly, the orthopaedic response to functional therapy has been questioned frequently on the basis of results published in the literature. Academic study is largely dependent on statistical analysis and evidence-based research. Inevitably, there is a time lag between the development of new clinical techniques, and their investigation and acceptance by scientific investigation, New research is providing convincing evidence to support the value of orthopaedic techniques using full time appliances to influence the functional environment of the developing dentition, and to produce significant improvements in the pattern of facial growth. One of the objectives in the second edition of this book is to update information on the effects of Twin Blocks on growth modification.

Functional orthopaedic techniques developed mainly in Europe during the twentieth century, and in the past Europeans have enjoyed wider experience of these techniques than colleagues in North America. At the beginning of a new millennium, however, it is relevant to note that the title of the *American Journal of Orthodontics* was altered in 1985 to include dentofacial orthopaedics, and the American Dental Association changed the name of the specialty to 'Orthodontics and Dentofacial Orthopedics'. This represents official recognition within the specialty, and in the dental profession as a whole, of the importance of orthopaedics within the field of orthodontics. The next step in the evolution of orthopaedic technique is to resolve any remaining doubts regarding the efficacy of an orthopaedic approach and to improve techniques in order to combine the benefits of orthodontic and orthopaedic treatment.

WILLIAM J. CLARK, 2002

Preface to the first edition

The opinions expressed in this book are based on the author's experience over 34 years in orthodontic practice. This is not intended to be a circumscribed view; the author acknowledges that other practitioners may differ in some respects but hopes that the material presented may help to integrate the orthodontic and orthopaedic objectives of our profession.

Abnormal musculoskeletal development is frequently the fundamental cause of dental malocclusion. The treatment objective in the growing child with a resultant skeletal discrepancy changes from an orthodontic approach, aiming to correct the dental irregularity, to an orthopaedic approach, where the objective is to correct the underlying skeletal abnormality. This difference in emphasis reflects the existence of two distinct schools of thought in evaluating the aims of orthodontic and dental orthopaedic treatment.

The purpose of this book is to advance the recognition of dentofacial orthopaedics as the treatment of choice for correction of malocclusion that results from abnormal skeletal development. The present philosophical basis of orthodontic and orthopaedic technique is examined with reference to current practice and research.

This book extends the armamentarium of dental orthopaedic treatment by introducing the Twin Block appliance system. Twin Blocks are designed for full-time wear in order to overcome problems associated with conventional functional appliances that were designed in one piece to fit the teeth in upper and lower dental arches. Twin Blocks are more comfortable, more aesthetic and more efficient than alternative functional appliances. The emphasis in this book is to provide practical advice and instruction that is of direct value to the teacher, practitioner and student of orthodontics.

The Twin Block technique is demonstrated in case reports to give guidance on diagnosis, treatment planning, and clinical management of the various types of appliances involved in the system. The clinical approach to treatment is supported by scientific investigation and analysis of patients treated consecutively, which evaluates the dentofacial changes that result from treatment with the Twin Block technique.

The purpose in presenting the material in this fashion is to provide both comprehensive analysis and instruction in a well-illustrated format that is easy to understand. Then the principles of diagnosis and therapy will in turn more readily provide a sound basis for clinical application of the techniques described.

WILLIAM J. CLARK, 1995

Acknowledgements

This book is based on a new approach to functional orthopaedics in clinical orthodontic practice. I wish to acknowledge first the cooperation of many excellent patients and their primary role in the development of the Twin Block technique, not least Colin Gove, the first patient I treated with Twin Blocks in 1977.

My dental technician, James Watt, has made my removable appliances for the past 35 years, and continues to do so. He made the first Twin Blocks and I should like to acknowledge his invaluable contribution and support in providing the expert technical help I needed to develop the Twin Block technique.

It has been interesting and challenging to travel and teach throughout the world, and to all the people who have offered their support and encouragement over the years I offer my sincere thanks. There are too many to mention individually in this short acknowledgement. My former partner, Ken Lumsden, currently Chairman of the British Orthodontic Society, was among the first to adopt the technique, and has always been unfailing in his support. I thank also my colleagues in the British Orthodontic Society.

I should also like to acknowledge those who offered support in the early days and helped to champion Twin Block therapy. Hans Eirew, former president of the British Association of Orthodontists and a leader in the cause of dentofacial orthopaedics, has been a great friend who offered unstinting and eloquent support over the years. He came to the first ever Twin Block course in 1979 with Peter Cousins, another past president and friend, who offered me my first position as assistant in orthodontic practice in 1961.

Jim McNamara, Tom Graber and Jim Broadbent are distinguished orthodontic teachers who have espoused the benefits of functional therapy, and I am grateful to them for their support over many years. Jim McNamara was the first orthodontist in America to express interest and to recognise the relationship of Twin Blocks to the animal research studies that have contributed so much to our knowledge of the biological processes involved in orthopaedic treatment. As a result he organised my earliest lecture tour of American Universities in 1983, when I also received support from Ram Nanda and Bill Profitt.

My first exposure to large audiences in North America and Canada was organised by John Witzig, culminating in 1991 with the first ever teleconference in orthodontics, when I presented a one day course to a live audience in Chicago that was broadcast by satellite to 25 cities throughout America and Canada. This was undoubtedly responsible for the wider adoption of the technique, and contributed to its subsequent worldwide popularity. The spread of new ideas is dependent on this type of initiative, and for that I am indebted to the late John Witzig.

In preparing the text of this book, including the first edition, I wish to thank Tom Graber, Jim McNamara, Hans Eirew, Terry Spahl and Ken Lumsden for their constructive criticism of the text. Jim Moss of University College, London was generous in providing illustrations of his excellent research on facial growth.

Tom Graber has been most generous in his support and is always a wise counsel in matters relating to functional orthopaedics. Tom was mainly responsible for changing the title of the *American Journal of Orthodontics* to include 'Dentofacial Orthopedics', recognising the importance of orthopaedics in the future development of the specialty of orthodontics. I thank him for his kind contribution of the foreword to this book.

In producing a second edition I am especially indebted to outstanding contributions from my professional colleagues. Christine Mills runs an excellent orthodontic practice in Vancouver, and has completed valuable research on the growth response to Twin Block therapy. Gordon Kluzak came to Scotland many years ago to learn about Twin Blocks, and was the first practitioner in the North American continent to adopt the technique in his orthopaedic practice in Calgary. His colleague and friend, Mel Taskey, duly applied Twin Blocks in the treatment of temporo-mandibular joint therapy in his practice in Edmonton, specialising in the treatment of all types of chronic TMD syndrome. Gary Baker is the fourth Canadian to offer a significant contribution, having developed an excellent approach in his dental practice in Vancouver to combine Twin Blocks with fixed appliances in an integrated orthodontic/ orthopaedic approach.

David Singh is a researcher with an excellent reputation in the study of facial growth and development using finite element analysis and similar techniques. We worked in collaboration in the University of Dundee to investigate mandibular growth changes, and to identify significant areas and mechanisms of growth related to Twin Block therapy. He has made a valuable contribution enabling us to understand better the effects of Twin Blocks on mandibular growth.

Last but not least, Forbes Leishman attended the first ever Twin Block course and subsequently emigrated to New Zealand, where he has successfully combined Twin Blocks with fixed appliances in his orthodontic practice in Auckland, producing some remarkable results. He is an experienced and consumate clinician, able to utilise the benefits of combination therapy.

In their own individual way all the contributors are expert on Twin Block technique in their environment of practice or research. I thank them sincerely for their contributions.

Technical support

Thanks are due to Martin Brusse and Rocky Mountain Orthodontics for their support in producing the Trombone and Lingual Arch Developer.

I am indebted to Lindsay Brehm and Steve Huff at Ortho Organizers for excellent technical support in designing the Trans Force series of lingual appliances for arch development, and for new initiatives in producing and testing prototypes for Fixed Twin Blocks.

I have enjoyed valuable contributions from Steve Franseen, an expert in all aspects of appliance design and development. Steve Franseen and Steve Huff are responsible for the design drawings of appliances which are undergoing clinical testing. They are the back-room boys of orthodontics, the engineers who design and manufacture products to our specification. These innovations are illustrated in Chapter 22, entitled 'New Horizons in Orthodontics'.

I am grateful for the assistance of Jim McDonald, in his capacity as Dental Dean of the Royal College of Surgeons, Edinburgh. We are currently engaged in a research programme for clinical testing of the Trans Force appliances, progressing to the development and testing of Fixed Twin Blocks.

Illustrations

The computerised diagrams and tracings in both editions of this book were prepared by Frank Dingwall, whose skill and dedication I wish to acknowledge in recognition of his patience and expertise. Frank is responsible for the composite profiles to illustrate growth changes relating to the facial profile during treatment and out of retention. He has a special talent, as can be seen from the many illustrations. Frank also taught me my computer skills, allowing me to convert all my presentations to computer. Several years ago he introduced me to digital photography; the photographs in the chapter on new horizons in orthodontics are therefore by digital camera.

Thanks are also due for the additional drawings in chapter 2 provided by William Brudon under the direction of Jim McNamara in the University of Michigan. The contributors mentioned above have provided photographs and cephalometric records, allowing us to compile the illustrations for their case reports.

Contents

Errata

p.87 1st column, line 10. The sentence should read, 'This is a disadvantage'.

p.338 Fig. 23.4B. The percentage in the scale should read 4%.

p.348 Fig. 24.4. T1-T4 = 54 months.

p.355 Table 24.7, 2nd column. Mandibular length of Twin Block should read 4.8 mm.

p.360 Ortholab. B.V., Netherlands does not hold a license for the design and construction of Twin Blocks.

CHAPTER 1

The Art of Orthodontics

INTRODUCTION

Orthodontics presents a philosophical challenge in that both art and science are of equal importance. A quotation of Edward Angle (1907), from the turn of the 20th century, is still pertinent today:

> *The study of orthodontia is indissolubly connected with that of art as related to the human face. The mouth is a most potent factor in making or marring the beauty and character of the face, and the form and beauty of the mouth largely depend on the occlusal relations of the teeth.*
>
> *Our duties as orthodontists force upon us great responsibilities, and there is nothing which the student of orthodontia should be more keenly interested than in art generally, and especially in its relation to the human face, for each of his efforts, whether he realises it or not, makes for beauty or ugliness; for harmony or inharmony; for perfection or deformity of the face. Hence it should be one of his life studies.*

Although orthodontics has gained wide recognition by the general public, it can be argued that the term 'orthodontics' is self-limiting and does not describe adequately the wider aesthetic and holistic aims of a speciality that is as concerned with harmonious facial balance as with a balanced functional occlusion.

The true art of the speciality lies in its pursuit of ideals in the arrangement and function of the dentition, but never at the expense of damaging facial aesthetics. Beauty is a precious, indefinable quality that is expressed in balanced facial proportions. Facial balance and harmony are goals of orthodontic treatment, of equal importance to a balanced functional occlusion.

Dental chess

Orthodontics may be thought of as the dental equivalent of chess. The analogy is appropriate in many respects. The game is played with 32 ivory pieces that are arranged symmetrically about the midline on a board in two equal and opposing armies.

The opening moves are crucial in determining the strategy of the game. From the outset, the game is won or lost depending on the strategy of development of the individual pieces. Indeed, these opening moves can determine whether the game is eventually won or lost.

It is a mistake in chess to become obsessed with the individual pieces. Rather, one must take a broader view and look at the game plan as a whole to maintain a balanced position of the pieces on the board in order to achieve mutual protection and support.

In dental chess, the board is analogous to the facial skeleton, which is of fundamental importance in supporting the individual pieces. As the orthodontic chess game progresses and the dental pieces are developed, the board may become overcrowded, with pieces converging upon each other, so that even the most experienced player may at times sacrifice pieces only to realise as the game develops that the gambit was miscalculated.

Only after the passage of time, on proceeding to the end game, can the success of the strategy be evaluated. Successful treatment is judged in terms of facial balance, aesthetic harmony and functional stability in the end result. One may conclude that the objectives of treatment have been achieved only when the final post-treatment balance of facial and dental harmony is observed.

Orthodontics and dental orthopaedics

An essential distinction exists between the terms 'orthodontics' and 'dental orthopaedics'. They represent a fundamental variance in approach to the correction of dentofacial abnormalities.

By definition, orthodontic treatment aims to correct the dental irregularity. The alternative term 'dental orthopaedics' was suggested by the late Sir Norman Bennett, and although this is a wider definition than 'orthodontics' it still does not convey the objective of improving facial development.

The broader description of 'dentofacial orthopaedics' conveys the concept that treatment aims to improve not only dental and orthopaedic relationships in the stomatognathic system but also facial balance. The adoption of a wider definition has the advantage of extending the horizons of the profession as well as educating the public to appreciate the benefits of dentofacial therapy in more comprehensive aesthetic terms.

A fundamental question that we must address in diagnosis is: 'Does this patient require orthodontic treatment or orthopaedic treatment, or a combination of both, and to what degree?' Alternatively, does the patient require dentofacial surgery, or to what extent can orthopaedic treatment be considered as an alternative to surgery?

An orthodontic approach aims to correct the dental irregularity and is inappropriate in the treatment of what are essentially skeletal discrepancies. By definition, orthodontics must either be combined with dentofacial orthopaedics or maxillofacial surgery in the correction of significant skeletal abnormality.

If the malocclusion is primarily related to a musculoskeletal discrepancy we should select an orthopaedic approach to treatment. It is in the treatment of muscle imbalance and skeletal disproportion that functional orthopaedic appliances come into their own. Functional appliances were developed to correct the aberrant muscle environment—the jaw-to-jaw relationship—and as a result restore facial balance by improving function. To achieve the best of both worlds it is necessary to combine the disciplines of fixed and functional appliance therapy.

THE PHILOSOPHICAL DIVIDE

In each succeeding generation the clinical approach to treatment is determined by the background of scientific research. The growth processes of the maxillofacial complex that control the response to treatment are of special significance. Since the beginning of the twentieth century, the pendulum of scientific opinion has swung back and forth in the evaluation of the 'form and function' philosophy in relation to the implementation of orthodontic and orthopaedic treatment. At the turn of the last century, a division occurred in the evolution of orthodontic technique that split treatment philosophy into the separate disciplines of fixed and functional appliance therapy.

The two schools of thought had a common origin in the 'form and function' philosophy as a basis to establish treatment objectives. The general goal was to correct arch-to-arch relationships, as defined by Angle (1907), while at the same time improving the skeletal relationships through the stimulation and guidance of adaptive remodelling of bone to support those corrected dental relationships.

This philosophical divide in treatment approach can be related to geographical factors as well as to differences in socio-economic development between the USA and Europe.

In his efforts at developing the foundations of modern US fixed appliance technique, Angle attempted to accommodate a full complement of teeth in every case, irrespective of the degree of crowding or lack of available underlying bony support. The following generation of orthodontists subsequently rejected Angle's 'form and function' philosophy as a basis for fixed appliance therapy, and discarded the functional concept of growth in favour of a concept of genetic control that dismissed the potential of environmental factors to influence growth. One dogmatic philosophy was replaced by another.

Provided skeletal development is within the range of normal, fixed appliances are ideally suited to detailing the occlusion by precise three-dimensional control of tooth movement. Fixed appliances are designed specifically to apply the optimum forces to move teeth, but they are less effective in the treatment of major muscle function imbalances or their companion jaw-to-jaw skeletal discrepancies.

THE GENETIC PARADIGM

In the development of orthodontic technique the concept of genetic control of the pattern of maxillofacial development was based on serial growth studies that came about as a byproduct of the development of the cephalostat by Broadbent (1948).

These studies formed the basis for an entire philosophical approach to orthodontic treatment, where the existing skeletal framework was accepted as genetically predetermined and therefore not subject to environmental factors.

In the literature there is scant evidence of significant growth changes showing increased mandibular growth as a result of an orthodontic as opposed to an orthopaedic approach to therapy. Other studies did confirm that auxilliary orthopaedic forces restricted downward and forward maxillary growth. As a result, maxillary dental retraction became commonly accepted as a reliable method of correcting Class II malocclusion overjet problems.

However, a strict interpretation of the genetic paradigm is called into question increasingly by current research, and is no longer the only valid basis for the practice of orthodontics combined with dentofacial orthopaedics. The present findings of modern research into bone growth represent a philosophical review that once again recognises the potential of improving the existing growth pattern by altering the muscle environment and/or functional environment of the developing dentition in an orthopaedic approach to treatment.

TREATMENT CONCEPTS

A fundamental difference in approach exists between orthodontic and orthopaedic schools of thought in relation to treatment philosophy and the management of malocclusion.

In the evolution of orthodontic technique, multiband fixed appliances were developed for treatment in the permanent dentition. It was customary to delay treatment until the permanent canines and premolars had erupted, at a stage when the malocclusion was already fully developed. The concept of treatment was to retract the upper arch using the perimeter of the orthodontically corrected, albeit retruded, lower arch as a template on which to rebuild the occlusion.

However, the majority of Class II malocclusions present a laterally contracted maxilla that is often related correctly to the cranial base but is associated with an underdeveloped mandible. The fundamental skeletal problem is not correctly addressed by an approach which is designed to retract a normal maxilla to match a deficient mandible.

A skeletal mandibular deficiency is well established at an early stage of dental and facial development. The orthopaedic approach to treatment endeavours to correct the skeletal relationship before the malocclusion is fully expressed in the permanent dentition. Early diagnosis and interceptive treatment aims to restore normal function, and thereby enable the permanent teeth to erupt into correct occlusal and incisal relationships.

The concept of functional therapy is to expand and develop the upper arch to improve archform, and to use the maxilla as a template against which to reposition the retrusive mandible in a correct relationship to the normal maxilla. The functional orthopaedic approach addresses the skeletal problem of a retrusive mandible, and the malocclusion is controlled at an earlier stage of development.

Class III malocclusion is also identified by early diagnosis, and may often respond to an interceptive approach to treatment which aims to reduce the skeletal discrepancy and restore normal function in order to promote normal growth and development.

Orthodontic force

Fixed appliances are designed to apply light orthodontic forces that move individual teeth. Schwarz (1932) defined the optimum orthodontic force as 28 g per square centimetre of root surface. By applying light forces with archwires and elastic traction, fixed appliances do not specifically stimulate mandibular growth during treatment.

A bracket or 'small handle' is attached to individual teeth. Pressure is then applied to those teeth by ligating light wires to the brackets. The resulting forces applied through the teeth to the supporting alveolar bone must remain within the level of physiological tolerance of the periodontal membrane to avoid damage to the individual teeth and/or their sockets of alveolar bone.

Smith & Storey (1952), investigating optimum force levels in the edgewise appliance, found that 150 g was the optimum force for moving canines, compared to 300 g for molars.

Allowance must be made, however, for frictional forces within the bracket slots themselves, in the region of 125–250 g, which must be overcome to move teeth along archwires.

Orthopaedic force

Orthopaedic force levels are not confined by the level of tolerance of the periodontal membrane but rather by the much broader tolerance of the orofacial musculature. An orthopaedic approach to treatment is not designed to move the teeth, but rather to change the jaw position and thereby correct the relationship of the mandible to the maxilla.

The forces of occlusion applied to opposing teeth in mastication are in the range of 400–500 g and these forces are transmitted through the teeth to the supporting bone. Occlusal forces form a major proprioceptive stimulus to growth whereby the internal and external structure of supporting bone is remodelled to meet the needs of occlusal function. This is effected by reorganisation of the alveolar trabecular system and by periosteal and endochondral apposition.

Considering the anteroposterior forces applied when the mandible is displaced forward in the presence of a Class II skeletal relationship, the investigations of Graf (1961, 1975) and Witt & Komposch (1971) have shown that for 1 mm of anterior displacement the forces of the stretched retractor muscles amount to approximately 100 g. A construction bite of 5–10 mm will therefore transmit considerable forces to the dentition through the functional receptors.

Orthopaedic forces would exceed the level of tolerance of the periodontal tissues if applied to individual teeth. However, these forces are spread evenly in the dental arches by appliances that are not designed to move individual teeth, but to displace the entire mandible and promote adaptation within the muscles of mastication. The muscles are the prime movers in growth, and bony remodelling is related to the functional requirements of muscle activity. The goal of functional appliances is to elicit a proprioceptive response in the stretch receptors of the orofacial muscles and ligaments, and as a secondary response to influence the pattern of bone growth correspondingly to support a new functional environment for the developing dentition.

DENTOFACIAL ORTHOPAEDICS

In contrast to the philosophical change that has accompanied the evolution of fixed appliance therapy, the form and function concept steadfastly remains the basic concept of functional therapy. The functional matrix theory of Moss (1968) supports the premise that function modifies anatomy.

By definition, the purpose of dentofacial orthopaedics is to modify the pattern of facial growth and the underlying bone structure of the face. The objective is to promote harmonious facial growth by changing the functional muscle environment around the developing dentition. The principle of functional therapy is to reposition a retrusive mandible to a forward position by constructing an appliance that effects a protrusive bite when the appliance is placed in the mouth. The mechanics are reversed to correct a retrusive maxilla, but the principle remains the same.

Functional appliances are designed to enhance forward mandibular growth in the treatment of distal occlusion by encouraging a functional displacement of the mandibular condyles downwards and forwards in the glenoid fossae. This is balanced by an upward and backward pull in the muscles supporting the mandible. Adaptive remodelling may occur on both articular surfaces of the temporomandibular joint to improve the position of the mandible relative to the maxilla.

In correction of mandibular retrusion, the mandible is held in a protrusive position by occlusal contact on the functional appliance. In this case a large 'handle' is attached to as many teeth as possible in both dental arches. The object of a functional appliance is not to move the individual teeth, but to displace the lower jaw downwards and forwards, and to increase the intermaxillary space in the anteroposterior and vertical dimensions. Repositioning the mandible stimulates a positive proprioceptive response in the muscles of mastication. The purpose is to encourage adaptive skeletal growth by maintaining the mandible in a corrected forward position for a sufficient period of time to allow adaptive skeletal changes to occur in response to functional stimulus.

Dentofacial orthopaedics, therefore, represents a positive approach to the treatment of craniofacial imbalance by addressing the underlying cause of the malocclusion, in an effort to maximise the natural potential for corrective growth.

REFERENCES

Angle, E.H. (1907). *Treatment of Malocclusion of the Teeth*, 7th edn. Philadelphia, S.S. White Dental Manufacturing Co.

Broadbent, B.H. (1931). *Practical Orthodontics*, ed. G.H. Anderson, 7th edn. St Louis, C.V. Mosby, p. 208.

Graf, H. (1961). In *Tecknik und Handhabung der Functionsregler.* Berlin, R. Frankel.

Graf, H. (1975). Occlusal forces during function. In *Proceedings of Symposium*, ed. N.H. Rowe. Ann Arbor, University of Michigan.

Moss, M.L. (1968). The primacy of functional matrices in profacial growth, *Dent. Pract.*, **19:** 65–73.

Schwarz, A.M. (1932). Tissue changes incidental to orthodontics. *Austral. J. Orthod.*, **18:** 331–52.

Smith, R. & Storey, E. (1952). The importance of forces in orthodontics. *Austral. J. Dent.*, **56:** 291–304.

Witt, E. & Komposch, G. (1971). Intermaxillare Kraftwirkung bimaxillarer gerate. *Gerate. Fortschr. Kieferorhop.*, **32:** 345–52.

FURTHER READING

Moyers, R.E. (1988). Force systems and tissue responses in orthodontics and facial orthopedics. In *Handbook of Orthodontics*. Chicago, Year Book.

Sinclair, P.M. (1991). The clinical application of orthopaedic forces: current capabilities and limitations. In *Bone Biodynamics in Orthodontic and Orthopaedic Treatment*, ed. Carlson, D.S. and Goldstein, S.A. Craniofacial Growth Series, University of Michigan, Vol. 27, pp. 351–88.

Witt, E. (1966). Investigations into orthodontic forces of different appliances. *Trans. Eur. Orthod. Soc.*, 391–408.

Witt, E. (1973). Muscular physiological investigations into the effect of bi-maxillary appliances. *Trans. Eur. Orthod. Soc.*, 448–50.

CHAPTER 2

Introduction to Twin Blocks

THE OCCLUSAL INCLINED PLANE

The occlusal inclined plane is the fundamental functional mechanism of the natural dentition. Cuspal inclined planes play an important part in determining the relationship of the teeth as they erupt into occlusion.

If the mandible occludes in a distal relationship to the maxilla, the occlusal forces acting on the mandibular teeth in normal function have a distal component of force that is unfavourable to normal forward mandibular development. The inclined planes formed by the cusps of the upper and lower teeth represent a servo-mechanism that locks the mandible in a distally occluding functional position.

Twin Block appliances are simple bite blocks that are designed for full-time wear. They achieve rapid functional correction of malocclusion by the transmission of favourable occlusal forces to occlusal inclined planes that cover the posterior teeth. The forces of occlusion are used as the functional mechanism to correct the malocclusion (Fig. 2.1 A,B).

PROPRIOCEPTIVE STIMULUS TO GROWTH

The inclined plane mechanism plays an important part in determining the cuspal relationship of the teeth as they erupt into occlusion. A functional equilibrium is established under neurological control in response to repetitive tactile stimulus. Occlusal forces transmitted through the dentition provide a constant proprioceptive stimulus to influence the rate of growth and the trabecular structure of the supporting bone.

Malocclusion is frequently associated with discrepancies in arch relationships due to underlying skeletal and soft-tissue factors, resulting in unfavourable cuspal guidance and poor occlusal function. The proprioceptive sensory feedback mechanism controls muscular activity and provides a functional stimulus or deterrent to the full expression of mandibular bone growth. The unfavourable cuspal contacts of distal occlusion represent an obstruction to normal forward mandibular translation in function, and as such do

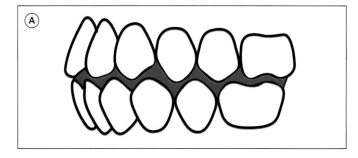

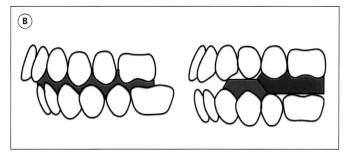

Fig. 2.1 A, B The occlusal inclined plane is the functional mechanism of the natural dentition. Twin Blocks modify the occlusal inclined plane and use the forces of occlusion to correct the malocclusion. The mandible is guided forwards by the occlusal inclined plane.

not encourage the mandible to achieve its optimum genetic growth potential.

Transverse maxillary development

Transverse maxillary development is restricted as a result of a distally occluding mandible. In a retrusive mandible the lower dentition does not offer support to the maxillary arch, therefore the maxillary intercanine width and interpremolar width is reduced accordingly. The constricted width of the maxillary dentition has the effect of locking the mandible in a distal occlusion and prevents normal mandibular development.

Functional appliance therapy aims to improve the functional relationship of the dentofacial structures by eliminating unfavourable developmental factors and improving the muscle environment that envelops the developing occlusion. By altering the position of the teeth and supporting tissues, a new functional behaviour pattern is established that can support a new position of equilibrium.

TWIN BLOCKS

The goal in developing the Twin Block approach to treatment was to produce a technique that could maximise the growth response to functional mandibular protrusion by using an appliance system that is simple, comfortable and aesthetically acceptable to the patient

Twin Blocks are constructed to a protrusive bite that effectively modifies the occlusal inclined plane by means of acrylic inclined planes on occlusal bite blocks. The purpose is to promote protrusive mandibular function for correction of the skeletal Class II malocclusion (Fig. 2.2).

The occlusal inclined plane acts as a guiding mechanism causing the mandible to be displaced downward and forward.

With the appliances in the mouth, the patient cannot occlude comfortably in the former distal position and the mandible is encouraged to adopt a protrusive bite with the inclined planes engaged in occlusion. The unfavourable cuspal contacts of a distal occlusion are replaced by favourable proprioceptive contacts on the inclined planes of the Twin Blocks to correct the malocclusion and to free the mandible from its locked distal functional position.

Twin Blocks are designed to be worn 24 hours per day to take full advantage of all functional forces applied to the dentition, including the forces of mastication. Upper and lower bite blocks interlock at a 70° angle when engaged in full closure. This causes a forward mandibular posture to an edge-to-edge position with the upper anteriors, provided the patient can comfortably maintain full occlusion on the

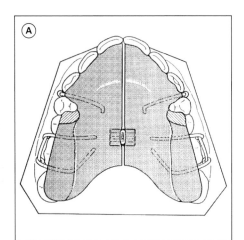
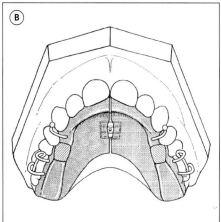
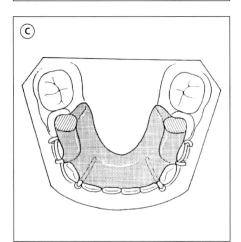
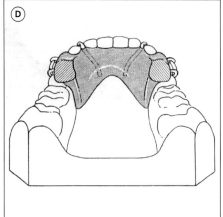
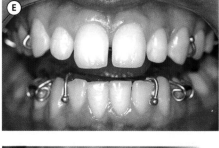
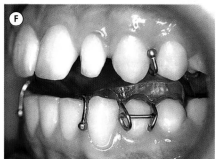

Fig. 2.2 E, F Twin Blocks.

Fig. 2.2 A, B Upper Twin Block – occlusal and frontal. **C, D** Lower Twin Block – occlusal and rear views. Courtesy of W. Brudon and J.A. McNamara Jr., University of Michigan.

appliances in that position. In treatment of Class II malocclusion, the inclined planes are positioned mesial to the upper and lower first molars with the upper block covering the upper molars and second premolars or deciduous molars, and the lower blocks extending mesially from the second premolar or deciduous molar region.

In the early stages of their evolution, Twin Blocks were conceived as simple removable appliances with interlocking occlusal bite blocks designed to posture the mandible forward to achieve functional correction of a Class II division 1 malocclusion. This basic principle still applies but over the years many variations in appliance design have extended the scope of the technique to treat a wide range of all classes of malocclusion. Appliance design has been improved and simplified to make Twin Blocks more acceptable to the patient without reducing their efficiency.

In the treatment of Class II division 2 malocclusion, appliance design is modified by the addition of sagittal screws

to advance the upper anterior teeth. Control of the vertical dimension is achieved by sequentially adjusting the thickness of the posterior occlusal inclined planes to control eruption (Fig. 2.3).

Treatment of Class III malocclusion is achieved by reversing the occlusal inclined planes to apply a forward component of force to the upper arch and a downward and distal force to the mandible in the lower molar region. The inclined planes are set at 70° to the occlusal plane with bite blocks covering lower molars and upper deciduous molars or premolars, with sagittal screws to advance the upper incisors (Fig. 2.4).

The first principle of appliance design is simplicity. The patient's appearance is noticeably improved when Twin Blocks are fitted. Twin Blocks are designed to be comfortable, aesthetic and efficient. By addressing these requirements, Twin Blocks satisfy both the patient and the operator as one of the most 'patient friendly' of all the functional appliances.

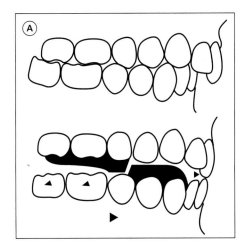
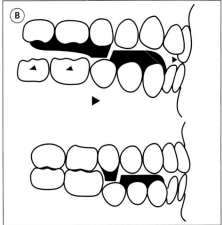
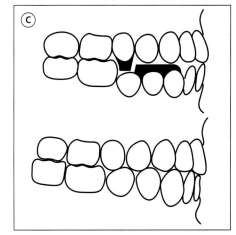

Fig. 2.3 Correction of Class II Division 2 malocclusion by advancing the mandible and proclining the upper incisors with sagittal screws.

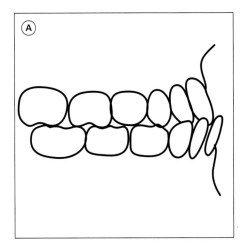
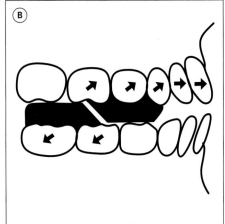
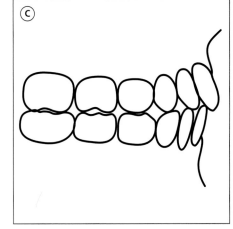

Fig. 2.4 Reverse Twin Blocks for correction of Class III malocclusion with sagittal screws to advance upper incisors.

DEVELOPMENT OF TWIN BLOCKS

CASE REPORT: C.G. AGED 7 YEARS 10 MONTHS

It is true that 'necessity is the mother of invention'. The Twin Block appliance evolved in response to a clinical problem that presented when a young patient, the son of a dental colleague, fell and completely luxated an upper central incisor. Fortunately, he kept the tooth, and presented for treatment within a few hours of the accident. The incisor was reimplanted and a temporary splint was constructed to hold the tooth in position (Fig. 2.5).

Before the accident the centre line was displaced to the right and the luxated incisor had a pronounced distal angulation with a central diastema of 3 mm. When the tooth was reimplanted the socket was enlarged to reposition the incisor as near as possible to the midline. Complete correction of the midline was not possible, recognising that enlarging the socket too much might reduce the prognosis for reattachment of the tooth.

After 6 months with a stabilising splint, the tooth had partially reattached, but there was evidence of severe root resorption and the long-term prognosis for the reimplanted incisor was poor.

The occlusal relationship was Class II division 1 with an overjet of 9 mm and the lower lip was trapped lingual to the upper incisors. Adverse lip action on the reimplanted incisor was causing mobility and root resorption. To prevent the lip from trapping in the overjet it was necessary to design an appliance that could be worn full time to posture the mandible forward. At that time no such appliance was available and simple bite blocks were therefore designed to achieve this objective. The appliance mechanism was designed to harness the forces of occlusion to correct the distal occlusion and also to reduce the overjet without applying direct pressure to the upper incisors.

The upper and lower bite blocks engaged mesial to the first permanent molars at 90° to the occlusal plane when the mandible postured forward. This positioned the incisors edge-to-edge with 2 mm vertical separation to hold the incisors out of occlusion. The patient had to make a positive effort to posture his mandible forward to occlude the bite blocks in a protrusive bite. Fortunately, the young patient was successful in doing this consistently to activate the appliance for functional correction. Had he not made this effort the technique may have been stillborn.

The first Twin Block appliances were fitted on 7 September 1977, when the patient was aged 8 years 4 months. The bite blocks proved comfortable to wear and treatment progressed well as the distal occlusion corrected and the overjet reduced from 9 mm to 4 mm in 9 months.

During the course of treatment radiographs confirmed that the reimplanted incisor had severe root resorption and an endodontic pin was placed to stabilise this tooth after 4 months of treatment. This was successful in stabilising the incisor.

At a later stage, in the permanent dentition, a simple upper fixed appliance was used to complete treatment. It was not possible to correct the centre line fully in replacing the luxated tooth, and the central incisor ankylosed during the process of reattachment. Consequently, a slight displacement of the centre line had to be accepted. The reimplanted incisor was crowned successfully, and the result is stable at age 25 years.

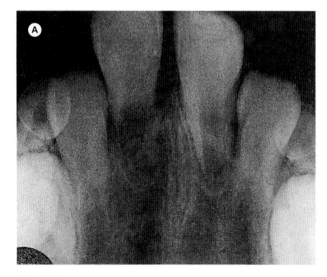
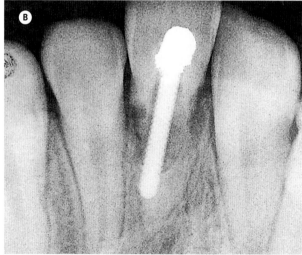

Fig. 2.5 Treatment:
A, B Before treatment: 1| was completely luxated and was reimplanted. An endodontic pin was fitted to stabilise the incisor. This was successful in achieving bony reattachment.

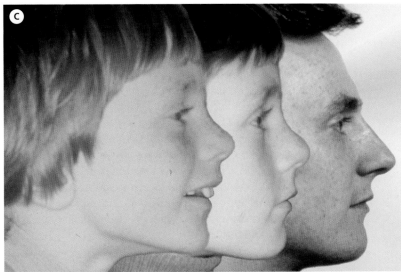

Fig. 2.5 Treatment (cont.):
C Profiles at ages 7 years 10 months (before treatment), 9 years 7 months (after 9 months of treatment) and 24 years.
D, E Dental views before treatment at age 7 years 10 months.
F After 9 months of treatment, the overjet has reduced, and the distal occlusion is corrected.
G, H The first Twin Blocks were simple bite blocks occluding in forward posture. The blocks were angled at 90° to the occlusal plane.
J A simple fixed appliance is used to improve alignment in permanent dentition. The damaged upper incisor is now ankylosed.
K, L, M The occlusion remains stable 5 years out of retention.

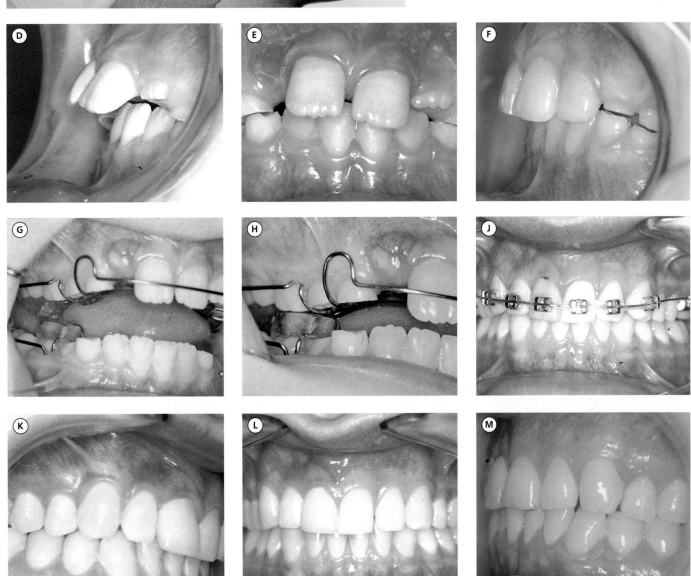

MODIFICATION FOR TREATMENT OF CLASS II DIVISION 2 MALOCCLUSION

CASE REPORT: A.K. AGED 11 YEARS

Two years later, having developed a protocol for Twin Block treatment of Class II division 1 malocclusion, attention was turned to Class II division 2 malocclusion. The first patient of this type presented a severe malocclusion with an excessive overbite and an interincisal angle approaching 180° (Fig. 2.6). As an indication of the depth of the overbite the intergingival height from the gingival margin of the upper incisors to the gingival margin of the lower incisors was 7 mm, suggesting that the upper incisors were impinging on the lower gingivae. The lower archform was good but the mandible was trapped in distal occlusion by the retroclined upper incisors.

The original Twin Block prototype appliances were modified from the standard design for correction of Class II division 1 malocclusion by the addition of springs lingual to the upper incisors to advance retroclined upper incisors. At the same time the mandible was translated forwards to correct the distal occlusion and the appliance was trimmed to encourage eruption of the posterior teeth to reduce the overbite.

The Class II division 2 Twin Blocks were worn for 6 months, at which stage brackets were fitted on the upper anterior teeth and activated with a sectional archwire to correct individual tooth alignment. This combination fixed/functional appliance treatment continued for 6 months. Completion of treatment was then effected with a simple upper fixed appliance.

CASE REPORT: A.K.

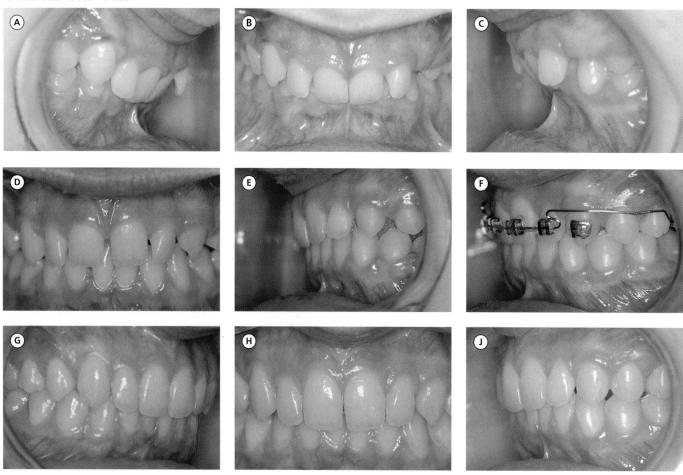

Fig. 2.6 The first patient (A.K.) with a Class II Division 2 malocclusion treated with Twin Blocks:
A, B, C Excessive overbite and severely retroclined incisors.
D, E After 8 months the distal occlusion is corrected and the overbite is reduced.

F A simple upper fixed appliance to correct alignment.
G, H, J The occlusion is stable 3 years later.
A diagrammatic interpretation of the treatment is given on page 11.

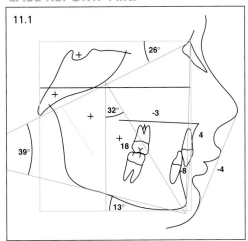

11.1

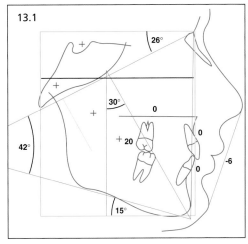

13.1

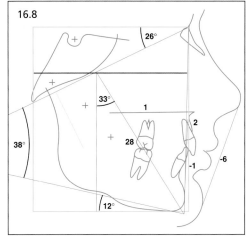

16.8

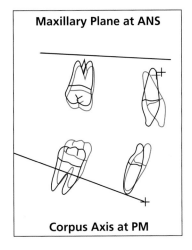

Maxillary Plane at ANS

Corpus Axis at PM

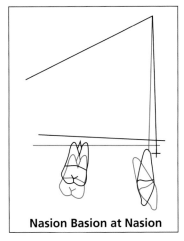

Nasion Basion at Nasion

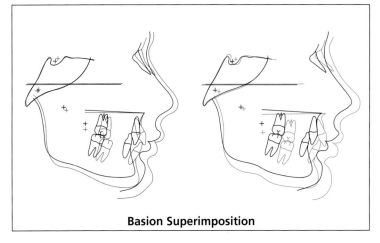

Basion Superimposition

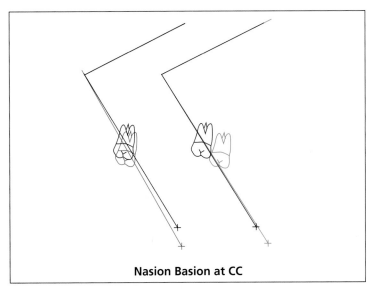

Nasion Basion at CC

A.K.	Age	11.1	13.1	16.8
Cranial Base Angle		26	26	26
Facial Axis Angle		32	30	33
F/M Plane Angle		13	15	12
Craniomandibular Angle		39	42	38
Maxillary Plane		-3	0	1
Convexity		4	0	2
U/Incisor to Vertical		-5	22	17
L/Incisor to Vertical		16	29	26
Interincisal Angle		169	129	137
6 to Pterygoid Vertical		18	20	28
L/Incisor to A/Po		-8	0	-1
L/Lip to Aesthetic Plane		-4	-6	-6

Angulation of the inclined planes

During the evolution of the technique, the angulation of the inclined plane varied from 90° to 45° to the occlusal plane, before arriving at an angle of 70° to the occlusal plane as the final compromise angle that proved most suitable in the majority of cases.

As previously stated, the earliest Twin Block appliances were constructed with bite blocks that articulated at a 90° angle, so that the patient had to make a conscious effort to occlude in a forward position. However, some patients had difficulty maintaining a forward posture and, therefore, would revert to retruding the mandible back to its old distal occlusion position, occluding the bite blocks together on top of each other on their flat occlusal surfaces. This was detectable at an early stage of treatment when it could be observed that the patient was not posturing forwards consistently. A significant posterior open bite was caused by biting on the blocks in this fashion. This complication was experienced in approximately 30% of the earliest Twin Block cases. It was resolved by altering the angulation of the bite blocks to 45° to the occlusal plane in order to guide the mandible forwards. This was immediately successful in eliminating the problem.

An angle of 45° to the occlusal plane applies an equal downward and forward component of force to the lower dentition. The direction of occlusal force on the inclined planes encourages a corresponding downward and forward stimulus to growth. After using a 45° angle on the blocks for 8 years, the angulation was finally changed to the steeper angle of 70° to the occlusal plane to apply a more horizontal component of force. It was reasoned that this may encourage more forward mandibular growth. If the patient has any difficulty in posturing forward, this is a sign that the activation should be reduced by trimming the inclined planes to reduce the amount of mandibular protrusion. It then becomes much easier for the patient to maintain a forward posture.

Bite registration

The Exactobite or Projet Bite Gauge (the name differs in the USA and the UK) is designed to record a protrusive interocclusal record or 'bite registration' in wax for construction of Twin Blocks (Fig. 2.7). Typically, in a growing child, an overjet of up to 10 mm can be corrected on the initial activation by registering an incisal edge-to-edge bite with 2 mm interincisal clearance (Fig. 2.8 A,B). This is provided that the patient can comfortably tolerate the mandible being protruded so the upper and lower incisors align vertically edge-to-edge. Larger overjets invariably require partial correction, followed by reactivation after the initial partial correction is accomplished.

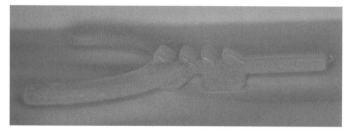

Fig. 2.7 Projet Bite Gauge.

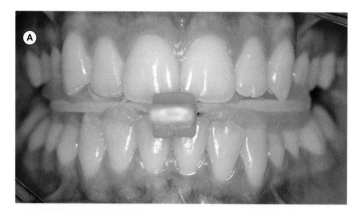

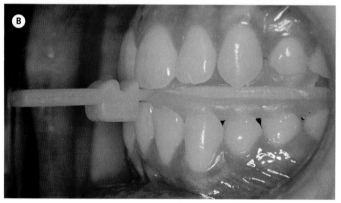

Fig. 2.8 A, B The blue bite gauge registers 2 mm vertical clearance between the incisal edges of the upper and lower incisors. This generally proves to be an appropriate interincisal clearance in bite registration for most Class division 1 malocclusions with increased overbite.

Appliance design – Twin Blocks for correction of uncrowded Class II division 1 malocclusion

It is usually necessary to widen the upper arch to accommodate the lower arch in the corrected protrusive position. The upper appliance incorporates a midline screw to expand the upper arch.

Delta clasps are placed on upper molars, with additional ball-ended clasps distal to the canines, or between the pre-molars or deciduous molars.

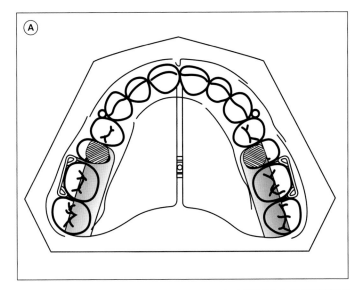

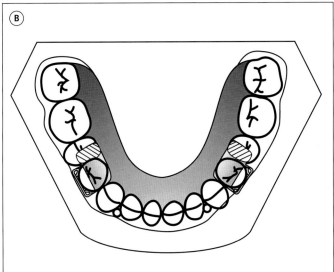

Fig. 2.9 Twin Blocks for correction of uncrowded Class II division 1.

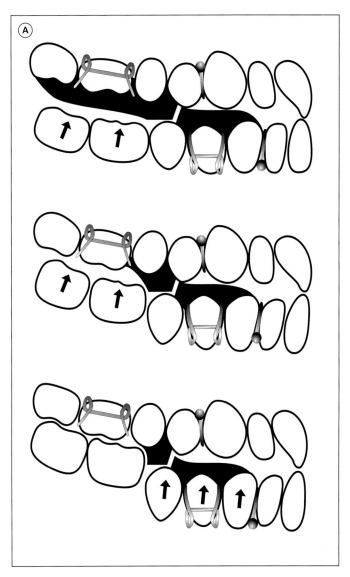

Fig. 2.10 Sequence of trimming blocks.

The lower appliance is a simple bite block with delta clasps on the first premolars and ball clasps mesial to the canines (Fig. 2.9).

THE TWIN BLOCK TECHNIQUE – STAGES OF TREATMENT

Twin Block treatment is described in two stages. Twin Blocks are used in the active phase to correct the anteroposterior relationship and establish the correct vertical dimension. Once this phase is accomplished, the Twin Blocks are replaced with an upper Hawley type of appliance with an anterior inclined plane, which is then used to support the corrected position as the posterior teeth settle fully into occlusion.

Stage 1: active phase

Twin Blocks achieve rapid functional correction of mandibular position from a skeletally retruded Class II to Class I occlusion using occlusal inclined planes over the posterior teeth to guide the mandible into correct relationship with the maxilla. In all functional therapy, sagittal correction is achieved before vertical development of the posterior teeth is complete. The vertical dimension is controlled first by adjustment of the occlusal bite blocks, followed by use of the previously mentioned upper inclined plane appliance.

In treatment of deep overbite, the bite blocks are trimmed selectively to encourage eruption of lower posterior teeth to increase the vertical dimension and level the occlusal plane (Fig. 2.10). Throughout the trimming sequence it is important not to reduce the leading edge of the inclined plane, so that adequate functional occlusal support is given until a three-point occlusal contact is achieved with the molars in occlusion.

The upper block is trimmed occlusodistally to leave the lower molars 1–2 mm clear of the occlusion to encourage lower molar eruption and reduce the overbite. By maintaining a minimal clearance between the upper bite block and the lower molars the tongue is prevented from spreading laterally between the teeth. This allows the molars to erupt more quickly. At each subsequent visit the upper bite block is reduced progressively to clear the occlusion with the lower molars to allow these teeth to erupt, until finally all the acrylic has been removed over the occlusal surface of the upper molars allowing the lower molars to erupt fully into occlusion.

Conversely, in treatment of anterior open bite and vertical growth patterns, the posterior bite blocks remain unreduced and intact throughout treatment. This results in an intrusive effect on the posterior teeth, while the anterior teeth remain free to erupt, which helps to increase the overbite and bring the anterior teeth into occlusion.

At the end of the active stage of Twin Block treatment the aim is to achieve correction to Class I occlusion and control of the vertical dimension by a three-point occlusal contact with the incisors and molars in occlusion. At this stage the overjet, overbite and distal occlusion should be fully corrected.

Stage 2: support phase

The aim of the support phase is to maintain the corrected incisor relationship until the buccal segment occlusion is fully interdigitated. To achieve this objective an upper removable appliance is fitted with an anterior inclined plane with a labial bow to engage the lower incisors and canines (Fig. 2.11).

The lower Twin Block appliance is left out at this stage and the removal of posterior bite blocks allows the posterior teeth to erupt. Full-time appliance wear is necessary to allow time for internal bony remodelling to support the corrected occlusion as the buccal segments settle fully into occlusion.

RETENTION

Treatment is followed by retention with the upper anterior inclined plane appliance. Appliance wear is reduced to night-time only when the occlusion is fully established. A good buccal segment occlusion is the cornerstone of stability after correction of arch-to-arch relationships. The appliance-effected advanced mandibular position will not be stable until the functional support of a full buccal segment occlusion is well established.

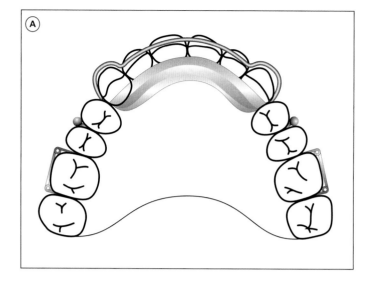

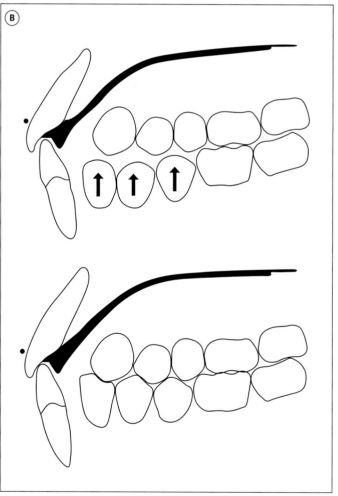

Fig. 2.11 A, B Support phase – anterior inclined plane.

Timetable of treatment: average treatment time

- Active phase: average time 6–9 months to achieve full reduction of overjet to a normal incisor relationship and to correct the distal occlusion.
- Support phase: 3–6 months for molars to erupt into occlusion and for premolars to erupt after trimming the blocks. The objective is to support the corrected mandibular position after active mandibular translation while the buccal teeth settle fully into occlusion.
- Retention: 9 months, reducing appliance wear when the position is stabilised.

An average estimate of treatment time is 18 months, including retention.

RESPONSE TO TREATMENT

Rapid improvements in facial appearance are seen consistently even during the first few months of Twin Block treatment. These changes are characterised by the development of a lip seal and a noticeable improvement in facial balance and harmony. Lip exercises are not necessary to achieve this change in soft-tissue behaviour. The patient develops a lip seal naturally as a result of eating with the appliances in the mouth. When the mandible closes in a forward position it is easier to form an anterior oral seal by closing the lips together than to support the lips with an anterior tongue thrust. In growing children, the facial muscles adapt very quickly to an altered pattern of occlusal function. The changes in appearance are so significant that the patients themselves frequently comment on the improvement in the early stages of treatment.

The facial changes are soon accompanied by equivalent dental changes and it is routine to observe correction of a full unit distal occlusion within the first 6 months of treatment. The response to treatment is noticeably faster compared to alternative functional appliances that must be removed for eating.

CASE REPORT: C.H. AGED 14 YEARS 1 MONTH

An example of treatment for a boy with an uncrowded Class II division 1 malocclusion with good archform and a full unit distal occlusion (Fig 2.12).

Diagnosis, skeletal classification:

- Moderate Class II.
- Facial type: moderate brachyfacial (horizontal growth).
- Maxilla: mild protrusion.
- Mandible: mild retrusion.
- Convexity = 6 mm.

Diagnosis, dental classification:

- Severe Class II division 1.
- Upper incisors: severe protrusion.
- Lower incisors: normal.
- Overjet = 12 mm.
- Overbite = 5 mm (deep).
- No crowding.

Treatment plan:

Functional correction to Class I occlusion by means of a combination of maxillary retraction and mandibular advancement, with reduction of overjet and overbite.

Bite registration:

The initial bite registration with the blue Exactobite aims to correct the overjet to edge-to-edge with a 2 mm interincisal clearance.

Appliances:

- Twin Blocks for correction of uncrowded Class II division 1 malocclusion.

CASE REPORT: C.H.

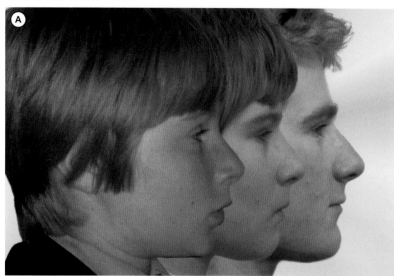

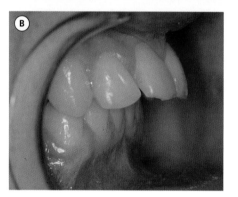

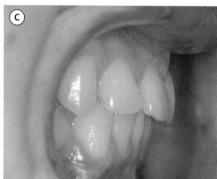

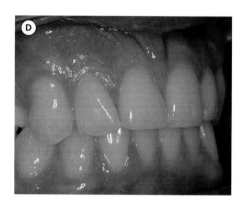

Fig. 2.12 Treatment:
A Profiles at ages 14 years 1 month (before treatment), 14 years 6 months (after 5 months of treatment) and 19 years 7 months.
B Occlusion before treatment at age 14 years 1 month.
C Occlusal change after 5 months of treatment, at age 14 years 6 months.
D Occlusion at age 19 years 7 months.
A diagrammatic interpretation of the treatment is given on page 17.

Clinical management

At the first adjustment visit 2 weeks after the appliance is fitted, it is noted that the patient is not always posturing forward, and is sometimes simply biting together on the flat occlusal surfaces of the blocks. This would tend to produce a posterior open bite, and it is important to avoid this complication by detecting this at an early stage in treatment. The problem is resolved simply by trimming the acrylic slightly from the anterior incline of the upper block until the patient bites comfortably and consistently on the inclined planes of the blocks. This reduces the initial forward activation to 7 mm with 2 mm interincisal clearance.

In spite of the slight upper block reduction, this activation reduces the overjet from 12 mm to 4 mm in 5 months. Nevertheless, as a general principle, if the overjet is greater than 10 mm it is usually necessary to correct the occlusion in a two-stage forward activation of the Twin Blocks.

After the initial partial correction, the Twin Blocks are reactivated to produce an upper to lower incisal edge-to-edge occlusion with 2 mm vertical clearance by adding cold cure acrylic to the anterior aspect of the upper inclined plane. This second activation by means of the longer upper block completes the mandibular correction to Class I occlusion. The blocks are trimmed occlusally as before to reduce the overbite and encourage vertical development.

Duration of treatment:

- Active phase: 8 months with Twin Blocks.
- Support phase and retention: 6 months.

Lower third molars were potentially impacted and on completion of treatment all four second molars were extracted to accommodate third molars, which subsequently erupted in good position.

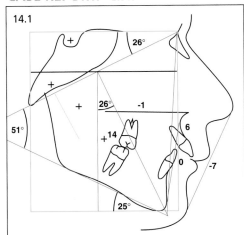

14.1

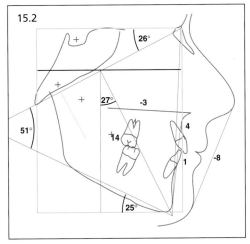

15.2

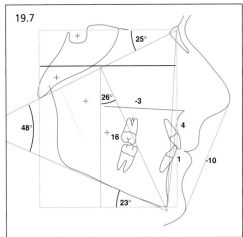

19.7

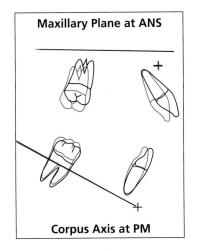

Maxillary Plane at ANS

Corpus Axis at PM

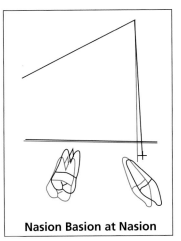

Nasion Basion at Nasion

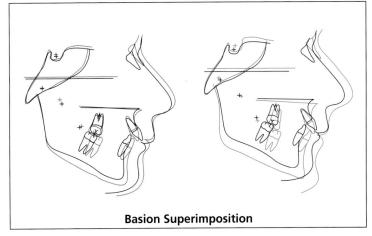

Basion Superimposition

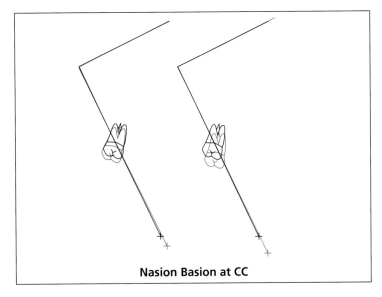

Nasion Basion at CC

C.H.	Age	14.1	15.2	19.7
Cranial Base Angle		26	26	25
Facial Axis Angle		26	27	26
F/M Plane Angle		25	25	23
Craniomandibular Angle		51	51	48
Maxillary Plane		-1	-3	-3
Convexity		6	4	4
U/Incisor to Vertical		38	26	27
L/Incisor to Vertical		31	30	30
Interincisal Angle		111	124	123
6 to Pterygoid Vertical		14	14	16
L/Incisor to A/Po		0	1	1
L/Lip to Aesthetic Plane		-7	-8	-10

CASE SELECTION FOR SIMPLE TREATMENT

In starting to use any new technique it is important to select suitable cases from which to learn the fundamentals of treatment without complications. This is especially important when the practitioner is not experienced in functional therapy. Case selection for initial clinical use of Twin Blocks should, therefore, display the following criteria:

- Angle's Class II division 1 malocclusion with good archform. It is easier to learn the management of the technique first by treating uncrowded cases before progressing to crowded dentitions.
- A lower arch that is uncrowded or decrowded and aligned.
- An upper arch that is aligned or can be easily aligned.
- An overjet of 10–12 mm and a deep overbite.
- A full unit distal occlusion in the buccal segments.
- On examination of the models in occlusion with the lower model advanced to correct the increased overjet, the distal occlusion is also corrected and it can be seen that a potentially good occlusion of the buccal teeth will result. A good buccal segment occlusion is the cornerstone of stability after correction of Class II arch relationships.
- On clinical examination the profile should be noticeably improved when the patient advances the mandible voluntarily to correct the overjet. This factor is fundamental in case selection for functional appliance therapy, and is a clinical indication that the Class II arch relationship is skeletal in origin.
- To achieve a favourable skeletal change during treatment, the patient should be growing actively. A more rapid growth response may be observed when treatment coincides with the pubertal growth spurt. Conversely, the response to treatment is slower if the patient is growing more slowly. Although the rate of growth will influence progress, it is not necessary to plan treatment to coincide with the pubertal growth spurt, as the Twin Block system is effective in mixed dentition, transitional dentition and permanent dentition.

In experienced hands, Twin Blocks are very effective in the treatment of complex malocclusions that are due to a combination of dental and skeletal factors. Twin Blocks integrate more easily with fixed appliances than any other functional appliance in a combined approach to orthopaedic and orthodontic treatment.

A girl with a Class II division 1 malocclusion and mild crowding in the upper labial segment due to narrowing of the upper arch (Fig. 2.13).

Diagnosis, skeletal classification:

- Moderate Class II.
- Facial type: mesognathic.
- Maxilla: slight protrusion, contracted laterally.
- Mandible: normal.
- Convexity = 6 mm.

Diagnosis, dental classification:

- Severe Class II division 1.
- Upper incisors: mild protrusion.
- Lower incisors: normal.
- Overjet = 9 mm.
- Overbite incomplete due to tongue thrust.

Treatment plan:

Slight functional protrusion of the mandible to reduce skeletal and dental Class II relationships.

Appliances:

- Twin Blocks with labial bow to align the upper incisors.
- Anterior guide plane to support the corrected occlusion and retain.

Bite registration:

The construction bite is registered with a blue Exactobite edge-to-edge with 2 mm vertical interincisal clearance.

Clinical management:

Progress in this case proved to be slow because the patient did not always posture forward. After 7 months the thickness of the blocks was increased slightly to discourage the patient from dropping out of contact with the inclined planes. This appliance adjustment was effective in completing the remaining skeletal correction and the overjet was fully reduced after 4 more months.

Duration of treatment:

- Active phase: 11 months with Twin Blocks.
- Support phase and retention: 5 months.

CASE REPORT: J.McL.

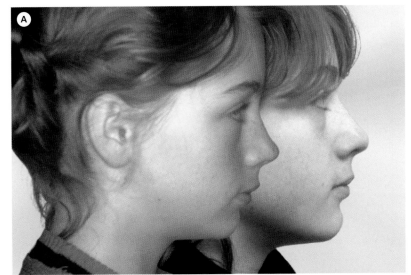

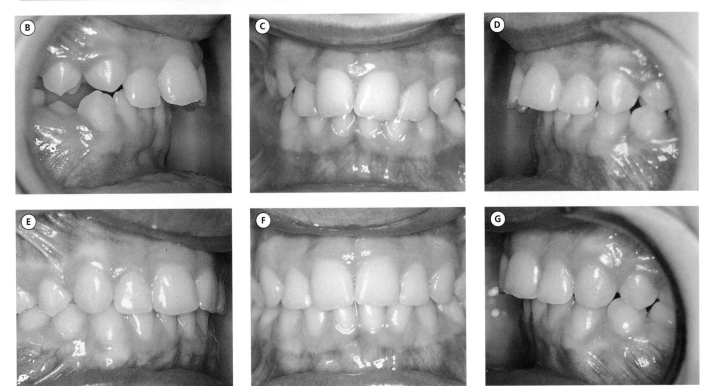

Fig. 2.13 Treatment:
A Profiles before treatment at age 12 years and 1 year out of retention at age 14 years 7 months.
B, C, D Occlusion before treatment.
E, F, G Occlusion 1 year out of retention.
A diagrammatic interpretation of the treatment is given on page 20.

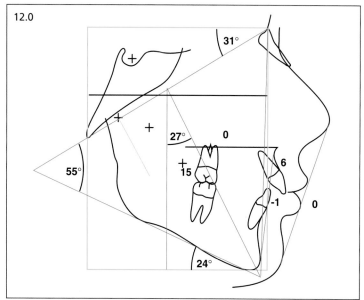

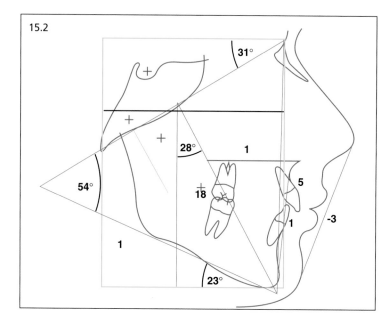

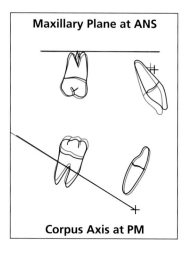

Maxillary Plane at ANS

Corpus Axis at PM

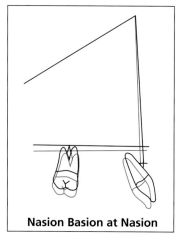

Nasion Basion at Nasion

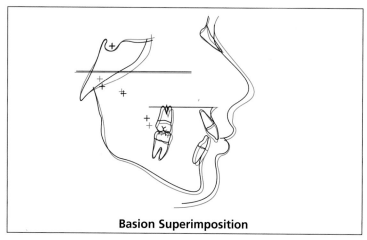

Basion Superimposition

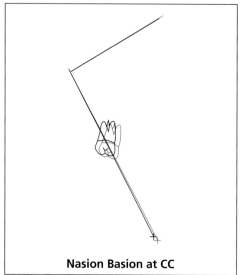

Nasion Basion at CC

J.McL.	Age 12.0	15.2
Cranial Base Angle	31	31
Facial Axis Angle	27	28
F/M Plane Angle	24	23
Craniomandibular Angle	55	54
Maxillary Plane	0	1
Convexity	6	5
U/Incisor to Vertical	33	28
L/Incisor to Vertical	27	25
Interincisal Angle	120	127
6 to Pterygoid Vertical	15	18
L/Incisor to A/Po	−1	1
L/Lip to Aesthetic Plane	0	−3

CHAPTER 3

Form and Function

DEVELOPMENT OF FUNCTIONAL TECHNIQUE

In the early part of the twentieth century, the 'form and function' philosophy was the fundamental basis for treatment in both fixed and functional schools of therapy. The objective of treatment was to achieve ideal correction of dental arch relationships as defined by Angle (1907) and, at the same time, improve the skeletal relationship by skeletal adaptation in response to correction of the dental relationship. However, from this common origin, fixed and functional techniques followed a divergent course of development.

Modern fixed appliance technique derives largely from the work of Angle, whose philosophy was based on the concept that compensatory growth would result from expanding the dental arches with multi-banded fixed appliances and archwires and placing the orthodontically corrected arches in perfect relationship to one another.

At the same time, a parallel development was occurring in Europe, where Pierre Robin (1902a,b) first described the monobloc as the forerunner of the modern functional appliance. This was closely followed by a parallel development from Viggo Andresen (1910), who developed the activator.

A philosophical division originated when Angle attempted to accommodate a full complement of teeth to the available jaw space in every case, regardless of tooth-to-bone size discrepancy, degree of crowding or the pattern of facial growth. Non-extraction techniques were used with fixed appliances to move teeth, without significantly influencing the underlying skeletal pattern. This was followed by relapse in a high proportion of crowded dentitions treated by fixed mechanics. Consequently, non-extraction therapy fell into disrepute.

The emergence of extraction therapy

By the middle of the twentieth century, the orthodontic philosophical pendulum had swung to the other extreme as Tweed (1944) and Begg (1954) gained acceptance for the use of extractions for the relief of crowding as an integral part of orthodontic treatment planning. Hence, a mechanical approach to treatment was adopted that accepted the extraction of first premolars as standard procedure in the majority of crowded cases. The lower labial segment was thought to be in a position of natural muscle balance before treatment, and the basal perimeter of the lower arch was therefore used as a template to position the upper dentition. However, this approach made no allowance for the potential to change abnormal muscle behaviour by functional therapy.

Therapeutic limitations of the genetic paradigm

The therapeutic limitations of a genetic paradigm are significant in the treatment of Class II malocclusion due to mandibular skeletal deficiency. A philosophy that does not accept the possibility of improving mandibular growth leaves only three options in the treatment of mandibular retrusion, all of which represent a biological compromise.

- **Maxillary retraction.** Reduction of forward maxillary growth by orthopaedic extraoral force has been well documented in the literature (Wieslander, 1963, 1974, 1975; Wieslander & Buck, 1974; Graber, 1969). A distal extraoral force applied to the maxillary molars by a Kloehn facebow is accompanied in some cases by a downward and backward rotation of the maxillary plane, and a secondary downward and backward rotation of the mandible. There is some evidence that maxillary expansion to free the occlusion combined with extraoral traction may help to promote mandibular growth in cases where the growth pattern is favourable. However, a distalising extraoral force is designed to retract the maxilla to match the position of a retrusive mandible and does not encourage a retrusive mandible to achieve its full genetic potential of growth.
- **Surgical correction of mandibular position.** The alternative is to correct arch alignment in a presurgical phase of treatment, followed by surgical correction to advance the mandible into correct relationship with the

maxilla. Finally, a postsurgical phase of orthodontic treatment is then needed to detail the occlusion. This approach has the disadvantages of being lengthy, traumatic, complex and expensive. The long-term effects on the temporomandibular joints are unpredictable. It is not a widely viable solution.

- **Dentoalveolar compensation.** An orthodontic approach to treatment offers a simpler compromise that aims for dentoalveolar compensation, while accepting that the result will not be ideal because the skeletal discrepancy is beyond the limits of orthodontic therapy.

An orthodontic approach to treatment is most efficient in correcting Class I malocclusion or mild skeletal discrepancies.

It is in correction of malocclusion due to skeletal discrepancies that functional appliances come into their own. The timing of treatment by functional appliances lends itself to the interception of malocclusion at an earlier stage of development, attempting to resolve skeletal and occlusal imbalance by improving the functional environment of the developing dentition before the malocclusion can become fully established in the permanent dentition.

As previously stated, in contrast to the philosophical change that has accompanied the evolution of fixed appliance therapy, the form and function philosophy remains the basic concept of functional appliance treatment. The 'functional matrix' concept of Melvin Moss (1968) is a contemporary evaluation supporting the premise that function modifies anatomy.

It is commonly postulated that patients will not necessarily achieve their full growth potential if environmental factors are unfavourable during development. Malocclusion is frequently associated with unfavourable occlusal contacts and aberrant muscle behaviour, which result in a negative proprioceptive stimulus to normal growth and development.

BONE REMODELLING IN RESPONSE TO FUNCTIONAL STIMULI

The internal and external structure of bone is continuously modified throughout life by the process of bony remodelling. The sensory feedback mechanism helps the bony remodelling process to address the changing requirements of function in dentofacial development. Occlusal forces transmitted by the muscles of mastication through the teeth to the underlying bone provide a proprioceptive stimulus to influence the external form and internal trabecular structure of the supporting bone.

Unlike other connective tissue, bone responds to mild degrees of pressure and tension by changes of this nature. These changes are achieved by means of resorption of existing bone and deposition of new bone. This may take place on the surface of the bone, under the periosteum or, in the case of cancellous bone, on the surfaces of the trabeculae.

In this respect, bone is more plastic and adaptive than any other connective tissue. The internal and external structure of bone is modified by functional requirements to enable it to withstand the physical demands made upon it with the greatest degree of economy of structure. This principle is exemplified in 'Wolff's law of transformation of bone'. The architecture of a bone is such that it can best resist the forces that are brought to bear upon it with the use of as little tissue as possible.

During mastication forces are transmitted through the teeth to the alveolar bone and to the underlying basal bone. Most of these forces are vertical, but some are transverse and anteroposterior. The external surface of the maxilla and mandible is modified precisely by function to absorb the forces of occlusion. Well-defined ridges of bone are specifically designed to absorb and transmit these force vectors.

Mastication is a function that involves the whole face, and even part of the cranium. Considerable forces are applied through the muscles of mastication to the teeth and the underlying bony structures to influence both the internal and external structure of the basal bone. It is this natural mechanism of bony remodelling by occlusal force vectors that forms the basis of functional correction by the Twin Block technique. The forces of occlusion that are applied during mastication are harnessed as an additional stimulus to growth.

Development of the temporomandibular joint

The relationship between form and function is exemplified exquisitely in the normal development of the craniofacial skeleton. As the patient matures, progressive adaptation of the intricate skeletal structures clearly exhibits the intimate relationship between skeletal form and function.

This relationship may be further demonstrated by examination of skulls to trace the stages of development of the temporomandibular joint from infancy to adulthood. Ide *et al.* (1991), in their *Anatomical Atlas of the Temporomandibular Joint*, describe the changes with age as follows:

> The size of the fossa increases by 1.2 to 1.3 times after eruption of the deciduous teeth compared to before and it increases again at the beginning of eruption of the permanent teeth. The degree of anterior inclination of the eminence changes drastically when the deciduous teeth erupt. Eventually it becomes steeper by three times in the permanent dentition than it was before the eruption of the deciduous teeth.

In the newborn child the mandible moves freely antero-posteriorly to develop suction in the primary function of breast feeding. At this stage of development the condyle is level with the gum pads, and the articular surface of the temporomandibular joint is relatively flat to allow complete freedom of movement during suckling. The form and function of the joint in the infant is similar to that of a herbivore, with flat articular surfaces that place no restriction on mandibular movement.

When a positive overbite develops as the deciduous central incisors erupt, it is then necessary for the mandible to take avoiding action by moving slightly downwards when performing a protrusive movement. This change in function is immediatly reflected in the shape of the articular surface of the temporomandibular joint. A small ridge appears that represents the first sign of an articular eminence when the deciduous incisors erupt into contact.

As yet there is no restriction on lateral movement in the joint and, at this stage, the child is still suckling. A change in function from suckling to eating solid food is related to further changes in the form and function of the temporomandibular joint to accommodate the corresponding change in masticatory function. When first deciduous molars erupt into occlusion, the form of the articular surface of the joint is modified by occlusion of the deciduous molars that now influence lateral guidance of the mandible.

As deciduous canines and molars erupt, the proprioceptive sensory feedback mechanism is responsible for continuing subtle changes in the form of the temporomandibular joint. Progressive modification of the shape of the joint articular surfaces relates to control of mandibular movement as the occlusion develops, and the joint adapts to altered function.

Still further modification of the shape of the temporomandibular articulation accompanies the transition from mixed to permanent dentition as the joint continues its adaptive development in response to the proprioceptive stimulus of a progressively more robust occlusion.

In the mature adult, the contours of the joint are fully developed and reflect the adaptive influences of the joint to the demands placed on it by the occlusion during the growth years. Occlusal guidance is directly related to condyle movement, and the shape of the joint articular surfaces in turn reflects the freedom of movement of the dentition in function. Malocclusion that presents occlusal interferences is related to restricted occlusal guidance with corresponding modification of the shape and function of the temporomandibular joint.

This correlation of form and function is also observed in the slope of the articular eminence as it relates to the occlusion. Restricted anterior movement is experienced in the Class II division 2 malocclusion, where the deep overbite necessitates a steep vertical movement of the mandible to allow the incisors to avoid occlusal interference in opening. There is an equivalent steep angulation of the articular eminence in this type of malocclusion that is related intimately to severely restricted mandibular movement in protrusive function.

Considering the aetiology of internal derangement of the temporomandibular joint, Hawthorn & Flatau (1990) observe:

> . . . displacement of the meniscus anteriorly with subsequent reciprocal click in many cases is the result of confinement of mandibular movement caused by deep anterior overbite. Further degeneration or confinement of mandibular movement is brought about by developmental changes that may occur in the occlusion during the mixed dentition stage, resulting in a restrictive functional tooth angle . . . it is necessary to release the mandible from a restrictive closing pathway. For long term success . . . it is also necessary to provide stable, bilateral occlusal support.

Most preactivated fixed appliances in present use are designed for treatment in the permanent dentition. Late treatment of malocclusion allows adverse occlusal guidance to influence the form of the developing temporomandibular joint. The relationship between malocclusion and the development of the temporomandibular joint supports the case for early interception of malocclusion.

Functional therapy, by interceptive treatment at an earlier stage of development, attempts to achieve freedom of movement in occlusal function and thereby encourage the development of healthy joints.

The form and function philosophy is a natural progression of normal development, where functional stimuli operate through the sensory feedback mechanism to influence bone growth. In the normal sequence of growth and development, occlusal function is related directly to the functional development of the temporomandibular joint.

Evolution of functional appliance technique

It was mainly due to socioeconomic reasons that the development of functional appliances occurred almost exclusively in Europe during the major part of the twentieth century.

In the early 1900s, parallel development began in the USA and Europe in fixed and functional techniques, respectively. The Atlantic Ocean formed a geographical barrier that restricted the sharing of knowledge and experience in the fixed and functional philosophies. Integration of the two disciplines was further restricted during the First and Second World Wars, after which both cultures were committed to treatment systems that reflected their economic state.

Construction and fitting of fixed appliances by hand was time consuming and expensive. The bands were formed on the teeth and welded before attaching brackets. This procedure was beyond the economic means and social circumstances of most Europeans at this stage.

The functional concept employs carefully designed removable appliances in an effort to achieve harmonious development of the dentofacial structures by eliminating unfavourable myofunctional and occlusal factors and improving the functional environment of the developing dentition. By altering the position of the teeth and supporting tissues, a new functional behaviour pattern is established to support a new position of equilibrium. This concept flourished in Europe and formed the basis of functional therapy for over a century, resulting in the development of a wide range of appliances.

The many variations in design of functional appliances that have been described since the beginning of the 20th century bear witness to their effectiveness in correcting malocclusion and improving facial balance and harmony in the developing dentition.

Significant progress has been made to improve the design of functional appliances, which were worn only at night for the first half of the twentieth century. There followed a steady process of evolution, whereby the bulk of the early monobloc and Andresen activator was reduced by removing acrylic in order to design a series of 'daytime activators', culminating in Balters Bionator, which was aptly described as 'the skeleton of the activator'.

Another avenue of development produced flexible functional appliances by substituting wire for acrylic. Bimler (1949) and Frankel & Frankel (1989) made excellent scientific contributions to the theory and practice of functional jaw orthopaedics using flexible appliances adapted for daytime wear.

Limitations of functional appliance design

All the functional appliances that have evolved from the monobloc share the limitation that the upper and lower components are joined together. As a result, the patient cannot eat, speak or function normally with the appliance in the mouth. It is also impossible to wear a one-piece functional appliance full time if it is attached to the teeth in both jaws, and the interruption to appliance wear can be a major disadvantage.

The early functional appliances were designed for night-time wear, which limited the response to treatment. It was also important to select patients who had a favourable growth pattern in order to improve the prognosis for correction, and to eliminate the uncertainty associated with night-time functional appliances. There is better potential for rapid mandibular growth when the patient has a favourable horizontal growth pattern than when the facial growth vector is more vertical.

The muscles are the prime movers that modify bone growth to meet the demands of function via the proprioceptive feedback mechanism. When the appliance is removed for eating the patient reverts to functioning with the mandible in a retrusive position. The strongest functional forces are applied to the dentition during mastication, and the proprioceptive functional stimulus to growth is lost if the appliance is removed for eating.

Comfort and aesthetics are crucial in appliance design. It is essential that the patient can speak clearly with the appliance in place to avoid embarrassment. A monobloc type of appliance that is designed to fit the teeth in both jaws simultaneously interferes with speech and limits normal function. These are important factors that influence patient motivation and compliance, and are closely related to success in treatment.

The Schwarz Double Plate

The Double Plate of Martin Schwarz (1956) attempted to combine the advantages of the activator and the active plate by constructing separate upper and lower acrylic plates that were designed to occlude with the mandible in a protrusive position. The Double Plate resembled a monobloc or activator constructed in two pieces.

The maxillary appliance for correction of Class II division 1 malocclusion carried lingual flanges that extended into the lower dental arch to articulate with the lower appliance on an inclined plane, causing a functional mandibular displacement on closure. There were two variations in appliance design that incorporated anterior or lateral lingual flanges, respectively, extending from the upper appliance to occlude in grooves fashioned in the lower appliance. The anterior lingual flange was used more commonly, and represented an extension of the principle of the anterior inclined plane, originally developed by Kingsley (1877). Graber & Neuman (1977) observed that in spite of the advantageous features of the double plates, they gained limited acceptance, as they were complicated to construct, and other competing appliances were more comfortable to wear.

A widely recommended variation in design was described by Muller (1962). The lateral wings were replaced by heavy gauge wires of 2 mm diameter, that extended downwards from the upper appliance at an angle of 70° to engage a groove in the lower appliance.

The anterior version of the double plate was later modified by F. G. Sanders using heavy wire extensions to replace the acrylic flanges.

The emergence of functional appliances for full-time wear, including for eating, is the next logical step in the evolution of functional jaw orthopaedics, thus taking advantage of the forces of mastication to provide an additional proprioceptive stimulus to growth by using the forces of occlusion to correct the malocclusion.

OBJECTIVES OF FUNCTIONAL TREATMENT

In the natural dentition a functional equilibrium is established under neurological control in response to repetitive tactile stimuli as the teeth come into occlusion. A favourable equilibrium of muscle forces between the tongue, lips and cheeks is essential for normal development of the dental arches in correct relationship.

Any persistent deviation from normal function is associated with malocclusion. Discrepancies in arch relationships due to underlying skeletal and soft-tissue factors result in unfavourable cuspal guidance and poor occlusal function.

The purpose of functional therapy is to change the functional environment of the dentition to promote normal function. Functional appliances are designed to control the forces applied to the dentition by the surrounding soft tissues and by the muscles that control the position and movement of the mandible. A new functional behaviour pattern is established to support a new position of equilibrium by eliminating unfavourable environmental factors in a developing malocclusion.

The natural occlusal forces acting on a mandible in distal occlusion do not favour mandibular development to the patient's full potential of growth. The mandible is locked in a distal position by an unfavourable or distal driving occlusion.

Conversely, in a Class III malocclusion the maxilla is locked in a distal relationship by unfavourable occlusal forces. Altered occlusal function in this type of malocclusion has the effect of restricting maxillary development and advancing the mandible.

Functional therapy aims to unlock the malocclusion and stimulate growth by applying favourable forces that enhance skeletal development. Growth studies on experimental animals support the view that altered occlusal function produces significant changes in craniofacial growth.

BITE REGISTRATION IN FUNCTIONAL THERAPY

Bite registration is a crucial factor in the design and construction of a functional appliance. The construction bite determines the degree of activation built into the appliance, aiming to reposition the mandible to improve the jaw relationship. The degree of activation should stretch the muscles of mastication sufficiently to provide a positive proprioceptive response. At the same time, activation must be within the physiological range of activity of the muscles of mastication and the ligamentous attachments of the temporomandibular joint. Bite registration should achieve a balance between these factors by providing the degree of

mandibular protrusion required to achieve the optimum functional stimulus to growth.

According to Woodside (1977, p. 293), in construction of the activator as described by Andresen (1910):

> A bite registration used commonly throughout the world registers the mandible in a position protruded approximately 3.0 mm distal to the most protrusive position that the patient can achieve, while vertically the bite is registered within the limits of the patient's freeway space.

In North America, a similar protrusive bite registration is made, except that the vertical activation is 4 mm beyond the rest position.

Roccabado (pers. comm.) quantifies normal physiological temporomandibular joint movement as 70% of total joint displacement. Beyond this point, the medial capsular ligamente begins to displace the disc by pulling the disc medially and distally off the condyle. This guideline allows us to measure the total mandibular displacement and relate the amount of activation to the freedom of movement of the joint for each individual patient.

Bite registration in Twin Block technique

Bite registration for Twin Blocks originally aimed for a single activation to an edge-to-edge incisor relationship with 2 mm intercisal clearance for an overjet of up to 10 mm. Allowance was made for individual variation if the patient had difficulty in maintaining an edge-to-edge position on registering the occlusion. This proved to be successful in correcting the overjet and reducing the distal occlusion in the majority of cases.

Where the overjet was greater than 10 mm, an initial advancement of 7 mm or 8 mm was followed by reactivation of the appliance after occlusion had corrected to the initial bite registration. Normally, a single further activation was sufficient to fully correct the overjet and distal occlusion.

In the early stages of using Twin Blocks it was noted that some patients had difficulty in maintaining the forward posture and occluding correctly on the inclined planes. These patients usually had a vertical growth pattern with weak musculature and were unable to maintain the forward mandibular posture consistently. They could be identified early in treatment as they tended to posture the mandible back and meet the blocks together behind the inclined planes. To overcome this problem the activation of the appliance was reduced slightly by trimming the inclined planes until the patient occluded comfortably and consistently in the forward position.

This difficulty can be avoided by relating bite registration to the patient's freedom of movement and by registering the protrusive path of the mandible. The George bite gauge has a millimetre gauge to measure the protrusive path of the mandible and to determine accurately the amount of activation registered in the construction bite.

The total protrusive movement is calculated by first measuring the overjet in centric occlusion and then in the position of maximum protrusion. The protrusive path of the mandible is the difference between the two measurements. Functional activation within normal physiological limits should not exceed 70% of the protrusive path (George, pers. comm.) (Fig. 3.1).

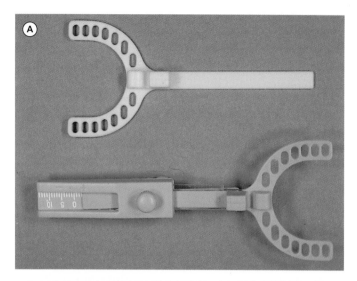

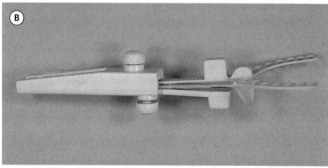

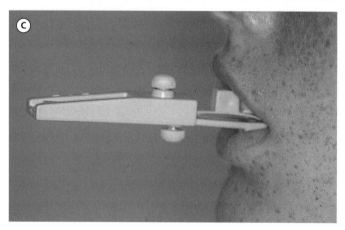

Fig. 3.1 A The George Bite Gauge has a millimetre gauge to measure the protrusive path of the mandible and to determine accurately the amount of activation registered in the construction bite.
B, C Lateral views to show method of bite registration.

By checking the protrusive path the adjustment may be related to the patient's physiological movements. The young patient usually has more freedom of movement while there is generally more restriction in the adult. In Class II division 1 malocclusion, young patients commonly have a protrusive path of 13 mm and will tolerate activation up to 10 mm. Beyond this range the muscles and ligaments cannot adapt to altered function and the patient will tend to posture out of the appliance. If the overjet is larger than 10 mm the initial activation should only partially reduce the overjet. The appliance is then reactivated during the course of treatment.

Vertical activation

The amount of vertical activation is crucial to the success of Twin Block treatment. The most common fault in Twin Block construction is to make the blocks too thin, so that the patient can posture out of the appliance, reducing the effectiveness of the treatment.

An important principle is that the blocks should be thick enough to open the bite slightly beyond the free-way space. This is necessary to ensure that the patient does not posture out of the appliance when the mandible is in the rest position.

On average the blocks are not less than 5 mm thick in the first premolar or first deciduous molar region. This thickness is normally achieved in Class II division 1 deep bite cases by registering a 2 mm vertical interincisal clearance.

In Class II division 2 malocclusion with excessive overbite it is sufficient to register an edge-to-edge incisal bite registration without the additional 2 mm interincisal clearance. This is normally sufficient in this type of malocclusion to accommodate blocks of the correct thickness.

In treatment of anterior open bite it is necessary to register bite with a greater interincisal clearance to make allowance for the anterior open bite. The projet or George bite gauge has thicker versions to accommodate an interincisal clearance of 4 or 5 mm. At bite registration a judgement should be made according to the amount of vertical space between the cusptips of the first premolars or deciduous molars to achieve the correct degree of bite opening to accommodate blocks of at least 5 mm thickness.

Single or progressive activation

Petrovic et al. (1981) found in animal experiments that a stepwise activation appeared to be the best procedure to promote orthopaedic lengthening of the mandible. Taking this into account, Falke & Frankel (1989) reduced initial activation for mandibular advancement to 3 mm, having previously registered an edge-to-edge bite unless the overjet was excessive. The concept of progressive activation for functional correction to achieve the optimum growth response has been investigated (De Vincenzo & Winn, 1989; Falke & Frankel, 1989) with differing results, and requires further investigation.

The latter study used occlusal bite blocks to investigate the relative effects of progressive activation compared to a single large activation. The study concludes that there is no difference in either orthodontic or orthopaedic variables between progressive 3 mm advancement and a single advancement averaging 5–6 mm. Continuous advancement by progressive 1 mm activations shows a diminished but still statistically significant response. Progressive activation is found to be time consuming with no measurable improvement in the response. These findings support the author's clinical experience that a single large activation is more efficient than smaller progressive activations.

However, Carmichael, Banks and Chadwick have described a screw advancement mechanism for progressive activation of Twin Blocks. Stepwise advancement may be beneficial in correction of larger overjets, or in the treatment of vertical growth patterns, where smaller adjustments may improve patient tolerance.

CONTROL OF THE VERTICAL DIMENSION

The mechanism of control of the vertical dimension differs in fixed and functional therapy. In fixed mechanics, the teeth remain in occlusion during the course of treatment, and the effect is limited to intrusion or extrusion of individual teeth to increase or decrease overbite and level the occlusal plane. The occlusal level is determined by occlusal contact with teeth in the opposing arch. Functional appliances have the advantage of influencing facial height to control the vertical dimension by covering the teeth with blocks or an occlusal table.

Functional appliances are designed to influence development in the anteroposterior and vertical dimensions simultaneously. Control of the vertical dimension is achieved by covering the teeth in the opposing arches and controlling the intermaxillary space. The management of the appliance differs according to whether the bite is to be opened or closed during treatment.

Opening the bite

Where a deep overbite is present it is necessary first to check that the profile is improved when the patient postures the mandible downwards and forwards. This confirms that the bite should be opened by encouraging eruption of the posterior teeth to increase the vertical dimension of occlusion.

This is achieved by placing an occlusal table between the teeth to encourage increased development of posterior facial height by growth of the vertical ramus. At the same time, the occlusion is freed between the posterior teeth to encourage selective eruption of posterior teeth to increase the vertical dimension of occlusion in the posterior quadrants.

In functional therapy anteroposterior correction is invariably achieved before vertical development in the buccal segments is complete. The overjet is reduced and the distal occlusion corrected before the buccal teeth have completely erupted into occlusion. It is common in functional therapy for a posterior open bite to develop as the overjet reduces. The upper and lower incisors come into occlusion before the posterior teeth erupt. Functional therapy should continue to encourage development in the vertical dimension until the occlusion of the posterior teeth is established to support the correction of the overbite and overjet.

If a functional appliance is removed for eating, the tongue often spreads laterally between the teeth and delays eruption. Full-time appliance wear with Twin Blocks prevents the tongue from spreading between the teeth and accelerates correction of deep overbite.

Closing the bite

Reduced overbite or anterior open bite is often related to a vertical facial growth pattern. The lower facial height is already increased, and the vertical dimension must not be encouraged to increase during treatment. It is necessary to close the anterior vertical dimension, and treatment should endeavour to reduce lower facial height by applying intrusive forces to the opposing posterior teeth.

An acrylic occlusal table is designed into the appliance to maintain contact on the posterior teeth throughout treatment. This occlusal contact results in a relative intrusion of the posterior teeth while the anterior teeth are free to erupt, thereby reducing the anterior open bite.

In the Twin Block technique the intrusive forces which close the bite are increased by wearing the appliances for

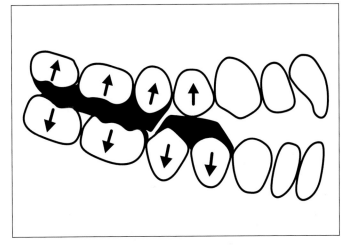

Fig. 3.2 Occlusal blocks contact posterior teeth to prevent eruption.

eating. In treatment of reduced overbite it is very important that the opposing acrylic occlusal bite block surfaces are not trimmed. All posterior teeth must remain in contact with the blocks throughout treatment to prevent eruption of posterior teeth (Fig. 3.2).

Manipulation of the occlusal table is an important aspect of functional appliance therapy. By separating the posterior teeth it is possible to adjust the dimensions of the intermaxillary space anteroposteriorly and vertically to correct skeletal discrepancies. The concept of using occlusal inclined planes as a functional mechanism to correct distal malocclusion is the next logical step in the evolution of functional appliance technique. The mechanics can be reversed, applying the same principles for correction of Class III malocclusion.

REFERENCES

Angle, E.H. (1907). *Treatment of Malocclusion of the Teeth*, 7th edn. Philadelphia, S.S. White Dental Manufacturing Co.

Andresen, V. (1910). Beitrag zur Retention. *Z. Zahnaerztl. Orthop.*, **3**: 121–5.

Begg, P.R. (1954). Stone Age man's dentition. *Am. J. Orthod.*, **40**: 298–312; 373–83; 462–75; 517–31.

Bimler, H.P. (1949) Die elastichen Gebissformer. *Zahnarzel. Welt.* **19**: 499–505

De Vicenzo, J.P. & Winn, M.W. (1989). Orthopaedic and orthodontic effects resulting from the use of a functional appliance with different amounts of protrusive activation. *Am. J. Orthod. Orthop.*, **96**: 181–190.

Falke, F. & Frankel, R. (1989). Clinical relevance of step by step mandibular advancement in the treatment of mandibular retrusion using the Frankel appliance. *Am. J. Orthod. Dentofac. Orthop.*, **96**: 333–41.

Frankel, R. & Frankel, Ch. (1989). *Orofacial Orthopedics with the Function Regulator*. Basel, Karger.

Graber (Ed.) (1969). *Dento-facial Orthopaedics. Current Orthodontic Concepts and Techniques*, Vol. 2. Philadelphia, W.B. Saunders.

Graber & Neumann (1977) *Removable Orthodontic Appliances*. Philadelphia, W.B. Saunders.

Hawthorn, R. & Flatau, A. (1990). Temporomandibular joint anatomy. In *A Colour Atlas of Temporomandibular Joint Surgery*, ed. J.E.DeB. Norman & P.E. Bramley. London, Wolfe Publishing.

Ide, Y., Nakazawa, K., Hongo, J. & Tateishi, J. (1991). *Anatomical Atlas of the Temporomandibular Joint*. Tokyo, Quintessence Publishing Co.

Kingsley, N.W. (1877). An experiment with artificial palates. *Dent. Cosmos.*, **19**: 231.

Moss, M.L. (1968). The primacy of functional matrices in profacial growth, *Dent. Practitioner*, **19**: 65–73.

Muller, G.H. (1962). Die Doppelplatte mit Oberkeifer-spornfuhrung. *Fortschr. Kieferorthop*, **23**: 245–50.

Petrovic, A.G., Stutzmann, J.J. & Gasson, N. (1981). The final length of the mandible: is it genetically determined? In *Craniofacial Biology*, ed. D.S. Carlson, Monograph No. 10. Center for Human Growth & Development, University of Michigan, pp. 105–26.

Robin, P. (1902a). Observation sur un nouvel appareil de redressement. *Rev. Stomatol.*, 9.

Robin, P. (1902b). Demonstration practique sur la construction et la mise en bouche d'un nouvel appareil de redressement. *Rev. Stomatol.*, 9.

Schwarz, A.M. (1956). *Lehrgang der Gebissregelung*, 2nd edn. Vienna, Urban & Schwarzenberg.

Tweed, C.H. (1944). Indications for the extraction of teeth in orthodontic procedure. *Am. J. Orthod. Oral Surg.*, August.

Wieslander, L. (1963). The effect of orthodontic treatment on concurrent development of the craniofacial complex. *Am. J. Orthod.*, **49**: 15–27.

Wieslander, L. (1974). The effect of force on cranio-facial development. *Am. J. Orthod.*, **65**: 531–8.

Wieslander, L (1975). Early or late cervical traction therapy in Class II malocclusion in the mixed dentition. *Am. J. Orthod.*, **67**: 432–9.

Wieslander, L. & Buck, D.L. (1974). Physiological recovery after cervical traction therapy. *Am. J. Orthod.*, **66**: 294–301.

Woodside, D.G. (1977). The activator. In *Removable Orthodontic Appliances*, ed. T.M. Graber & B. Neumann. Philadelphia, W.B. Saunders.

FURTHER READING

Broadbent, J.M. (1987). Crossroads: acceptance or rejection of Functional Jaw Orthopedics. *Am. J. Orthod.*, **92**: 75–8.

Carmichael, G.J., Banks P.A., Chadwick S.M. (1999). A modification to enable controlled progressive advancement of the Twin Block Appliance. *Br. J. Orthodon.*, **26**: 9–14.

George, P.T. (1992). A new instrument for functional appliance bite registration. *J. Clin. Orthod.*, **26**: 721–3.

Wolff, J. (1892). *Das Gesets der transformation der Knochen*. Berlin, Hirschwald.

CHAPTER 4

Growth Studies in Experimental Animals

HISTOLOGICAL RESPONSE TO ORTHODONTIC AND ORTHOPAEDIC FORCE

During the first half of the twentieth century animal research established the basis for orthodontic tooth movement. Classic histological studies by Sandstedt (1904, 1905), Oppenheim (1911), Schwarz (1932) and Reitan (1951) defined the ground rules for orthodontic treatment. Dogs were used as experimental animals to determine the tissue response to the application of force to individual teeth, and Reitan made comparative studies in human subjects. Thus the role of osteoclasts and osteoblasts in the remodelling of alveolar bone was described and optimum force levels determined for efficient movement of teeth through alveolar bone. The findings of this research remain of fundamental importance in clinical orthodontic practice today, and indeed established the ground rules for orthodontic treatment.

During the second half of the twentieth century as the emphasis of research moved from orthodontic to orthopaedic treatment, histological examination has revealed the mechanism of bony remodelling in the condyle and, of equal importance, in the glenoid fossa in response to the application of orthopaedic forces by functional mandibular protrusion. Experiments in monkeys and rodents used full-time appliances with occlusal inclined planes to demonstrate the biological response to functional mandibular protrusion. Animal research is again important in providing scientific evidence as the basis to establish guidelines for orthopaedic treatment in a similar pattern to the investigation of orthodontic treatment. The present state of knowledge of the biological response to orthopaedic treatment is similar to our perception of orthodontic treatment during the first half of the twentieth century.

Animal experiments to investigate the biological response to orthodontic and orthopaedic techniques provide a basis for comparison with clinical experience, when we apply similar techniques in the treatment of patients. Many researchers have reached similar conclusions regarding the effects of functional mandibular protrusion on the growth of the condyle and bony remodelling in the glenoid fossa. The findings of current research into the mechanisms that control bone growth are now examined.

The results of recent growth studies on experimental animals suggest consistently that skeletal form is adaptable to functional stimulus (Charlier et al., 1969; Moyers et al., 1970; Petrovic et al., 1971; Stockli & Willert, 1971; Elgoyhen et al., 1972; McNamara, 1972).

Experiments have shown that condylar cartilage is highly responsive to mechanical stimuli (Stockli & Willert, 1971) and to hormonal and chemical agents (Petrovic & Stutzmann, 1977).

Hinton (1981) reviews temporomandibular joint function to clarify past misconceptions. Clinical, experimental and biochemical data strongly suggest that the temporomandibular joint is an articulation to which forces are transmitted during normal dental function, and one that undergoes adaptive remodelling in response to these forces.

Harvold (1983) commented on research started in the University of California in 1965 to examine the changes that occur in the internal structure of bone in response to functional stimulus:

> The pilot studies demonstrated that an alteration in pressure distribution on the maxilla caused rapid resorption of the existing trabecular system within two months. Another few months were necessary before the stabilised pressure distribution was manifested in a new, functionally orientated trabecular system. These pilot experiments indicated that only stimuli that were relatively uniform for a period of several months could contribute to the development of a trabecular system.

THE OCCLUSAL INCLINED PLANE IN ANIMAL EXPERIMENTS

Moss (1980), investigating the effects of the inclined plane in six adult ferrets, concluded:

> The results of this simple experiment illustrate the profound effect that a biting force on an inclined plane can have on the whole of the dental arch, including the condylar head, the muscle attachments and teeth remote from the tooth being moved. Even in the adult animal, the whole of the stomatognathic system, including the soft tissues, adapts to re-establish an efficient masticatory system.

FUNCTIONAL REGULATION OF CONDYLAR CARTILAGE GROWTH RATE

The theory of functional regulation of condylar cartilage growth rate is supported by recent evidence from animal experiments (Stutzmann & Petrovic, 1979; McNamara 1980).

Fixed occlusal inclined planes have been used to alter the distribution of occlusal forces in animal experiments investigating the effects of functional mandibular displacement on mandibular growth and on adaptive changes in the temporomandibular joint (Stutzmann & Petrovic, 1979; McNamara, 1980). Results have demonstrated improved mandibular growth in experimental animals compared to control animals (Fig. 4.1).

A fundamental study of the relationship between form and function was carried out in animal experiments at the University of Michigan, and the results were summarised by McNamara (1980). The studies evaluated changes in muscle function and related changes in bone growth in the rhesus monkey by a comparison of experimental and control animals as monitored by electromyographic (EMG), cephalometric and histological studies. McNamara concluded:

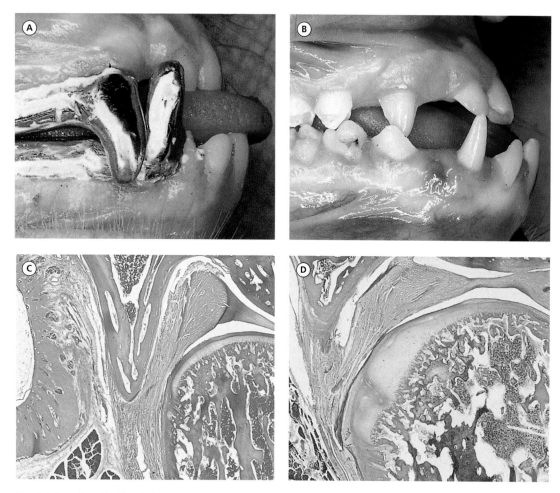

Fig. 4.1 A, B Fixed inclined planes produced a Class III dental relationship in monkeys.
C, D Proliferation of condylar cartilage in experimental animals demonstrated compared to controls.
Courtesy of J.A. McNamara Jr.

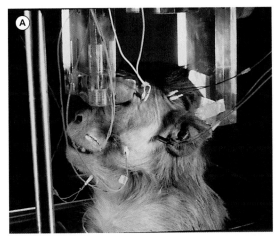 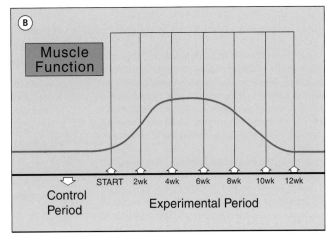

Fig. 4.2 A, B Electromyographic study shows the cycle of change in muscle behaviour. *Courtesy of J.A. McNamara Jr.*

These studies demonstrated the close relationship between the functional and structural components of the craniofacial region.

The findings were based on the use of fixed occlusal inclined planes that were designed to cause a forward postural displacement of the mandible in all active and passive muscle activity. The pattern of muscle behaviour during the experimental period showed a cyclical change in response to functional mandibular propulsion. Each animal was used as its own control to register muscle activity by a series of control records prior to appliance placement. This established the level of muscle activity before treatment.

Initial placement of the appliance produced an increase in the overall activity of the muscles of mastication as the animal sought to find a new occlusal position. A distinct change in muscle activity occurred within 1–7 days. This was characterised by a decrease in the activity of the posterior head of temporalis, an increase in activity of the masseter muscle, and most significantly an increase in function of the superior head of the lateral pterygoid muscle.

After 3 weeks a new plateau of muscle activity was reached at a higher level of activity than the pretreatment record. This level of activity persisted for 4 weeks before a further decline in muscle activity over a period of 4 weeks to the level recorded before treatment. The cycle of changes was completed in a 3-month period (Fig. 4.2).

These changes are consistent with an equilibrium of muscle activity before treatment which is disturbed by placement of the appliance. The level of muscle activity increases accordingly until, after a period of adjustment, a new equilibrium is reached at a higher level of activity. Further adaptation within the muscles over a period of time results in a reduction of muscle activity when a new equilibrium is again established at the same level that existed before treatment.

A similar experimental study at the University of Toronto came to different conclusions on the effect of placement of a functional appliance on muscle activity (Sessle *et al.*, 1990). This study used chronically implanted EMG electrodes to identify a statistically significant decrease in postural EMG activity of the superior and inferior heads of the lateral pterygoid, and the superficial masseter muscles, which persisted for 6 weeks and returned to pretreatment levels during a subsequent 6-week period. Progressive mandibular advancement of 1.5–2 mm every 10–15 days did not prevent the decrease in postural EMG activity.

The clinical implication of these differing results is that the question of activation of a functional appliance by a single large mandibular displacement or a progressive series of smaller activations is still to be resolved.

It is not established whether active muscle contraction or passive muscle tension is the primary stimulus to growth in functional therapy.

CENTRAL CONTROL OF ADAPTIVE RESPONSE

Neuromuscular and skeletal adaptations

In principle, the muscles are the prime movers in promoting skeletal adaptation in response to proprioceptive sensory stimulus. Adaptive skeletal changes in the structure and form of bone are a secondary response to alterations in sensory and muscle function. Essentially, skeletal changes occur to support the alteration in load and functional requirements, assuming that the alterations in occlusal function are within the biological limits of tolerance of the organism.

McNamara (1980) summarises the adaptive responses observed in functional protrusion experiments as follows:

> The placement of the appliance results in an immediate change in the stimuli to the receptors in the orofacial region, particularly those in the tongue, gingiva, palate, dentition and temporo-mandibular joint region. This alteration in stimuli is transmitted to the central nervous system that . . . mediates changes in muscle activity. This alteration in muscle function leads to a forward positioning of the jaw. These muscular changes are very rapid and can be measured in terms of minutes, hours and days.
>
> Structural adaptations are more gradual in nature. Structural adaptations occur throughout the craniofacial region … As structural balance is restored during the weeks and months following appliance placement, the need for altered muscle activity is lessened, and there is a gradual return to more typical muscle patterns. This experimental model provides a clear illustration of the relationship between form and function in the growing individual.

McNamara concluded that a rapid neuromuscular response is followed by a more gradual skeletal adaptation. Structural harmony can be restored by a combination of mechanisms including dentoalveolar movement or condylar growth. The exact nature of the skeletal adaptations depends upon the age of the animal.

In growing monkeys, increased growth of the mandibular condyle is shown following functional protrusion. As a result of mandibular hyperpropulsion, the dental relationship changed in the experimental animals from normal to Class III occlusion.

The following factors may all contribute to the development of a Class III molar relationship:

- Restriction of maxillary skeletal growth.
- Inhibition of downward and forward migration of maxillary dentition.
- Mesial migration of mandibular dentition.
- Increased mandibular skeletal growth.
- Adaptations in other regions.

The study concluded that the Class III dental relationship could not be explained by adaptations in any single craniofacial structure or region, but was a result of both pronounced and subtle adaptations throughout the structures of the craniofacial complex.

ADAPTATION IN BONE GROWTH IN RESPONSE TO FUNCTIONAL STIMULUS

Research on bone growth at the University of Toronto has examined adaptive changes in bone in response to functional stimulus. Woodside *et al.* (1983) hypothesised that the movement of bone into new positions within a muscle system results in rearrangement of the stress distribution and reorganisation of shape and internal structure. To test the hypothesis, clinical and animal experiments involving the use of posterior occlusal bite blocks, Herbst appliances and temporal and masseter muscle stimulation were undertaken. This study concluded:

> Chronic or continuous alteration in mandibular position within the neuromuscular environment with the posterior occlusal bite block and the Herbst appliance in a sample of monkeys produced extensive condylar remodelling and change in mandibular size.

These experiments demonstrate the principle that:

> consistent changes in bone shape and internal structure are obtained when the alteration in neuromuscular activity is continuous and that changing the muscle activity will affect the bone morphology.

THE INFLUENCE OF FUNCTIONAL APPLIANCE THERAPY ON GLENOID FOSSA REMODELLING

In further experiments Woodside *et al.* (1987) examined: 'The influence of functional appliance therapy on glenoid fossa remodeling', following a period of progressively activated and continuously maintained advancement using the Herbst appliance. They concluded:

> In adult, adolescent and juvenile primates, continuous and progressive mandibular protrusion produces extensive anterior remodelling of the glenoid fossa. In all experimental animals, including, most importantly, the mature adult, a large volume of new bone had formed in the glenoid fossa, especially along the anterior border of the postglenoid spine. With this bone formation, and the resorption along the posterior border of the postglenoid spine, the glenoid fossa appeared to be remodelling anteriorly.
>
> Expert histopathologists agreed that the newly forming bone had a normal appearance. The new bone formation appeared to be localised in the primary attachment area of the posterior fibrous tissue of the articular disc. The deposition of the finger-like woven bone seemed to correspond to the direction of tension exerted by the stretched fibres of the posterior part of the disc.

This study further concluded that the proliferation of condylar tissue may be age- or sex-related, and was seen only in the juvenile primate. Proliferation of the posterior part of the fibrous articular disc was also described, splinting the condyle eccentrically in the glenoid fossa. The skeletal jaw relationship may be altered by both glenoid fossa remodelling and condylar extension in young primates, and thereafter by glenoid fossa relocation. This result may be related to age, sex and the amount of mandibular protrusion. Deposition of new bone on the posterior wall of the glenoid fossa is even more significant than thickening of the condylar cartilage, and is a major factor in the repositioning of the mandible (Fig. 4.3).

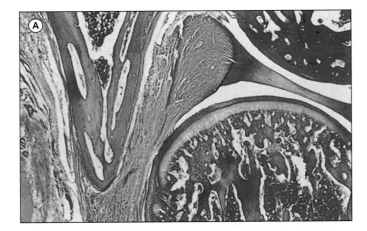

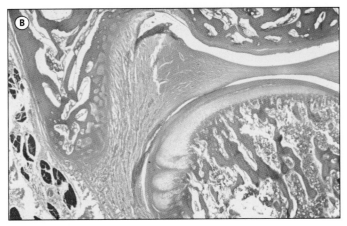

Fig. 4.3 A, B Adaptive changes in the glenoid fossa.

A REVIEW OF THE PARADIGM OF GENETIC CONTROL

It is never too late to give up your prejudices (Henry David Thoreau)

The paradigm of strict genetic control of growth mechanisms is reviewed in a paper by Petrovic *et al.* (1981), entitled: 'The final length of the mandible: is it genetically predetermined?':

> Our concept of orthopaedically modulable growth in the mammalian condylar cartilage was confirmed by Stockli & Willert (1971); McNamara *et al.* (1975); Graber (1975) and Komposh & Hocenjos (1977). Only experiments by Gaumond (1973, 1975) in the rat fail to support the possibility that the mandible can be lengthened by orthopaedic forces.
>
> The orthodontic community began to accept the idea that it is possible to change not only growth direction, but also growth rate (Graber, 1972; Linge, 1977). The idea that the final length of the mandible is 'genetically preprogrammed' has been the prevalent concept for the past 40 years, even if not specifically substantiated (Brodie, 1941; Ricketts, 1952; Bjork, 1955; Hiniker & Ramfjord, 1964; Harvold, 1968; Joho, 1968). Indeed, this concept is widely accepted as part of the doctrine underlying fixed appliance ideology.

Petrovic *et al.* (1981) conclude:

- Appropriate orthopaedic appliances placing the rat mandible in a forward position increase the condylar cartilage growth rate, and growth amount, i.e. the mandible becomes longer than that of control animals. … No genetically predetermined length of the mandible could be detected in these experiments.
- When the appliance was removed after the growth of the animal was completed, no relapse was observed. When the appliance was removed before growth was completed no significant relapse was detected if a good intercuspation had been achieved during the experimental phase; if a good intercuspation had not been achieved, the 'comparator' of the servosystem imposed an increased or decreased condylar growth rate until a state of intercuspal stability was established.
- Appliances used in the child and aimed to produce effects similar to those produced in the rat should be appropriate.

A comparison of Twin Block response with animal experiments

The clinical response observed after fitting Twin Blocks is closely analogous to the changes observed and reported in animal experiments using fixed inclined planes. Harvold (1983) confirms from histological study in animal experiments that rapid adaptive changes occur in the tissues surrounding the condyle when a full-time functional appliance is fitted:

> The placement of appliances results in an immediate change in the neuromuscular proprioceptive response . . . the resulting muscular changes are very rapid, and can be measured in terms of minutes, hours and days. Structural alterations are more gradual and are measured in months, whereby the dentoskeletal structures adapt to restore a functional equilibrium to support the altered position of muscle balance.

Harvold has demonstrated in animal experiments the tissue changes that occur as a result of altered occlusal function. When the mandible postures downwards and forwards a vacuum is not created distal to the condyle. Above and behind the condyle is an area of intense cellular activity described as a 'tension zone' that is quickly invaded by proliferating connective tissue and capillary blood vessels, when the mandible functions in a protrusive position. These changes occur within hours and days, rather than weeks and months of the appliance being fitted.

These tissue changes are reflected in the clinical signs after fitting Twin Blocks. The patient experiences adaptation of muscle function immediately on insertion of the appliances, in response to altered occlusal function. When an occlusal inclined plane is fitted, a rapid initial conscious adaptation occurs to avoid traumatic occlusal contacts.

Within a few days the patient experiences pain behind the condyle when the appliance is removed. From the studies of histological changes in animal experiments, it may be deduced that retraction of the condyle results in compression of connective tissue and blood vessels and that ischaemia is the principal cause of pain.

A new pattern of muscle behaviour is quickly established whereby the patient finds it difficult and later impossible to retract the mandible into its former retruded position. After a few days, it is more comfortable to wear the appliance than to leave it out. This change in muscle activity has been described by McNamara as the 'pterygoid response' which results from altered activity of the medial head of the lateral pterygoid muscle in response to mandibular protrusion. It is extremely rare for such a response to be observed with functional appliances that are not worn full time.

The initial response to functional mandibular protrusion is, therefore, a change in the muscles of mastication to establish a new equilibrium in muscle behaviour. Volumetric changes behind the condyle result in cellular proliferation at this stage. When the altered muscle function is established the proprioceptive sensory mechanism initiates compensatory bone remodelling to adapt to the altered function.

The muscles are the prime movers in growth, followed by bone remodelling as a secondary response to altered muscle function. Muscle function must be altered over a sufficient period of time to allow adaptive bone remodelling changes to occur to reposition the condyle in the glenoid fossa.

Muscle response to the Twin Block appliance – an electromyographic study

Research on a group of patients treated with Twin Blocks in India (Aggarwal *et al.*, 1999) provides important information on the adaptive changes during treatment. Bilateral EMG activity of elevator muscles of the mandible (i.e. anterior temporalis and masseter) was monitored longitudinally with bipolar surface electrodes to determine changes in postural, swallowing and maximum voluntary clenching activity during an observation period of 6 months. The muscle activity was measured at the start of treatment, within 1 month of Twin Block insertion, at the end of 3 months, and at the end of 6 months.

The results revealed a significant increase in postural and maximum clenching EMG activity in masseter ($P < 0.01$) and a numerical increase in anterior temporalis activity during the 6-month period of treatment. The increased activity can be attributed to an enhanced stretch (myotatic) reflex of the elevator muscles, contributing to isometric contractions. The main corrective force for Twin Block treatment appears to be

provided through increased active tension in the stretched muscles and not through passive tension.

The 3-month registration appears crucial for analysing the neuromuscular changes occurring with functional appliance treatment, indicating a strong possibility that sagittal repositioning of a retruded mandible in Class II division 1 cases takes place approximately within 3 months of initiating functional appliance treatment. The increased EMG activity during posture and maximum voluntary clenching supports active reflex contractions (motor unit stimulation) to play a dominant role in the neuromuscular changes with Twin Block treatment and not passive tension due to viscoelasticity of the muscles. The results of this study reaffirm the importance of full-time wear for functional appliances to exert their maximum therapeutic effect by way of neuromuscular adaptation.

This study supports the view that repeated contact between the inclined planes during posture and clenching leads to uninterrupted stretch on the muscle spindles and repeated stimulation of the stretch receptors (Fig. 4.4).

Effects of Twin Block therapy on protrusive muscle functions

Further research in the University of Adelaide, Australia (Chintakanon *et al.*, 2000a,b) combines the study of protrusive muscle function with magnetic resonance imaging to evaluate the functional adaptation of the condyles within the glenoid fossae during Twin Block treatment.

"Fatiguing the protrusive muscles did not alter mandibular position in the Twin Block group after 6 months treatment. The findings suggest a lack of habitual forward posture." In other words, none of the children demonstrated dual bite or 'Sunday bite' as a result of treatment with Twin Blocks, as confirmed by a protrusive muscle fatigue test.

A prospective study of Twin Block appliance therapy assessed by magnetic resonance imaging (Chintakanon *et. al.*, 2000b)

The use of magnetic resonance imaging (MRI) to demonstrate temporomandibular joint (TMJ) adaptation during functional appliance therapy (Herbst appliance) has recently been reported by Ruf & Pancherz (1998, 1999). However, their studies did not include control groups for comparison. Ruf and Pancherz demonstrated an increase in MRI signal at the postero-superior border of the condyle and at the anterior surface of the postglenoid spine of the fossa that has not been demonstrated previously. This increase in MRI signal was interpreted as being associated with remodelling, and the effects on the condyle were more prominent than on the

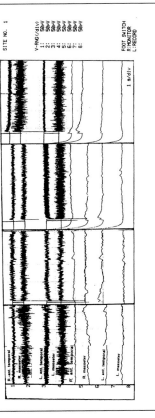

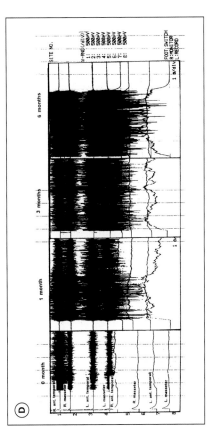

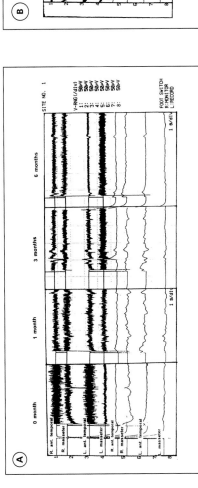

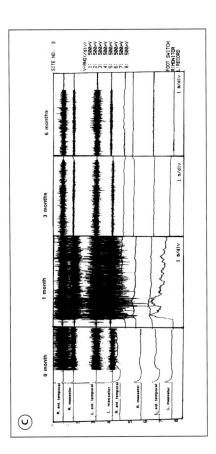

Fig. 4.4

A Representative sections of EMG during postural position of the mandible without Twin Block.

B Representative sections of EMG during postural position of the mandible with Twin Block. (**A** and **B**, *Tracings 1, 2, 3,* and *4* represent raw EMGs, and *5, 6, 7,* and *8* are integrated EMGs.)

C Representative sections of EMG during maximal voluntary clenching without Twin Block.

D Representative sections of EMG during maximal voluntary clenching with Twin Block. (**C** and **D** *Tracings 1, 2, 3,* and *4* represent raw EMGs, and *5, 6, 7,* and *8* are integrated EMGs.) (Reproduced from American Journal of Orthodontics and Dentofacial Orthopedics Vol. 118: 407–408, Mosby, St Louis 1999, with permission)

fossa. The increase in MRI signal was found only after 6 to 12 weeks of therapy, but could not be seen at the end of treatment (7 months).

In the present study, no increase in the MRI signal was seen. It is possible that the MRI obtained after 6 months of treatment may have missed this remodelling process. Periodic MRI at shorter intervals is needed to clarify this phenomenon.

Comparison between controls and Twin Block groups suggested that reduction of the condylar axis angle represents a feature of untreated Class II growth patterns, whereas axial angle stability with Twin Block therapy may suggest alteration of condylar growth direction. Condyles that were positioned at the crest of the eminence at the beginning of treatment had reseated back into the glenoid fossa after 6 months. However, 75% of the condyles were more anteriorly positioned in successfully treated Twin Block cases. There was no clear evidence of remodelling of the glenoid fossa at the eminence as a result of Twin Block treatment. Twin Block therapy had neither positive nor negative effects on disc position.

This research underlines the significance of the direction of growth of the condylar axis, which may result in forward repositioning of the mandible, as an important factor in the adjustment of the maxillo-mandibular relationship in correction of a retrusive mandible. Increasing evidence is emerging to confirm that the condyle is repositioned in the glenoid fossa after 6 months of therapy with a full-time functional mechanism.

SUMMARY

Over the past 30 years many animal experiments investigating the orthopaedic effects of functional mandibular protrusion have come to consistent conclusions. Electromyographic, cephalometric and histological studies in animal experiments provide a better understanding of the biological changes that result from orthopaedic technique. Controlled experiments confirm that the mandibles of monkeys and rats are responsive to functional stimuli, and that bone remodelling occurs in the glenoid fossa, and in muscles and ligaments and their attachments at sites which are remote from the dentoalveolar areas normally associated with a response to orthodontic treatment.

The conclusions drawn from these experiments differ from traditional views relating to orthodontic treatment, and only serve to underline that different mechanical systems do not produce an identical biological response.

Animal growth studies are of direct relevance to clinical practice. As one evaluates the biological and histological changes produced by appliance mechanisms in experimental animals, a better understanding is gained of the changes observed clinically in patients. The growth response in animals has been measured through full-time appliances using inclined planes as the functional mechanism. It is now possible to conduct equivalent growth studies for patients with an identical appliance mechanism using the occlusal inclined plane. Growth studies of consecutively treated patients against untreated control values form a basis for comparison with the results of animal growth studies.

A visco-elastic hypothesis

Voudouris and Kuftinec (2000) present a further explanation to account for growth changes in Twin Block and Herbst treatment, following recent research in Toronto. They observe that it was previously thought that increased activity in the postural masticatory muscles was the key to promoting condyle–glenoid fossa growth. By analysing results from several studies they postulate a non-muscular hypothesis as a result of radiating viscoelastic forces on the condyle and fossa in treatment and long term retention.

'This premise is based on three specific findings: significant glenoid fossa bone formation occurs during treatment that includes mandibular displacement; glenoid fossa modification is a result of the stretch forces of the retrodiscal tissues, capsule, and altered flow of viscous synovium; observations that glenoid fossa bone formation takes place at a distance from the soft tissue attachment. This latter observation is explained by transduction or referral of forces. . . . The impact of the viscoelastic tissues may be highly significant and should be considered along with the standard skeletal, dental, neuromuscular, and age factors that influence condyle–glenoid fossa growth with orthopedic advancement.'

REFERENCES

Aggarwal, P., Kharbanda, O.P., Mathur R., Ritu Duggai, & Parkash, H. (1999). Muscle response to the Twin-block appliance: an electromyographic study of the masseter and anterior temporalis muscles. *Am. J. Orthod. Dentofac. Orthop.*, **116**: 405–14.

Brodie, A.G. (1941). On the growth pattern of the human head from the third month to the eighth year of life. *Am. J. Anatomy*, **68**: 209–62.

Bjork, A. (1955). Facial growth in man studied with the aid of metallic implants. *Acta Odont. Scand.*, **13**: 9–34.

Charlier, J.P., Petrovic, A. & Stutzmann, J. (1969). Effects of mandibular hyperpropulsion on the prechondroblastic zone of the young rat condyle, *Am. J. Orthod.*, **55**: 71–4.

Chintakanon, K., Turker, K.S., Sampson, W., Wilkinson, T. & Townsend, G.(2000a). Effects of Twin-block therapy on protrusive muscle functions. *Am. J. Orthod. Dentofac. Orthop.*, **118**: 392–396.

Chintakanon, K., Turker, K.S., Sampson, W., Wilkinson, T. & Townsend, G.(2000b). A prospective study of Twin-block appliance therapy assessed by magnetic resonance imaging. *Am. J. Orthod Dentofac. Orthop.*, **118**: 494–504.

Elgoyhen, J.C., Moyers, R.E., McNamara, Jr, J.A. & Riolo, M.L. (1972). Craniofacial adaptation to protrusive function in juvenile Rhesus monkeys. *Am. J. Orthod.*, **62**: 469–80.

Gaumond, G. (1973). Les effets d'une force extraorale de traction sur la croissance mandibulaire de jeunes rats. *L'Orthodontie Française*, **44**: 213–27.

Gaumond, G. (1975). Effets d'un sopareil d'hyperpropulsion fonctionelle sur la croissance mandibulaire de jeunes rats. *L'Orthodontie Française*, **46**: 107–28.

Graber, T.M. (1972). *Orthodontics: Principles and Practice*, 3rd edn. Philadelphia, W.B. Saunders.

Graber, L.W. (1975). The alterability of mandibular growth. In *Determinants of Mandibular Form and Growth*, ed. J.A. McNamara Jr, Monograph No. 4, Craniofacial Growth Series. University of Michigan, pp. 229–41.

Harvold, E.P. (1968). The role of function in the etiology and treatment of malocclusion. *Am. J. Orthod.*, **54**: 883.

Harvold, E.P. (1983). Altering craniofacial growth: force application and neuromuscular–bone interaction. In *Clinical Alteration of the Growing Face*, Monograph 14, Craniofacial Growth Series. University of Michigan.

Hiniker, J.J. & Ramfjord, S.P. (1964). Anterior displacement of the mandible in adult rhesus monkey. *J. Dent. Res.*, **43**: suppl., 811.

Hinton, R.H. (1981). Form and function in the temporomandibular joint. In *Craniofacial Biology*, ed. D.S. Carlson, Monograph 10, Craniofacial Growth Series. University of Michigan.

Joho, J.P. (1968). Changes in the form of the mandible in the orthopaedically treated Macaca virus (an experimental study). *Eur. Orthod. Soc.*, **44**: 161–73.

Komposh, G. & Hocenjos, Cl. (1977). Die Reaktionsfahigkeit des temporomandibularen Knorpels. *Fortschr. Kieferorthopadie*, **38**: 121–32.

Linge, L. (1977). Klinishe Relevanz tierexperimenteller Untersuchungen (Korreferat Zum Vortrag Petrovic). *Fortschr. Kieferorthopadie*, **38**: 253–60.

McNamara, Jr, J.A. (1972). *Neuromuscular and Skeletal Adaptations to Altered Function in the Orofacial Region*. Monograph No. 1, Craniofacial Growth Series. University of Michigan.

McNamara, Jr, J.A. (1980). Functional determinants of craniofacial size and shape. *Eur. J. Orthod.*, **1**: 131–59.

McNamara, Jr, J.A., Connelly, T.G. & McBride, M.C. (1975). Histological studies of temporomandibular joint adaptations. In *Control Mechanisms in Craniofacial Growth*, ed. J.A. McNamara Jr. University of Michigan, pp. 209–27.

Moss, J.P. (1980). The soft tissue environment of teeth and jaws. *Br. J. Orthod.*, **7**: 127–37, 205–16.

Moyers, R.E., Elgoyhen, J.C. & Riolo, M.L. (1970). Experimental production of class III malocclusion in Rhesus monkeys. *Trans. Eur. Orthod. Soc.*, **46**: 61.

Oppenheim, A. (1911). Tissue changes, particularly of the bone, incident to tooth movement. *Eur. Orthodont. Soc. Trans.*, 303–359.

Petrovic, A. & Stutzmann, J. (1977). Further investigations into the functioning of the 'comparator' of the servosystem (respective positions of the upper and lower dental arches) in the control of the condylar cartilage growth rate and of the lengthening of the jaw. In *The Biology of Occlusal Development*, ed. J.A. McNamara Jr, Monograph No. 6, Craniofacial Growth Series. Center for Human Growth & Development, University of Michigan, pp. 225–91.

Petrovic, A., Stutzmann, J. & Lavergne, J. (1971). Mechanisms of craniofacial growth and modus operandi of functional appliances: a cell-level and cybernetic approach to orthodontic decision making. In *Cranofacial Growth Theory and Orthodontic Treatment* ed. D.S. Carlson, Monograph, Cranial Growth Series, University of Michigan.

Petrovic, A.G., Stutzmann, J.J. & Gasson, N. (1981). The final length of the mandible: is it genetically determined? In *Craniofacial Biology*, ed. D.S. Carlson, Monograph No. 10. Center for Human Growth & Development, University of Michigan, pp. 105–26.

Reitan, K. (1951). The initial tissue reaction incident to orthodontic tooth movement. *Acta. Odontol. Scand.*, **9**: suppl. 6.

Ricketts, R.M. (1952). A study of the changes in temporomandibular relations associated with the treatment of Class II malocclusion (Angle). *Am. J. Orthod.*, **38**: 918.

Ruf, S. & Pancherz, H. (1998). Temporomandibular joint growth adaptation in Herbst treatment: a prospective magnetic resonance imaging and cephalometric roentgenographic study. *Eur J. Orthod.*, **20**: 375–88.

Ruf, S. & Pancherz, H. (1999) Long term TMJ effects of Herbst treatment: a clinical and MRI study. *Am. J. Orthod. Dentofac. Orthop.*, **114**: 375–88.

Sandstedt, C. (1904). Einige Beitrage zur Theorie der Zahnregulierung. *Nord. Tand.Tidskr.*, **5**: 236.

Sandstedt, C. (1905). Einige Beitrage zur Theorie der Zahnregulierung. *Nord. Tand.Tidskr.*, **6**: 1.

Schwarz, A.M. (1932). Tissue changes incidental to orthodontic tooth movement. *Int. J. Orthodont.*, **18**: 331–352.

Sessle, B.J. *et al.* (1990). Effect of functional appliances on jaw muscle activity. *Am. J. Orthod. Dentofac. Orthop.*, **98**: 222–30.

Stockli, P.W. & Willert, H.G. (1971). Tissue reactions in the temporomandibular joint resulting from the anterior displacement of the mandible in the monkey. Am. J. Orthod., **60**: 142–55.

Stutzmann, J. & Petrovic, A. (1979). Intrinsic regulation of condylar cartilage growth rate. *Eur. J. Orthod.*, **1**: 41–54.

Voudouris, J.C. & Kuftinec, M.M (2000). Improved clinical use of Twin Block and Herbst as a result of radiating viscoelastic tissue forces on the condyle and fossa in treatment and long-term retention: growth relativity. *Am. J. Orthod. Dentofac. Orthop.*, **117**: 247–266.

Woodside, D.G., Altuna, G., Harvold, E. & Metaxas, A. (1983). Primate experiments in malocclusion and bone induction. *Am. J. Orthod.*, **83**: 460–8.

Woodside, D.G., Metaxas, A. & Altuna, G. (1987). The influence of functional appliance therapy on glenoid fossa remodelling. *Am. J. Orthod. Dentofac. Orthop.*, **92**: 181–98.

FURTHER READING

McNamara, Jr, J.A. & Bryan, F.A. (1987) Long-term mandibular adaptations to protrusive function: an experimental study in *Macaca mulatta*. *Am. J. Orthod. Dentofac. Orthop.*, **92**: 98–108.

McNamara, Jr, J.A. & Carlson, D.S. (1979) Quantitative analysis of temporomandibular joint adaptations to protrusive function. *Am. J. Orthod.*, **76**: 593-611.

McNamara, J.A. Jr, Hinton, R.J. & Hoffman, D.L. (1982). Histological analysis of temporomandibular joint adaptation to protrusive function in young adult rhesus monkeys (*Macaca mulatta*). *Am. J. Orthod.*, **82**: 288–98.

Pancherz, H., Ruf, S. & Thomalske-Foubert, C. (1999) Mandibular articular disc position changes during Herbst treatment: a prospective longitudinal MRI study. *Am. J. Orthod. Dentofac. Orthop.*, **116**: 207–14

CHAPTER 5

Diagnosis and Treatment Planning

CLINICAL EXAMINATION

What you see is what you get

Clinical examination provides the fundamental guideline in case selection for functional therapy. A retrusive mandible can be detected by examining the profile and the facial contours with the teeth in occlusion. The patient is then instructed to close the incisors in normal relationship by protruding the mandible, with the lips closed lightly together. The change in facial appearance is a preview of the anticipated result of functional treatment. If the profile improves with the mandible advanced, this is a clear indication that functional mandibular advancement is the treatment of choice. Clinical diagnosis has the advantage of providing an accurate prediction of the three-dimensional change in the facial contours as a result of mandibular advancement, and is more important than the diagnostic profiles defined by lines and angles drawn on a cephalometric x-ray. This does not negate or diminish the value of cephalometric analysis, but adds a three-dimensional view to support and confirm the diagnosis (Fig.5.1). Important clinical guidelines in treatment planning for Class II division 1 malocclusion are now considered.

Photographic records

Facial and dental photographs are an invaluable diagnostic aid to establish the objectives of treatment and to monitor progress.

Photographs are used to predict the change in facial appearance that will result from treatment. Profile and full-face photographs with the mandible in the retrusive position show the appearance before treatment, and are repeated with the mandible advanced to give the projected optimum improvement in facial appearance.

An additional set of photographs for the patient, from a simple polaroid camera, improves motivation by allowing the patient to observe the rapid improvement in appearance during the first few months of treatment.

CASE REPORT: S.W. AGED 14 YEARS 2 MONTHS

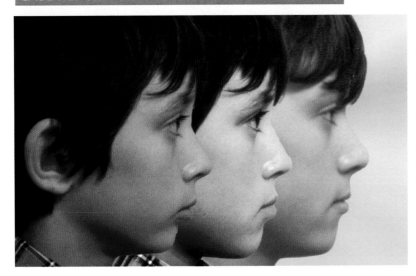

Fig. 5.1 Treatment:
A The profile far left shows a retrusive mandible at age 14 years 2 months (before treatment). The middle profile is also taken before treatment with the mandible protruded to bring the incisors into normal relationship, showing a preview of the anticipated changes from functional treatment. The profile far right at age 15 years 1 month confirms that the appearance after treatment is very close to the predicted result.

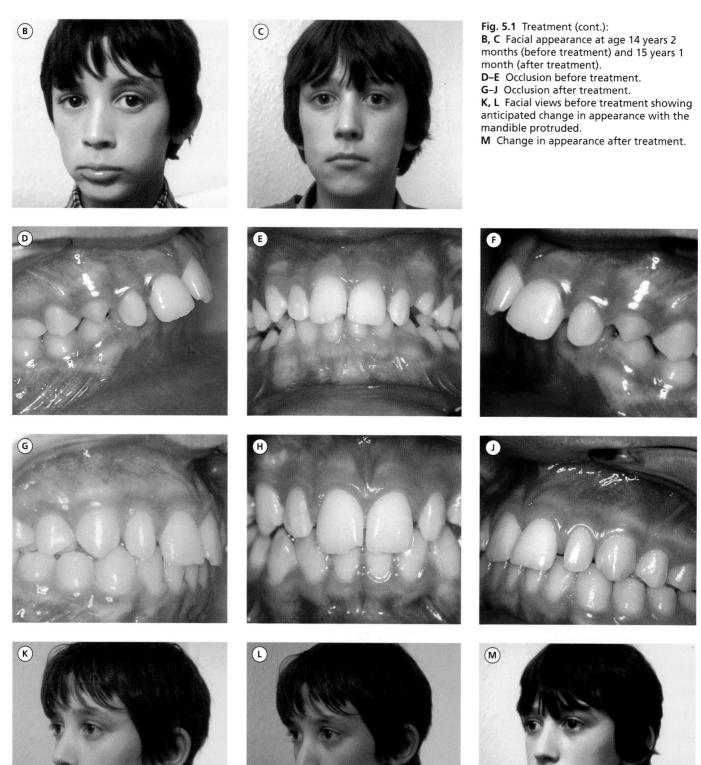

Fig. 5.1 Treatment (cont.):
B, C Facial appearance at age 14 years 2 months (before treatment) and 15 years 1 month (after treatment).
D–E Occlusion before treatment.
G–J Occlusion after treatment.
K, L Facial views before treatment showing anticipated change in appearance with the mandible protruded.
M Change in appearance after treatment.

Orthodontic records

Successful orthodontic treatment is dependent on a disciplined approach to record taking and diagnosis, as well as careful monitoring of progress in treatment. Inadequate records may reflect a poor standard of treatment. In general the standard of orthodontic care is directly related to the quality of the orthodontic records.

The essentials for orthodontic records are a diagnostic report supported by study models, x-rays and photographs to establish the condition of the case before treatment and to record progress during treatment.

Radiographic examination is necessary to identify and locate all unerupted teeth. This is accomplished routinely by a panoral x-ray with intraoral films if required for individual teeth. Temporomandibular joint x-rays are also extremely important, especially in today's litigious society, to establish the condition of the joint before treatment. Cephalometric analysis of a lateral skull x-ray gives detailed information to support clinical diagnosis.

EXAMINATION OF MODELS

An equally simple guideline helps to predict occlusal changes by checking the occlusion resulting when the mandible postures downwards and forwards to reduce the overjet. This can be observed directly in the mouth, but is best confirmed on study models by sliding the lower model forwards and observing the articulation of the mandibular dental arch with that of the upper model.

In an uncrowded Class II division 1 malocclusion with an overjet of 10 mm or more, it can be seen that a good buccal segment occlusion will result from advancing the mandible and, at the same time, laterally expanding the maxilla to match the width of the mandibular dental arch in the projected advanced position.

If the arches are crowded with irregular teeth, the upper and lower models will often not fit when the lower model is advanced. Depending on the degree of irregularity, a first phase of arch development may be necessary to correct archform before the mandible can be advanced to correct the occlusion. Alternatively, appliance design may be modified to improve archform during the Twin Block phase, if the irregularity is less severe.

If the upper incisors prevent the lower model from advancing into a Class I buccal segment occlusion, provision must be made to advance the upper incisors with springs or screws to accommodate the mandible in correct occlusion (Fig. 5.2). This often applies in a Class II malocclusion when an overjet of less than 9 mm is present with a full unit distal occlusion. It is necessary to procline the upper incisors to release the mandible forwards. The same restriction applies in Class II division 2 malocclusion, and appliance design must be modified accordingly.

CASE REPORT: G.D. AGED 14 YEARS

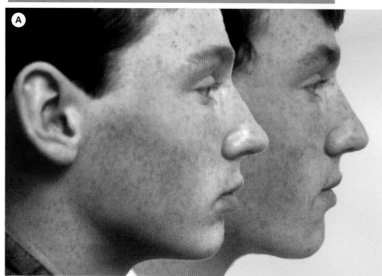

Fig. 5.2 Treatment:

A Profiles at ages 14 years (before treatment) and 15 years (after treatment).

B, C, D Retroclined incisors must be proclined with springs or screws on the upper Twin Block to release the mandible forwards.

E Aesthetic design. Light Class II elastics are optional.

F, G Anterior inclined plane to support the corrected incisor relationship and to allow the lower premolars and canines to erupt into occlusion.

H, J, K After 12 months the occlusion has settled and the same appliance serves as a retainer.

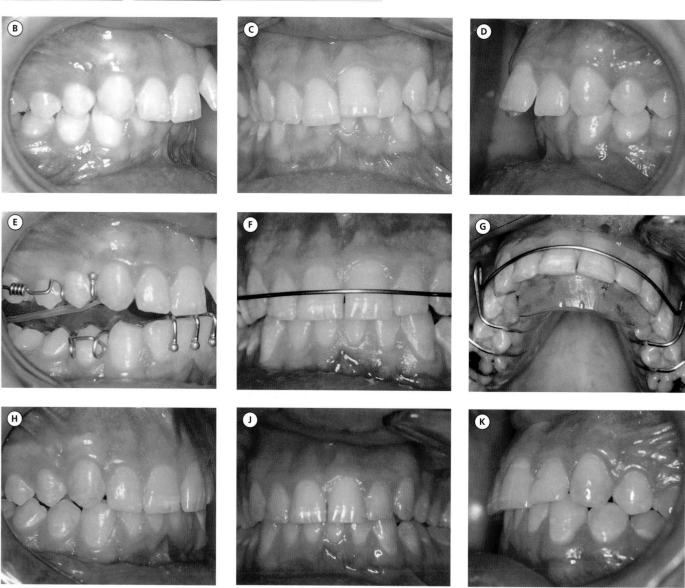

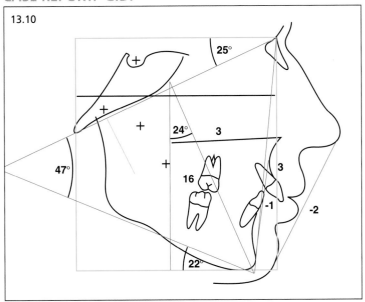

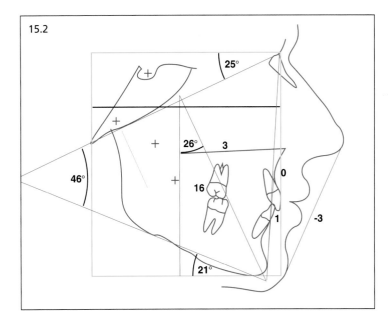

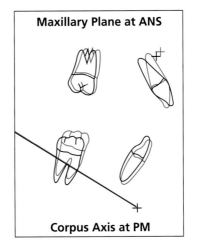

Corpus Axis at PM

Maxillary Plane at ANS

Nasion Basion at Nasion

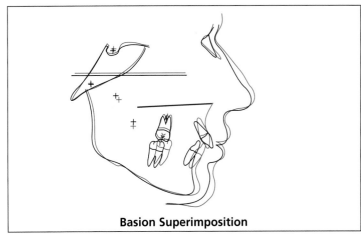

Basion Superimposition

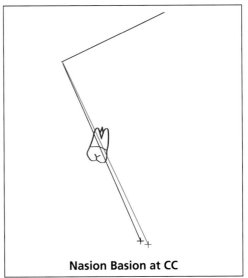

Nasion Basion at CC

G.D.	Age 13.10	15.2
Cranial Base Angle	25	25
Facial Axis Angle	24	26
F/M Plane Angle	22	21
Craniomandibular Angle	47	46
Maxillary Plane	3	3
Convexity	3	0
U/Incisor to Vertical	36	20
L/Incisor to Vertical	32	33
Interincisal Angle	112	127
6 to Pterygoid Vertical	16	16
L/Incisor to A/Po	-1	1
L/Lip to Aesthetic Plane	-2	-3

DIFFERENTIAL DIAGNOSIS

Extraction or non-extraction therapy

Throughout the twentieth century, the pendulum swung back and forth between extraction and non-extraction therapy. At the beginning of the century, Angle believed unconditionally that all 32 teeth should be accommodated in every case, regardless of the growth pattern or the relationship of the size of the teeth to the basal bone. His philosophy insisted that if the teeth were moved into normal interdigitation, functional stimulation would result in compensatory basal bone growth to accommodate the teeth in their corrected position. It was heresy for a disciple of Angle even to think about extraction of teeth as a part of orthodontic therapy.

As a student of Angle, Tweed practised non-extraction therapy for 6 years and observed a high percentage of relapse by reappearance of crowding in cases with a tooth/supporting tissue discrepancy. In edgewise mechanics, correction of a Class II dental relationship in permanent dentition by intermaxillary traction was accompanied by forward movement of the lower dentition. He related lack of harmony in facial contour to the extent to which the denture was displaced mesially into protrusion and concluded that the orthodontist must find a means of accurately predetermining the anterior limits of stability of the denture in functional balance.

Tweed (1966) gained acceptance for premolar extraction therapy and established an entire orthodontic treatment philosophy based on the concept that facial balance and harmony are dependent on the mandibular incisors being upright over basal bone. He expressed a mean angulation of the lower incisor to the Frankfort plane of $65° \pm 5°$ as a position of balance.

Tweed differentiated facial growth trends into three basic types to account for patients who exhibited balanced growth, vertical growth and horizontal growth patterns. He believed that extractions were mandatory in vertical growth patterns for patients with high ANB angles, anticipating that point B would always drop down and back in treatment. He observed that lower incisors often had to be proclined in treating patients with vertical growth patterns to compensate for skeletal discrepancies, but as a rule these teeth then remained stable and devoid of rotations after treatment. Conversely, in patients with horizontal growth patterns, the mandible grows forwards faster than the maxilla, resulting in lingual tipping of the lower incisors and development of crowding in the lower labial segments.

Begg (1965) was also a student of Angle who later developed the Light Wire Technique using round wires in a vertical slot bracket to achieve a one-point contact on the archwire. The Begg Technique incorporated auxilliary springs to tip and torque the teeth using differential forces to control tooth movements. Begg based his philosophy on Stone Age man's dentition after studying the attritional occlusion observed in a series of aboriginal skulls in Australia. Begg reasoned that the amount of interproximal attrition in the permanent teeth due to aboriginal dentition was sufficient to accommodate third molars. By comparison, modern man has a refined diet which does not require chewing, therefore interproximal attrition does not occur which results in a high incidence of late crowding due to mesial migration of the dentition prior to eruption of third molars. Begg was a strong advocate of routine extraction of premolars, and indeed in some cases advised the extraction of all first molars in addition to the first premolars. The Begg school introduced the concept of interdental stripping to help resolve crowding of mandibular incisors by flattening the interproximal contacts in the lower labial segment. Sheridan (1985) extended this procedure to the buccal segments by air rotor stripping, as an alternative to extraction.

In developing the 'bioprogressive philosophy', Ricketts et al. (1979) moved away from a dogmatic approach to extraction therapy. Ricketts related treatment planning to facial aesthetics and the pattern of facial growth. Relating treatment to facial form gives further guidance in case selection for extraction or non-extraction therapy. Brachyfacial or mesofacial growth patterns are more suited to non-extraction techniques for relief of crowding than the vertical growing dolichofacial type.

Studies of the long-term results of treatment were carried out by the bioprogressive group, assisted by Rocky Mountain Data Systems (Ricketts et al., 1979). This resulted in improved methods of differential diagnosis for the selection of extraction or non-extraction therapy. These studies also provided a foundation for computerised growth prediction based on average increments of growth. Ricketts defined parameters in cephalometric analysis to assist more accurate treatment planning related to facial aesthetics.

The position of the lower incisor relative to the anterior limit of the skeletal base is crucial in facial aesthetics. The principle of relating lower incisor position to the skeletal apical base by means of linear measurements was originally described by Downs (1948) and elaborated by Ricketts (1960). The A–Po line joins point A and pogonion, the anterior points on the maxillary and mandibular skeletal bases, respectively. This line defines the anterior limit of the skeletal base.

The Begg school were the first to relate lower incisor stability to the position of the lower incisor relative to the A–Po line. Raleigh Williams, in his cephalometric appraisal of the Light Wire Technique in Begg's book, observed:

> The incisal edge of the lower incisor reaches a final position very close to the AP line, a very critical position if upper and lower lip balance is to be achieved. This simple measurement of dental–skeletal relationship has a profound influence on a harmonious soft tissue balance in the lower third of the face.

In dental prosthetics we follow the principle of placing the lower incisors upright over the ridge to stabilise a lower denture. Positioning the incisors too far labially results in an unstable denture and placing them too far lingually encroaches on tongue space. The same principle applies in the natural dentition.

Lower incisor position is always reflected in the position of the lower lip and has a significant influence on the profile and, therefore, on facial aesthetics. Ricketts recommends positioning the tip of the lower incisor at +1 to +3 mm relative to the A–Po line for the best aesthetic result (Fig. 5.3). This positions the lower incisor over basal bone close to the anterior limit of the skeletal base, and gives a pleasing contour to the lower lip in profile related to the nose and chin.

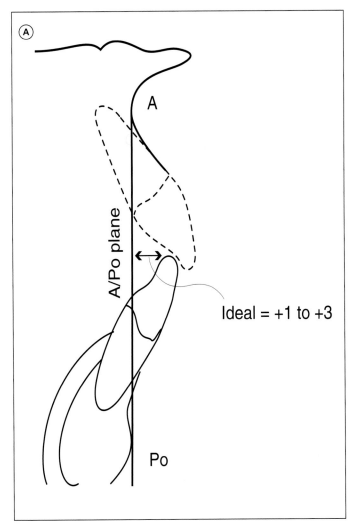

Fig. 5.3 The distance from the tip of lower incisor to the A–Po line. For the best aesthetic result the range is +1 to +3 mm.

Arch length discrepancy

Arch length discrepancy defines the amount of crowding present in the dental arch by comparing the space available with the space required to accommodate all the teeth in the arch in correct alignment. The degree of crowding is determined by examining the models from the occlusal aspect, starting at the mesial contact point of the first permanent molar on one side and estimating the amount of crowding at each contact point, passing round the arch to the mesial contact point of the first molar on the opposite side. The summation of crowding at each contact point gives the arch length discrepancy in millimetres. Allowance may also be made for potential crowding of second or third molars. The same calculation in the mixed dentition is referred to as a mixed dentition analysis and, if space is maintained by holding the position of the first molars after loss of second deciduous molars, provision should be made for an additional 4 mm of arch length during the transition to permanent dentition.

The 'Richter Scale'

It is helpful in treatment planning to classify the degree of difficulty of the malocclusion as mild, moderate or severe. In arch length discrepancy:

- Mild crowding is in the range 1–3 mm.
- Moderate crowding is classified as 4–5 mm.
- Severe crowding is 6 mm or more.

This is a sliding scale (the author describes it as the 'Richter scale') expressing degree of difficulty for dental correction by non-extraction therapy. The higher the value, the more difficult it is to resolve crowding permanently without extractions.

Two factors improve the prognosis for non-extraction therapy in moderate or severely crowded dentitions:

- First, early treatment by arch development to increase arch width before permanent premolars and canines erupt.
- Second, lingual positioning of the lower dentition relative to the skeletal base requires a non-extraction approach.

The 'Richter scale' can also be applied when the measure of convexity is used to determine the skeletal discrepancy:

- A skeletal convexity of 1–3 mm is within the range of normal.
- 4–5 mm convexity is a moderate Class II skeletal discrepancy.
- 6 mm or more is severe Class II.

The higher the convexity, the more likely that functional orthopaedics is indicated to improve the skeletal relationship.

TREATMENT PLANNING IN CROWDED DENTITIONS

Ricketts' parameters for a lower incisor position relative to the A–Po line serve as a baseline from which to plan the treatment of crowding. The degree of crowding in the lower arch is related to the labiolingual position of the lower incisor as a guide to determine a differential diagnosis for extraction or non-extraction therapy.

Assessing arch length discrepancy and lower incisor position determines whether the lower incisors can be advanced to a stable position relative to the skeletal base after treatment. This depends on the degree of protrusion or retrusion of the lower incisors related to the degree of crowding in the lower arch. Before moving the lower incisors it should be established that good bony support is available to accommodate the proposed movement.

If the lower incisors are retroclined and positioned lingual to the A–Po line, arch length can be increased by advancing the lower incisors. As a guide, proclination of the lower incisors by 1 mm increases arch length by 2 mm (equivalent to a gain of 1 mm on each side).

Conversely, if lower incisors are proclined and positioned too far labial to the A–Po line they should be retracted to improve facial aesthetics. Each 1 mm of retraction will reduce total arch length by 2 mm.

According to the position of the lower incisors before treatment, the space required to correct crowding can be calculated by repositioning the tip of the lower incisors within the range of +1 to +3 mm to the A–Po line. This is a reliable guideline to relate treatment to facial aesthetics in extraction and non-extraction therapy (Fig. 5.4).

One other factor should be taken into account. Functional mandibular advancement carries pogonion forward and invariably results in a relative forward movement of the lower incisors as the A–Po line becomes more upright. The lower incisor position should therefore be reviewed after functional therapy when the occlusion has settled.

LIP CONTOUR

The fullness of the lips provides an additional aesthetic guideline for extraction or non-extraction therapy. The angulation of the upper lip is a crucial factor in facial aesthetics. Ideally the upper lip should be angled between 20° and 30° to the nasion vertical for the best aesthetic appearance. If the angle between the upper lip and the undersurface of the nose is more than 90°, the patient's appearance in profile is progressively less aesthetic as the naso-labial angle becomes more obtuse. Labial movement of the upper incisors is indicated to restore better balance

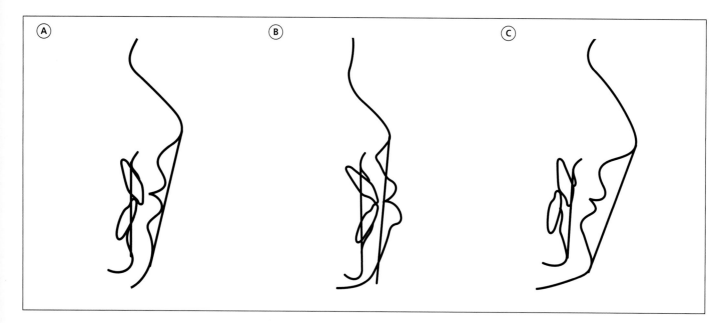

Fig. 5.4 Diagram of three profiles to show the relationship of lip position to lower incisor position.
A The profile on the left shows good facial balance. Nonextraction treatment is preferred to maintain balance.
B The middle profile shows the lower incisor positioned significantly forward to the skeletal base (+7 mm to the A–Po line). Extraction therapy is indicated to improve the lip position.
C The profile on the right shows the lower incisor positioned significantly lingual to the skeletal base (–5 mm to the A–Po line). Extraction therapy is contraindicated and nonextraction therapy should aim to advance the upper and lower labial segments to improve the profile.

between the nose and the upper dento-alveolar structures aiming to improve the aesthetic result by advancing the upper lip to reduce the naso-labial angle.

Extraction of premolars should be avoided at all costs if the lips are a thin red line and the lower lip lies well behind the aesthetic line (tangent to the nose and chin). The resulting loss of lip support would cause further damage to the facial appearance, and may compromise temporomandibular joint function.

When the lip contour is good before treatment it is important not to destroy good facial balance and premolar extractions should be avoided. In an ideal profile the lower lip lies fractionally behind the aesthetic line (2 mm in the child and 4 mm in the adult). The characteristic flattening of the profile that occurs in the late teens should be taken into account when planning treatment for a young patient. A flat profile in a young child will become retrusive as the child grows into adulthood.

When the lips extend beyond the aesthetic line this reflects a labial position of the lower incisors. Crowding associated with bimaxillary protrusion is an indication for extraction of premolars.

NON-EXTRACTION THERAPY

Non-extraction therapy has become a popular misnomer because it refers to non-extraction of premolars. Crowding may still be relieved by extraction of second or third molars after a period of non-extraction therapy. This approach lends itself to early intervention to combine arch development and functional therapy in a first phase of interceptive treatment, followed by an orthodontic phase for detailed finishing in the permanent dentition.

Extraction of second molars

Extraction of second molars has long been recognised as an effective alternative to premolar extraction in gaining arch length in the lower arch without the disadvantage of sacrificing lip support and damaging facial aesthetics (Wilson, 1964, 1966, 1971; Liddle, 1977; Witzig & Spahl, 1987). Reporting on 500 cases where second molars had been

extracted, Wilson (1974) noted that 87% showed the third molars erupted in an acceptable position. Richardson (Richardson & Mills, 1990; Richardson & Burden, 1992) followed the effects of extraction of second molars and found that extraction of second molars is effective in reducing the incidence of late lower arch crowding and third molar impaction.

When examining the effect of second molar extraction in the treatment of lower premolar crowding it was concluded that up to 4 or 5 mm of lower premolar crowding can be successfully treated by extraction of lower second molars, with or without the use of simple orthodontic appliances. Early extraction of lower second molars, before second premolar eruption, seems to create the most favourable conditions for spontaneous premolar alignment.

Richardson & Richardson (1993), investigating lower third molar development subsequent to second molar extraction, found that 99% of third molars upright mesiodistally, but few became as upright as the second molars they replaced. Model analysis showed that 96% of the lower third molars erupted in good and acceptable positions.

CONTRAINDICTIONS FOR TWIN BLOCK THERAPY

Careful case selection is the most important aspect of diagnosis and treatment planning in order to achieve a successful outcome. Besides selecting suitable cases by an orthopaedic approach, it is equally important to recognise features that contraindicate treatment by functional mandibular protrusion. Factors that are unfavourable for correction by Twin Blocks include cases with vertical growth and crowding that may require extractions.

Although the majority of Class II malocclusions are suitable for correction by Twin Blocks, there are some exceptions. The same guidelines as those described to define indications for treatment can be used to assess contraindications. Examination of the profile is the most important clinical guideline. If the profile does not improve when the mandible is advanced, this is a clear contraindication for functional mandibular advancement, and an alternative approach should be considered.

CASE REPORT: C.H. AGED 11 YEARS 4 MONTHS

This girl presents in early permanent dentition with a severe skeletal discrepancy and convexity of 10 mm. The maxilla is correctly related to the cranial base, while the mandible is small and severely retrusive. Moderate crowding is present in the lower arch with mesial drift of lower canines with the molars in Class I relationship. The lower incisors are advanced by 3 mm relative to the A-Po line, causing the lower lip to be protrusive.

A severe vertical growth pattern is confirmed by cephalometric analysis as the facial axis angle is 17° and the Frankfort mandibular plane angle is 39°. An upward cant of 4° on the maxillary plane further increases the lower facial height. While it may seem advisable to advance the retrusive mandible, this would not improve the facial appearance, as confirmed by clinical and cephalometric examination. This patient was treated by extraction of four premolars to relieve crowding, followed by fixed appliances to reduce the protrusion of the dentition, with an acceptable improvement in the profile. (Fig. 5.5)

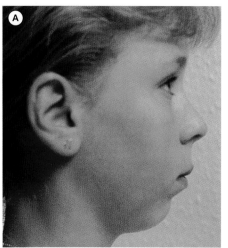
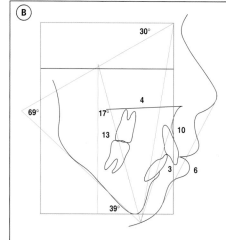
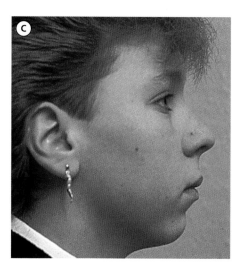

Fig. 5.5 Treatment:
A, B Profile and tracing before treatment.
C Profile after treatment.

CASE REPORT: K.J. AGED 13 YEARS

This boy presents another example of a protrusive profile, but in this case, a convexity of 11 mm is due to maxillary protrusion. A vertical growth tendency again limits the improvement observed in the profile when the mandible is advanced as the degree of convexity would not be compensated by predicted mandibular growth. The profile and facial appearance improved following extraction of four premolars and fixed mechanics by the Bioprogressive Technique. (Fig. 5.6)

CASE REPORT: K.I. AGED 11 YEARS 8 MONTHS

A Class II Division I malocclusion is associated with bimaxillary dental protrusion, in this case, with upper and lower labial crowding. The lower incisors are 4 mm ahead of the A-Po line resulting in the protrusive lower lip. Maxillary protrusion is also a factor in the protrusive profile. Differential diagnosis again depends on evaluating the profile change when the mandible is advanced. Bimaxillary dental protrusion often does not respond well to mandibular advancement, as the profile remains protrusive. The crowding cannot be resolved by advancing incisors which are already proclined. Extraction of premolars was followed by fixed appliances to relieve the anterior crowding with a resulting improvement in the profile. (Fig. 5.7)

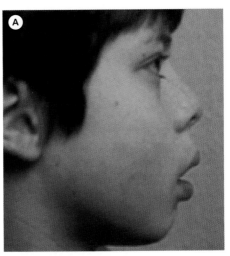
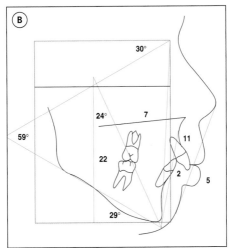
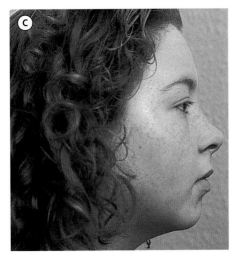

Fig. 5.6 Treatment:
A, B Profile and tracing before treatment.
C Profile after treatment.

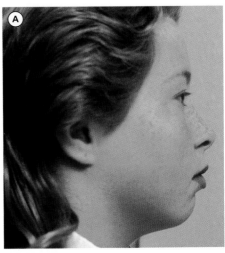
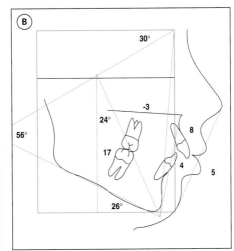
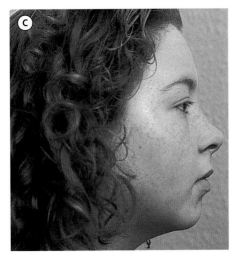

Fig. 5.7 Treatment:
A, B Profile and tracing before treatment.
C Profile after treatment.

CASE REPORT: J.S. AGED 13 YEARS 7 MONTHS

In this case, the Class II Division I malocclusion occurs on a class I skeletal base relationship with both mandible and maxilla prognathic relative to the cranial base. The patient presents a severe brachyfacial growth pattern with a strong horizontal growth component in the mandible. Cephalometric analysis confirms a mandibular plane angle of 10°, while the facial axis angle is 36°. This accounts for the prognathic mandible with a well developed chin, clearly contra-indicating further mandibular advancement. The maxillary dental protrusion should be corrected by an orthodontic approach to treatment. (Fig. 5.8)

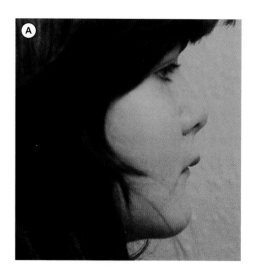

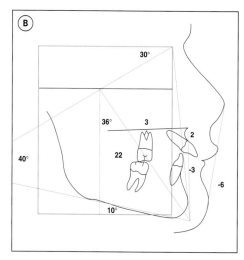

Fig. 5.8 Treatment:
A, B Profile and tracing before treatment.

REFERENCES

Begg, P.R. (1965). *Begg Orthodontic Theory and Technique.* W.B.Saunders Company, Philadelphia.

Downs, W.B. (1948). Variations in facial relationship: their significance in treatment and prognosis. *Am. J. Orthod. Oral Surg.,* **34:** 812.

Liddle, D.W. (1977). Second molar extraction in orthodontic treatment. *Am. J. Orthod.,* **72:** 599–616.

Richardson, M.E. & Burden, D.J. (1992). Second molar extraction in the treatment of lower premolar crowding. *Br. J. Orthod.,* **19:** 299–304.

Richardson, M.E. & Mills, K. (1990). Late lower arch crowding. The effect of second molar extraction. *Am. J. Orthod. Dentofac. Orthop.,* **98:** 242–6.

Richardson, M.E. & Richardson, A. (1993). Lower third molar development subsequent to second molar extraction. *Am. J. Orthod. Dentofac. Orthop.,* **104:** 566–74.

Ricketts, R.M. (1960). A foundation for cephalometric communication. *Am. J. Orthod.,* **46:** 330–57.

Ricketts, R.M. *et al.* (1979). *Bioprogressive Therapy.* Denver, Rocky Mountain Orthodontics.

Sheridan, J.J. (1985). Air rotor stripping. *J.Clin. Orthod.,* **19:** 43 –59.

Sheridan, J.J. (1987). Air rotor stripping update. *J.Clin. Orthod.,* **21:** 781–8.

Tweed, C.H. (1966) *Clinical Orthodontics.* C.V. Mosby, Saint Louis, MO.

Wilson, H.E. (1964). Extraction of second molars in treatment planning. *Orthod. Fr.,* **25:** 61–7.

Wilson, H.E. (1966). The extraction of second molars as a therapeutic measure. *Eur. Orthod. Soc.,* 141–5.

Wilson, H.E. (1971). Extraction of second molars in orthodontic treatment. *Orthodontist,* **3:** 1–7.

Wilson, H.E. (1974). Long term observation on the extraction of second molars. *Eur.Orthod. Soc.,* **50:** 215–21.

Witzig, J.W. & Spahl, T.J. (1987). The great second molar debate. In *The Clinical Management of Basic Maxillofacial Orthopedic Appliances,* Vol. 1–*Mechanics,* pp. 155–216. Massachusetts, PSG.

CHAPTER 6

The Clark Cephalometric Analysis

You who wish to describe by words the form of man and all aspects of the ways his parts are put together, drop that idea. For the more minutely you describe, the more you will confuse the mind of the reader and the more you will prevent him from the knowledge of that which you describe. So it is necessary to draw and describe.

(Leonardo Da Vinci, *Notebooks*. Translation by Robert E. Moyers)

THE JIGSAW PUZZLE

The jaw bone's connected to the head bone. (Popular song)

Consider the jigsaw puzzle: the aim is to assemble all the pieces into a recognisable pattern, but the method of achieving this objective is rather haphazard. We examine the shape and form of each piece of the puzzle as a separate entity. By concentrating our attention on the detail of the individual pieces we may fail to recognise the underlying pattern. Only when all the pieces are assembled in a unified framework can we clearly understand the puzzle. Current methods of cephalometric analysis resemble a jigsaw puzzle.

Cephalometric analysis attempts to define the pattern of craniofacial growth by examining the angular and linear relationships of clearly defined skeletal landmarks on cephalograms. Having defined a series of reference points and planes, the most common analytical method is to compare a series of unrelated measurements with means and standard deviations to evaluate the diagnostic significance of areas of deficient or excessive craniofacial growth in the aetiology of malocclusion. The lack of correlation of measurements makes it more difficult to arrive at a clear perception of the diagnostic significance of each factor in order to resolve the puzzle.

No existing method of analysis correlates all the linear and angular measurements in a common framework. There is no specific orientation of reference points in space. Current methods of analysis essentially examine each piece of the jigsaw puzzle as a separate entity without attempting to assemble the component parts into a unified pattern to define the relationship of the pieces. It is impossible to isolate the component parts of the craniofacial skeleton, and the principle of analysis by fragmentation is of limited value as a means of illustrating the pattern of craniofacial growth.

An alternative approach is to examine reciprocal relationships in the pattern of craniofacial development by a correlative method of cephalometric analysis. The logical basis for this approach is that the component parts of the craniofacial complex are mutually interdependent so that variation of one component has a reciprocal effect on the others. If a reliable registration framework is established using horizontal and vertical axes it is then possible to observe reciprocal variations in the pattern of craniofacial growth of the individual, with less dependence on unrelated corporate or average values.

A new approach to cephalometric analysis is derived from principles expressed in three previous analytical methods. These are the Ricketts (1960), McNamara (1984) and Bimler (1977) analyses. Having used and studied these analyses the author has adapted features of these methods to arrive at a system which aims to simplify and clarify the analytical method for diagnostic purposes.

Since the early cephalometric studies of Broadbent (1948) and Brodie (1940, 1941, 1946), the teaching of cephalometric analysis has been based largely on the concept that the face grows downwards and forwards from the base of the skull along the Y-axis or facial axis. Structures in the anterior cranial base were selected for superimposition of serial cephalometric tracings to demonstrate growth changes.

Assessment of facial growth by superimposition in the anterior cranial base is equivalent to judging the growth of a tree by sitting in its branches. This would give the impression that the earth grows downwards. Only when we stand away from the tree do we realise from a new perspective that the tree grows upwards. This analogy applies with equal logic to our concepts of facial growth.

Coben (1955) has spent 40 years of research on cephalometric analysis, with particular reference to growth of the cranial base. Coben observes that superimposition of tracings in the anterior cranial base has the major disadvantage of ignoring growth at the primary growth site in the base of the skull, the spheno-occipital synchondrosis, which has a fundamental influence on facial growth. The growth and angulation of the cranial base inevitably affects the structure of the face. Growth of the head is observed more accurately by superimposition at basion as recommended by Coben.

The head is suspended on the vertebral column and grows in a radial direction from its fulcrum of attachment. Basion is the closest point to this fulcrum that can be used in cephalometric analysis as a base point to establish growth of the face. Superimposition at basion gives a new perspective on growth of the face, and this represents an improved interpretation of our present concepts of facial growth.

Coben (1961) retraced the tracings used in the Bolton growth study (Broadbent, 1937) to show growth changes from childhood to adulthood. Comparison with Bolton tracings reveals a more regular pattern of facial growth, illustrated by superimposing the tracings at the basion with the Frankfort plane horizontal. This is a more accurate method of evaluating growth vectors in facial development.

Coben's concept of facial growth is that the wedge of the face opens by growth upwards and forwards along the cranial base, and downwards and forwards along the mandibular plane. The opening of the facial wedge increases facial height to accommodate growth in height of the nasal sinuses and to accommodate the successional teeth from deciduous to permanent dentition. Frankel & Frankel (1989) subsequently used Coben's concept in his book to analyse the results of treatment with the function regulator. Superimpositions are made at the basion with the Frankfort plane horizontal.

The Clark analysis lends itself well to the expression of Coben's interpretation of facial growth by horizontal orientation of the head and evaluation of growth changes from basion. The same method of superimposition has been selected to demonstrate facial growth changes with Twin Block treatment in this book, using basion as a fulcrum point for analysis of growth changes in the facial rectangle, with the Frankfort plane horizontal.

VISION, BALANCE AND POSTURE

Our perception of the world is based on horizons that are dependent on a highly developed mechanism of vision, balance and posture. To demonstrate this clearly, we need only tilt our head to one side, or forwards or back, to realise that we cannot function comfortably for long in this posture. While freedom of movement is necessary in function, in more prolonged postural activity it is necessary that the face is directed approximately to the front in a vertical plane to maintain anatomical and physiological balance. A limited range of visual acuity ensures that body posture is adapted accurately to our area of attention.

It is no accident that the facial plane lies approximately in the vertical plane. This is a necessary physiological feature in humans as an accommodation to an upright stature. A similar principle applies in the midsagittal plane of the head, which approximates

to the vertical plane, and also to the midtransverse plane which passes through the head and down through the shoulders. These characteristics ensure that in normal posture the eyes lie in a horizontal plane, and are directed forwards, in the same direction as the feet, to assist in balance and locomotion. The weight of the head is evenly balanced on the vertebral column with the minimum of muscular effort. Vertical and horizontal axes therefore represent an important adaptation in anatomical and physiological function to allow humans to adopt an erect posture.

Facial architecture

In cephalometric analysis, the significance of horizontal and vertical reference planes in relation to facial balance, and the resulting implications in treatment planning, have not yet been fully realised. Visual appreciation of aesthetic balance is clearly evident in good architectural design. The architect, who is involved in planning the construction of inanimate objects, makes constant reference to horizontal and vertical planes in order to achieve structural balance. The same principle applies in the analysis of facial form and the planning of reconstructive treatment of the face.

In many respects, the orthodontist is a facial architect who can alter the structure and balance of the face. Orthodontic and dentofacial orthopaedic techniques have the potential to produce dramatic changes in facial appearance that may be beneficial or detrimental according to the quality of treatment planning. Successful treatment depends on accurate analysis of the facial growth pattern before treatment, and prediction of the future growth trend to select the appropriate technique to produce the best long-term functional and aesthetic result within the growth potential of the individual patient.

PARALLELISM IN DENTOFACIAL DEVELOPMENT

A major advantage of a correlative approach using horizontal and vertical axes is the resulting simplification in the interpretation of results. The existence of parallelism in dentofacial development transforms a complex subject. It immediately becomes easier to teach and understand.

Parallelism has been referred to before in cephalometric analysis. Bimler (1957) and others have noted the parallel relationship that often exists between the Frankfort and maxillary planes. Similarly, Ricketts (1960) referred to the parallel development of the facial axis, the condyle axis and the upper incisor. Ricketts recommended that the upper incisor should be positioned parallel to the facial axis for stability and balance after treatment. These features may be interpreted as indicating harmony in facial development, and are usually evident in aesthetically pleasing, well-balanced faces (Fig 6.1).

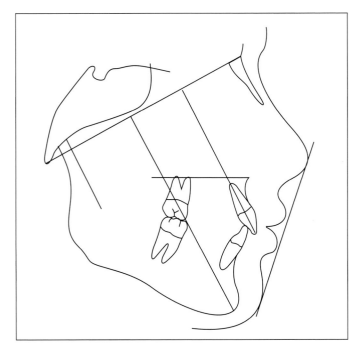

Fig. 6.1 Tracing (P.G.) to show facial axis, condyle axis and upper incisor parallel, indicating balance in facial development.

Ricketts expressed the view that growth and development followed the fundamental rules of physics, resulting in the recurrence of the divine proportion in facial development. This can be illustrated using a device to measure the proportions of the face and the facial features. The principle of incremental archial growth was described to account for the natural balance in facial contours. A balanced relationship of form and function in facial development is expressed in aesthetic harmony.

A REGISTRATION FRAMEWORK FOR CEPHALOMETRIC ANALYSIS

The jigsaw concept of cephalometric analysis has the disadvantage that the component parts of the puzzle are not correlated. This complicates both the understanding and the teaching of the principles of analysis, which remain incomprehensible to a large proportion of the profession.

To return to the jigsaw puzzle, the best technique in assembling a puzzle is first to establish the outer framework, usually a rectangle, by constructing the edges to define the outer limits of the puzzle. This provides a guide as a basis for examination and definition of structures within the framework.

The fundamental principle of framing an object in order to define balance and contour is well exemplified in the world of art. The concept is of equal value in examining facial contours, and as a means of evaluating the underlying skeletal structures

in aesthetic and scientific terms. Essentially, the principles of cartography are applied to cephalometric analysis to study the relationship of the craniofacial structures.

On a cephalogram the face is represented in simple terms as a wedge-shaped triangle superimposed on a rectangle. In the upright position, the facial features lie approximately in the anterior vertical plane. A rectangle provides an ideal framework to examine the position and dimensions of the craniofacial structures in cephalometric analysis.

Ricketts triangle: the facial wedge

The Ricketts triangle defines the face in profile as a wedge-shaped triangle attached to the undersurface of the cranial base (Fig. 6.2):

- The base of the triangle extends from basion to nasion and defines the cranial base plane.
- The facial plane extends from nasion tangent to the chin at the pogonion to define the angulation of the face in the anterior plane.
- The mandibular plane is the third leg of the triangle defining the angulation of the lower border of the mandible.
- The triangle is bisected by the facial axis, extending from pterygoid to gnathion to define the direction of growth of the chin.

The facial wedge defined by the Ricketts triangle is superimposed on the facial rectangle to provide a good visual

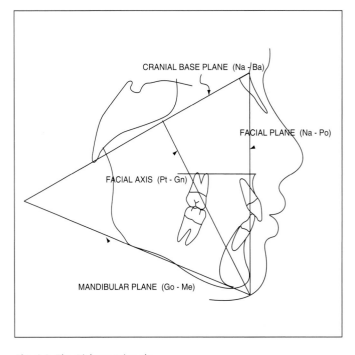

Fig. 6.2 The Ricketts triangle.

representation of the face with the component parts orientated in a common framework. A few key angular measurements define the pattern of craniofacial growth and the relationship of the cranial, maxillary and mandibular structures. It is easy to identify correlations that exist within the craniofacial complex by visual reference to the facial rectangle.

THE FACIAL RECTANGLE

A facial rectangle is formed to frame the face. The formation of a facial rectangle helps to define the relative position and angulation of cranial, maxillary, mandibular and dentoalveolar structures. The rectangular framework makes it easier to identify areas where growth departs from normal in the facial pattern. Perhaps the most obvious feature of the analysis is the visual simplification of the underlying pattern that results from placing the face in a rectangle. It is easier to recognise the pattern of the jigsaw puzzle when the pieces are fitted together in a recognisable framework.

The same principle lends itself to three-dimensional analysis.

Horizontal registration plane

The facial rectangle is constructed to define the upper, lower, anterior and posterior limits of the face. No single anatomical plane consistently relates exactly to the true horizontal in every case. Either a skeletal plane or the true horizontal may be selected to construct the upper registration plane of the facial rectangle (Fig. 6.3).

For practical purposes in most cases the Frankfort horizontal is suitable, except where porion or orbitale cannot be identified clearly, or when the Frankfort plane diverges significantly from the true horizontal. The true horizontal may be selected as an alternative when the cephalogram is taken in the natural head position. The selected plane is used as a horizontal baseline to construct the facial rectangle. The following description uses the Frankfort plane as the registration plane.

Frankfort plane: porion to orbitale

The Frankfort horizontal has the advantage that it can be located on external examination of the face, and it may be defined on a photograph. This is increasingly important as we relate analysis of the underlying bony strucures to the facial contours in computer-imaging technology. A further significant advantage of the Frankfort plane is that it has been widely taught and so it is familiar to the majority of the profession.

Nasion horizontal

A line is drawn through nasion parallel to the Frankfort plane. This defines the upper limit of the face and the anterior point of union with the cranium.

Menton horizontal

This is a tangent through menton on the lower border of the symphysis parallel to the Frankfort plane. It defines the lower limit of the face.

Nasion vertical

A perpendicular line is drawn to the Frankfort plane through nasion. This line defines the anteroposterior relationship of the maxilla and the mandible relative to the anterior cranial base.

Basion vertical

A perpendicular through basion defines the posterior limit of the face. Basion is an important anatomical point in the midline on the foramen magnum, marking the anterior point of union between the cervical column and the base of the skull.

Pterygoid vertical

A perpendicular line to the Frankfort plane through the pterygoid point. This midfacial perpendicular line was selected by Ricketts because it is in a stable area of growth, being close to the point of emergence of the trigeminal nerve from the base of the skull.

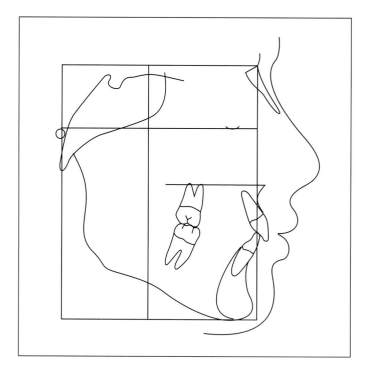

Fig. 6.3 The facial rectangle.

The facial rectangle now defines the upper, lower, anterior and posterior limits of the face, with the addition of a mid-facial vertical line. This construction facilitates measurement of all factors relative to vertical and horizontal axes. The spatial relationship of the key structures in facial development can now be observed and related to common vertical and horizontal axes.

BALANCED FACIAL PROPORTIONS

If the structure of the face is superimposed on a rectangular framework with horizontal and vertical axes, certain consistent criteria must be fulfilled in order to achieve the harmonious facial balance that is characteristic of the classical straight profile. Excellent facial balance results in the face growing correctly into the facial rectangle, so that the facial features relate closely to the anterior vertical (Fig. 6.4).

To achieve ideal facial proportions, the integral parts of the facial structure must be well related in size, shape and position. In well-balanced faces the Frankfort and maxillary planes are approximately parallel to the upper maxillary plane and optic plane, and relate closely to the true horizontal in the natural head position. This signifies parallel development of the anterior cranial base and the floor of the nose. Functional balance of the craniofacial and cervical components may be expressed in a favourable equilibrium of muscle forces acting on the underlying skeletal structures to produce a balanced growth response to the forces of gravity and

posture. By comparison, divergence of the horizontal planes is an expression of functional imbalance in facial development that can be recognised in cephalometric analysis, and is significant in the aetiology and treatment of malocclusion.

The relative angulation of the upper incisor, the facial axis, the axis of the condyle and the nasal outline are easily compared as they are all related to the vertical axis. A direct comparison of these measurements is useful in evaluating the aetiology of the malocclusion in structural and positional terms, and is helpful in diagnosis and treatment planning. In a well-balanced face with a good occlusion these structures show approximately parallel development. In treatment, one aims to align these structures to improve facial balance.

A unique feature of this method of analysis is the close correlation of the mean values of key factors involved in the determination of facial type. The mean values express balance and harmony in facial proportions, and departure from the mean is often related to occlusal imbalance of skeletal origin in the aetiology of malocclusion. Significant deviation from a mean of 27° in key factors may be used to identify areas where the pattern departs from the norm. Disproportion in one area is reflected in reciprocal changes in other areas when we examine facial proportions in the facial rectangle. When we assemble all the pieces within a unified framework a pattern in the jigsaw puzzle begins to emerge.

The means referred to in this chapter are based on cephalometric values for caucasian faces and should be modified for different racial and facial groups. Irrespective of the racial group, the mean values for a cross-section of the population differ from values representing ideal facial proportions.

In a predominantly caucasian population the mean values are biased towards mild Class II skeletal pattern, reflecting the higher proportion of Class II skeletal patterns compared to a small proportion of Class III skeletal patterns. There is invariably a difference between the mean values and the ideal values observed in patients with excellent facial balance and aesthetics. For key factors this is expressed in the difference between the mean and ideal values.

Skeletal planes

A further construction is now made to define the main facial and dental characteristics by defining points (Fig. 6.5) and planes:

- **Cranial base plane:** nasion (N) to basion (Ba).
- **Mandibular base plane:** menton (ME) to gonion (Go).
- **Facial plane:** nasion to pogonion (P).
- **Facial axis:** pterygoid point (Pt) to gnathion (Gn).
- **Condyle axis:** centre of the condyle to Xi-point.
- **Maxillary plane:** anterior nasal spine (ANS) to posterior nasal spine (PNS).
- **A to Po:** A-point to pogonion (P).

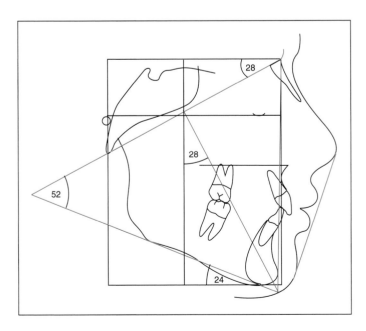

Fig. 6.4 Patient P.G. showing a mesognathic pattern with good facial balance.

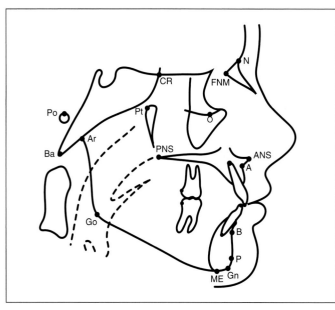

Fig. 6.5 Location of points. See text above for key.

Dental planes

- **Functional occlusal plane:** distal the intersection of the first molars to the intersection of the first premolars.
- The long axis of the upper incisor.
- The long axis of the lower incisor.

Soft-tissue planes

- **Nasal plane:** the outline of the nose from root to tip.
- **Aesthetic plane:** the tangent to the nose and chin.

A CORRELATIVE CEPHALOMETRIC ANALYSIS

Measurement relative to common vertical and horizontal axes reveals a surprising consistency in the mean angulation of key structures in cephalometric analysis. This confirms the structural interdependence between key parts of the craniofacial skeleton that leads to balanced facial development.

Angular analysis

Cranial base angle:
Cranial base plane to horizontal registration plane.
Norm = 27°; clinical deviation ± 3°; ideal = 29–30°.

The angulation of the cranial base to the horizontal is of fundamental importance in determining facial type.

Mandibular plane angle:
Angle of mandibular plane to horizontal.
Norm = 26°; clinical deviation ± 4°.
A measure of vertical or horizontal growth potential.

Craniomandibular angle:
Angle of cranial base plane to mandibular base plane.
Norm = 53°; clinical deviation + 5°.
A measure of facial height.
Equals the sum of the cranial base angle and the mandibular base angle.

Facial plane angle:
Angulation of facial plane to nasion vertical.
Norm = –3°; clinical deviation = 3°.
Determines the degree of mandibular prognathism or retrognathism.

Facial axis angle:
Facial axis to pterygoid vertical.
Norm 27°; clinical deviation ± 3°; ideal = 29–30°.
Determines the direction of growth of the chin.
An important indicator for prognosis related to growth direction.

Condyle axis angle:
Condyle axis to pterygoid vertical.
Norm = 27°; clinical deviation ± 4°.
Relate to the facial axis angle for balance in facial development.

Mandibular arc:
Angulation of condyle axis to body of mandible (Xi to Pm).
Norm = 26° at age 8; clinical deviation = 4°.
Increases by 0.5° per year.
High angles > square mandible/deep bite/prognathic.
Low angles > open bite/retrognathic.

Craniomaxillary angle:
Cranial base plane to maxillary plane.
Norm = 27°; clinical deviation = 3°.
Relates the cranial base angle to maxillary deflection.

Maxillary deflection:
Angulation of maxillary plane to horizontal.
Norm = 0°; clinical deviation ± 3°.
Determines the proportions of upper and lower facial height.

Dental analysis

The dental relationship may be defined by the following measurements:

The upper and lower incisors are related to the anterior vertical

Upper incisor angle:
Upper incisor to anterior vertical.
Norm = 25°; clinical deviation ± 7°.

Lower incisor angle:
Lower incisor to anterior vertical.
Norm = 25°; clinical deviation ± 4°.
This is equivalent to 65° to the Frankfort horizontal in the Tweed analysis.

Interincisal angle:
Angle between upper and lower incisal axes.
Norm = 128°; clinical deviation = 6°.

Position of dentition

Position of upper dentition:
Distal of upper molar to pterygoid vertical.
Norm = patient's age + 3 mm.
Indicates whether or not to distalise upper molars.

Position of lower dentition:
Lower incisor to A–Po line.
Norm = +1 mm; clinical deviation + 2 mm.
An important indicator of stability of the lower incisor position.
A key guideline for extraction or non-extraction therapy.
Determines the position of the lower incisors relative to the anterior limit of the skeletal base.
Functional therapy advances the lower incisors relative to the A–Po line.
It is necessary to review the lower incisor position relative to the A–Po line after functional therapy before completing treatment.

Linear factors

Convexity: A-point to facial plane:
Mean = 2.5 mm at age 8; decreases by 0.1 mm per year.
Increased convexity is Class II skeletal; decrease is Class III skeletal.

Maxillary position: A-point to nasion vertical:
Mean = 0 mm in mixed dentition; mean = +1 mm in adult.
Positive values measure maxillary protrusion.
Negative values measure maxillary retrusion.

Mandibular position: pogonion to nasion vertical:
Mean = –10 mm at age 8; decreases by 0.75 mm per year.

Soft tissue analysis

Nasal angle:
Angulation of nose to anterior vertical.
In a harmonious face, the nasal plane is nearly parallel to the facial axis.

Lower lip to E-plane:
Distance of lower lip from a line tangent to nose and chin.
Norm –2 mm at age 8; decreases by 0.2° per year.
Determines the degree of protrusion or retrusion of the lips.

Key factors in diagnosis and treatment planning

The pattern of facial growth is largely determined by the relative size and growth vectors of the cranial base, the maxilla and the mandible. Key angular factors express the contribution of these components to the growth pattern.

Three key angles can be used to express the basic pattern of facial growth as determined by the basal components. (Fig. 6.4):

- Cranial base angle.
- Facial axis angle.
- Mandibular plane angle.

The mean values for the cranial base/facial axis/mandibular plane angles are: 27/27/26. These angles express the basic form of the face.

The cranial base angle represents the degree of flexion of the cranial base as measured to the horizontal axis, while the mandibular plane angle measures the flexion of the mandibular base to the horizontal axis. High or low cranial or mandibular plane angles have a significant effect on the facial pattern.

The craniomandibular angle is the sum of the cranial base angle and the mandibular plane angle, because they are measured to a common horizontal axis. The mean craniomandibular angle is 53°. This angle measures the total facial height.

A high craniomandibular angle indicates increased facial height, with vertical growth and a dolichofacial growth pattern, which may be associated with anterior open bite. Conversely a low craniomandibular angle indicates horizontal growth and a brachyfacial growth pattern with deep overbite and a skeletal closed bite.

Brachyfacial and mesofacial growth patterns are favourable for functional correction, whereas dolichofacial patterns are not favourable, as the growth is expressed vertically, and increased vertical growth does not improve the facial appearance or the profile.

The gradient of growth of the chin

The facial axis angle measures the gradient of growth of the chin relative to the vertical axis. The direction of growth of the chin does not vary significantly during growth, with or without orthodontic or orthopaedic treatment. This angle is therefore an important indicator of the prognosis for correction of the profile by functional mandibular advancement. In mathematical terms the gradient of the facial axis can be used to express the number of millimetres of horizontal growth relative to vertical growth of the chin. This proportion determines whether or not it is possible to improve the profile by advancing the mandible. In a straight profile which is neither prognathic nor retrognathic the ideal facial axis angle is in the region of 29° to 30°. In a caucasian population with a higher proportion of Class II malocclusions (30–35%) and a small proportion of Class III (3%) a mean facial axis angle of 27° expresses mild mandibular retrusion. As the facial axis angle reduces to the mid or low twenties, or even into the teens, the degree of mandibular retrusion increases accordingly, and the growth pattern becomes progressively more vertical, and less favourable for functional correction.

Different racial and facial types are characterised by different means of the facial axis angle, expressing different facial patterns. For example the mean facial axis angle for Japanese is 25°, whereas Hispanic is 29° and Black is 26°.

Vertical growth results in a downward translation of the mandible and the profile does not improve, whereas horizontal growth results in a forward mandibular translation, with a corresponding improvement in a retrusive mandible. The facial axis angle may be used to support clinical diagnosis in case selection for functional orthopaedic treatment. The facial axis angle is influenced by the relative flexion of the cranial and mandibular base planes. A high mandibular plane angle with a low facial axis angle may indicate a poor prognosis for functional correction by mandibular advancement. The profile should be examined carefully before treatment to determine the effect of forward mandibular posture. If the profile does not significantly improve, the prognosis for functional correction is poor.

Conversely as the facial axis angle increases into the thirties the direction of growth becomes more horizontal, expressing mandibular prognathism when pogonion moves ahead of the nasion vertical.

The facial axis angle is therefore a useful indicator of the pattern of facial growth. It should be viewed together with the cranial base angle and mandibular plane angle to determine the prognosis for functional correction by mandibular advancement.

Maxillary convexity

Convexity is a measure of the anteroposterior skeletal relationship. The position of the maxilla relative to the cranial base and the mandible is measured as the distance from A-point to the facial plane. Thus A-point, the anterior point on the maxilla, is assessed relative to nasion and pogonion, the anterior points on the cranial base and mandible respectively. The range of normal convexity is +1 to +3 mm. Increased convexity is an indication of maxillary protrusion or mandibular retrusion. The relative position of the maxilla and mandible is confirmed by reference to the nasion vertical. The maxilla is correctly related to the cranial base when A-point lies on the nasion vertical. The maxilla is protrusive when A-point is ahead of the vertical, and retrusive when it lies behind the nasion vertical. The position of the mandible is assessed by the distance of the chin point (pogonion) to the nasion vertical.

Position of the upper dentition

The position of the upper dentition can be assessed with reference to the first permanent molars or incisors. According to Ricketts the upper first molar may be related to the pterygoid vertical. The norm for the individual is determined as the age of the patient plus 3 mm, and this applies only until growth is complete. This measurement helps to determine whether distalising forces should be applied to the molar. The molar position is usually related to the position of the maxilla as indicated by A-point relative to the nasion vertical. A protrusive maxilla will normally be related to a mesially positioned upper molar, indicating that the molar can be moved distally. Conversely, a retrusive maxilla is more likely to be related to a distally positioned molar relative to the pterygoid vertical. This would contraindicate distal movement of the molar.

Upper incisor position may be assessed either by angular or linear measurement. The mean upper incisor angle to the nasion vertical is 25°. McNamara determines the position of the tip of the upper incisor relative to the nasion vertical, with a normal range of +4 to +6 mm.

A combination of all factors relating molar and incisor position should be viewed with reference to the position of the maxilla as a primary aetiological factor in determining the position of the upper dentition.

Position of the lower dentition

The position of the lower dentition may be assessed by relating the tip of the lower incisors to the A–Po line. The A–Po line represents the anterior limit of the skeletal base, as it joins the most anterior points on the maxilla and mandible. This line is an important diagnostic indicator in determining whether or not the lower incisors should be moved labially or lingually during treatment. The aim of treatment is to position the lower incisors in a stable position over basal bone at the end of treatment. The ideal position for the tip of the lower incisors in a caucasian population is +1 to +3 mm ahead of the A–Po line. This position gives the best aesthetic profile by supporting the lower lip. Ricketts described a broad range of acceptability for this factor from –1 to +3 mm.

It must be appreciated that where an anteroposterior or vertical discrepancy exists in the mandibular position, a functional mandibular advancement alters the relationship of the lower incisors to the A–Po line. As a general rule the lower incisors are advanced relative to the A–Po, and an adjustment must be made to allow for this. A second tracing of the mandible may be made and positioned so that the overjet and overbite are corrected to give an estimated correction of the lower incisor after treatment. Alternatively a second cephalogram may be taken to review the position after functional correction (Fig. 6.6).

The position of the lower incisors influences the outline of the lower lip in profile. Lingually positioned lower incisors behind the A–Po line are normally associated with a retrusive lip, which may be trapped lingual to the upper incisors, while labially positioned lower incisors are related to protrusive lips. In some facial patterns lip protrusion is the norm, and is an expression of bimaxillary protrusion, which is often a racial characteristic. The normal range for lower incisor position relative to the A–Po line in black populations is 4–6 mm, while the norm for hispanic populations is 3–5 mm. In general, functional treatment is less effective in correction of bimaxillary protrusion, and may be contraindicated, depending on the effect of mandibular advancement on the profile.

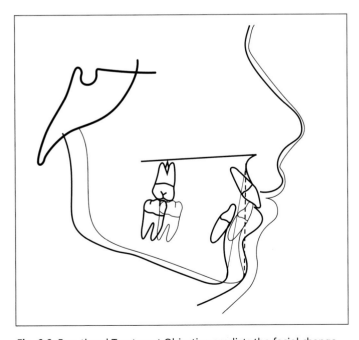

Fig. 6.6 Functional Treatment Objective predicts the facial change that will result from mandibular advancement. The lower incisor translates forward relative to the A–Po line.

DESCRIPTIVE TERMS IN CEPHALOMETRIC ANALYSIS

Definition of facial type

Mesognathic
A normal relationship of the maxilla and mandible to the cranial base.

Prognathic
Prominence of jaw position relative to the cranial base.

Retrognathic
Retrusion of jaw position relative to the cranial base.

Where the relationship of the maxilla and mandible to the cranial base is not the same, the terms normal, protrusive and retrusive are used to describe the individual jaw relationship.

Mesofacial
Describes a well-balanced face with harmonious musculature and a pleasant soft-tissue profile.

Brachyfacial
The face is typically short and square with a reduced mandibular plane angle and strong musculature. It describes a horizontal growth pattern (Ricketts, 1960) with a deep overbite of skeletal origin. A mild brachyfacial tendency is favourable for normal dental development. A strong brachyfacial growth pattern is accompanied by retrusion of the lips in the profile. Anchorage is good and non-extraction therapy is indicated.

Dolichofacial
The face is typically long and narrow with a high mandibular plane angle and weak musculature. It describes a vertical growth pattern (Ricketts, 1960) with an anterior open bite tendency. Patients are likely to exhibit naso-respiratory problems with incompetent or strained lip musculature. The alveolar processes are long and thin due to increased lower facial height. There is frequently dental crowding associated with narrow archform. Natural anchorage is poor and these patients present difficulties in treatment. Extraction therapy may be indicated for relief of crowding.

Note. Confusion arose in terminology when Bimler (1977) used the anthropological terms dolichoprosopic and leptoprosopic to relate facial depth to facial height, while Ricketts combined Latin and Greek roots in his terminology. A detailed explanation of the origin of this confusion is given by Witzig & Spahl (1989) (see Chapter 3, pp. 118–31).

To avoid further confusion, because of the use of Ricketts' triangle in the Clark analysis, the terminology used in this book is as defined by Ricketts.

FACIAL CHANGE IN TWIN BLOCK TREATMENT

This section illustrates examples of the treatment of uncrowded Class II division 1 malocclusion in different facial types with Twin Blocks to compare the response to treatment.

CASE REPORT: K.H. AGED 9 YEARS 7 MONTHS

This girl was treated in early permanent dentition and presented a severe Class II division 1 malocclusion with an overjet of 10 mm and a full unit distal occlusion. Cephalometric analysis indicates a mild Class II skeletal pattern with a brachyfacial growth pattern, indicating horizontal growth. There is a prognathic tendency in the maxilla with convexity of 5 mm due to maxillary protrusion. However, clinical examination confirms that the profile improves when the mandible is advanced slightly. When the patient postures downwards and forwards, the resulting change in the profile is a preview of the change which will be produced by functional therapy. Clinical guidelines therefore indicate a functional approach to treatment. Guiding the mandible forwards to match the slightly protrusive position of the maxilla will improve the profile in this case (Fig. 6.7).

Twin Blocks – 5 months
Support appliance – 3 months
Treatment time – 8 months, including retention.

Treatment is uncomplicated thanks to good archform, and the response to treatment is rapid due to the strong horizontal skeletal growth pattern. As a general rule the profile will continue to straighten as the patient matures when there is a brachyfacial pattern with horizontal growth.

CASE REPORT: K.H.

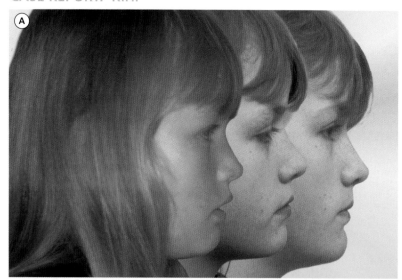

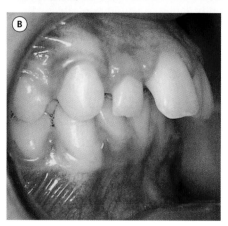

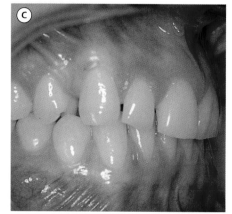

Fig. 6.7 Treatment:
A Profiles at ages 9 years 7 months (before treatment), 11 years 3 months (after treatment) and 14 years 7 months (out of retention).
B Occlusion before treatment at 9 years 7 months.
C Occlusion 3 years out of retention at age 14 years 7 months.

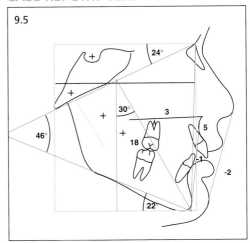

9.5

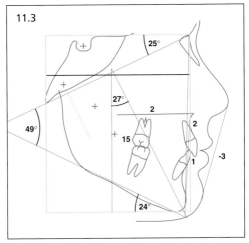

11.3

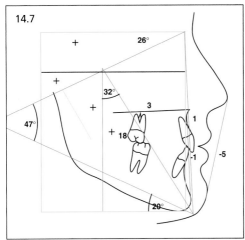

14.7

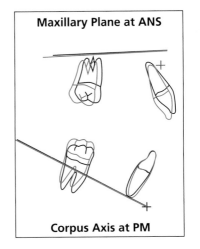

Maxillary Plane at ANS

Corpus Axis at PM

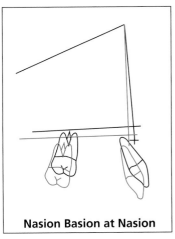

Nasion Basion at Nasion

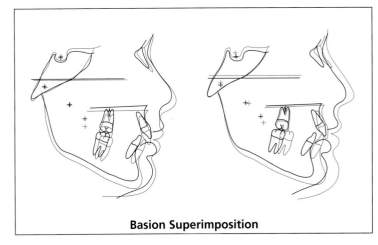

Basion Superimposition

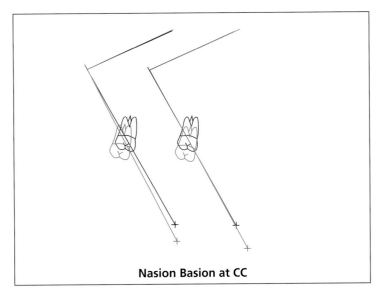

Nasion Basion at CC

K.H.	Age	9.5	11.3	14.7
Cranial Base Angle		24	25	26
Facial Axis Angle		30	27	32
F/M Plane Angle		22	24	20
Craniomandibular Angle		46	49	47
Maxillary Plane		3	2	3
Convexity		5	2	1
U/Incisor to Vertical		29	19	22
L/Incisor to Vertical		32	29	26
Interincisal Angle		119	132	132
6 to Pterygoid Vertical		18	15	18
L/Incisor to A/Po		−1	1	−1
L/Lip to Aesthetic Plane		−2	−3	−5

CASE REPORT: M.E. AGED 13 YEARS

This boy presents a severe Class II division 1 malocclusion with an overjet of 13 mm and an excessive overbite. Cephalometric analysis indicates a severe class II skeletal pattern with 8 mm convexity due to a combination of maxillary protrusion and mandibular retrusion. The growth pattern is brachyfacial and the upper central incisors are proclined by a trapped lower lip. The favourable growth pattern again produces a rapid response to treatment. The overjet reduces from 11 mm to 2 mm in 3 months and the distal occlusion is corrected by the initial activation of the Twin Blocks (Fig. 6.8).

Twin Blocks: 6 months
Support phase: 4 months
Retention: 4 months
Treatment time: 14 months
Final records: 2 years 10 months out of retention at age 17 years.

CASE REPORT: M.E.

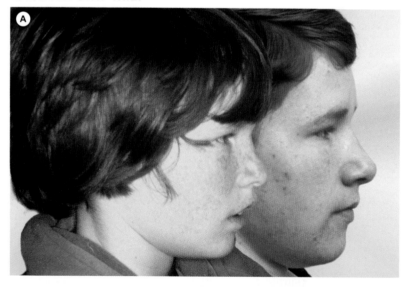

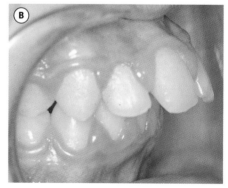

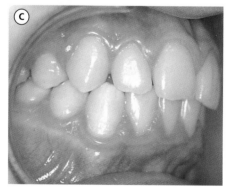

Fig. 6.8 Treatment:
A Profiles at ages 13 years (before treatment) and 17 years (out of retention).
B Occlusion before treatment.
C Occlusion after treatment.

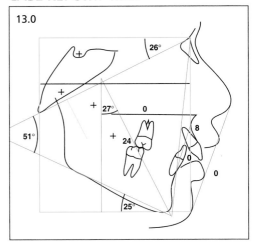

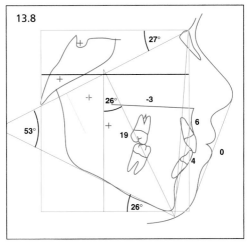

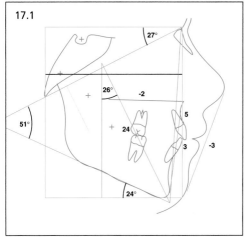

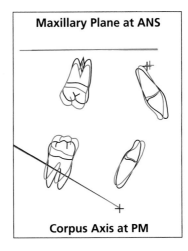

Maxillary Plane at ANS

Corpus Axis at PM

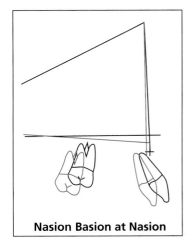

Nasion Basion at Nasion

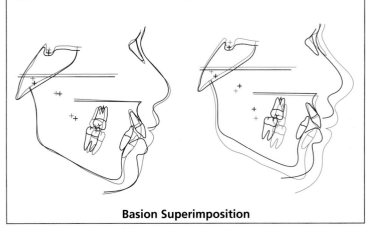

Basion Superimposition

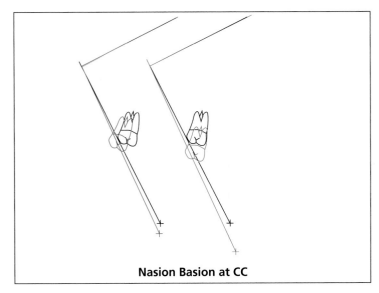

Nasion Basion at CC

M.E.	Age	13.0	13.8	17.1
Cranial Base Angle		26	27	27
Facial Axis Angle		27	26	26
F/M Plane Angle		25	26	24
Craniomandibular Angle		51	53	51
Maxillary Plane		0	−3	−2
Convexity		8	6	5
U/Incisor to Vertical		31	22	24
L/Incisor to Vertical		26	36	26
Interincisal Angle		123	122	122
6 to Pterygoid Vertical		24	19	24
L/Incisor to A/Po		0	4	3
L/Lip to Aesthetic Plane		0	0	−3

CASE REPORT: P.McL. AGED 11 YEARS 6 MONTHS

This girl has a Class II division 1 malocclusion on a Class I skeletal base relationship with only 2 mm convexity. An incomplete overbite is associated with a forward tongue thrust, causing severe proclination of the upper incisors and an overjet of 11 mm. Slight facial asymmetry is eliminated by correcting the centre lines in the bite registration so as to encourage unilateral activation to improve the asymmetry. A tongue guard and spinner are effective in controlling the tongue thrust (Fig. 6.9).

Twin Blocks: 7 months
Support phase: 5 months
Retention: 9 months
Total treatment time: 21 months.

CASE REPORT: P.McL.

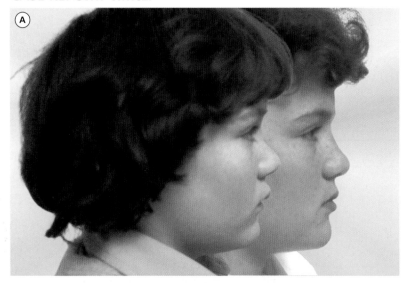

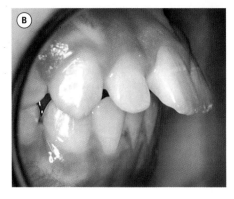

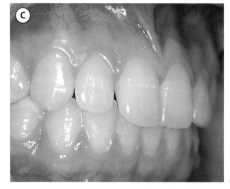

Fig. 6.9 Treatment:
A Profiles at ages 11 years 6 months (before treatment) and 13 years (after treatment).
B Occlusion before treatment.
C Occlusion after treatment.

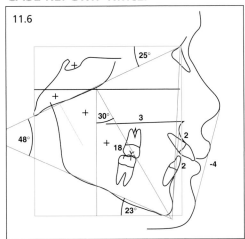

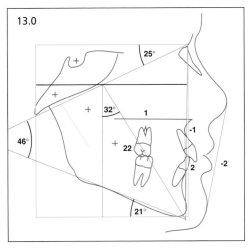

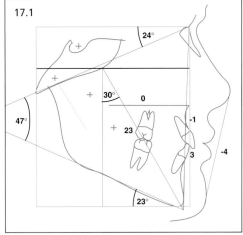

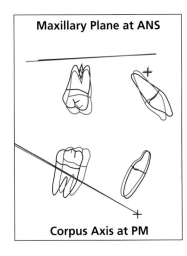

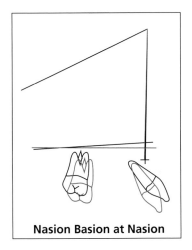

Maxillary Plane at ANS

Corpus Axis at PM

Nasion Basion at Nasion

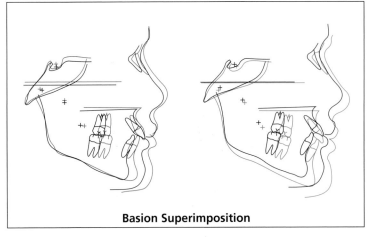

Basion Superimposition

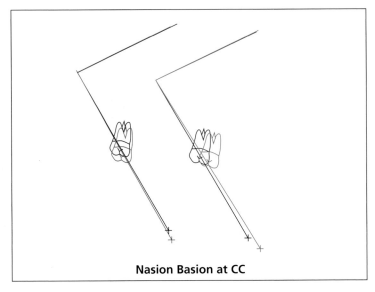

Nasion Basion at CC

P.McL.	Age	11.6	13.0	17.1
Cranial Base Angle		25	25	24
Facial Axis Angle		30	32	30
F/M Plane Angle		23	21	23
Craniomandibular Angle		48	46	47
Maxillary Plane		3	1	0
Convexity		2	−1	−1
U/Incisor to Vertical		44	31	31
L/Incisor to Vertical		28	28	28
Interincisal Angle		108	121	121
6 to Pterygoid Vertical		18	22	23
L/Incisor to A/Po		2	2	3
L/Lip to Aesthetic Plane		−4	−2	−4

CASE REPORT: E.F. AGED 12 YEARS 9 MONTHS

A girl with good archform and mild crowding in the lower arch and impaction of a lower second premolar. A moderate Class II skeletal base with a convexity of 5 mm is due to mandibular retrusion, with a favourable brachyfacial growth pattern. An overjet of 14 mm and excessive overbite is partially corrected by an initial activation of 8 mm, before reactivating to edge-to-edge to complete the correction (Fig. 6.10).

Twin Blocks: 14 months
Support and retention: 12 months
Treatment time: 26 months.

CASE REPORT: E.F.

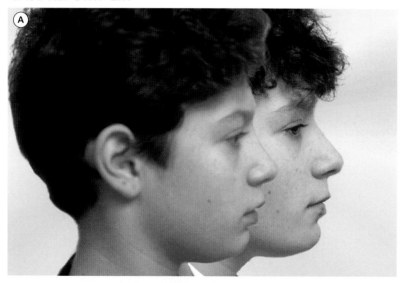

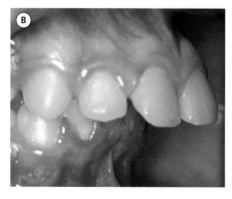

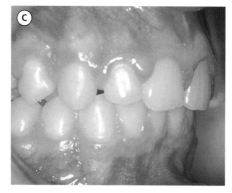

Fig. 6.10 Treatment:
A Profiles at ages 12 years 9 months (before treatment) and 15 years (after treatment).
B Occlusion before treatment.
C Occlusion after treatment.

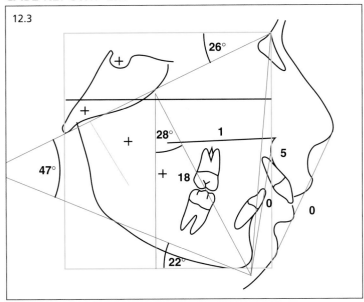

12.3

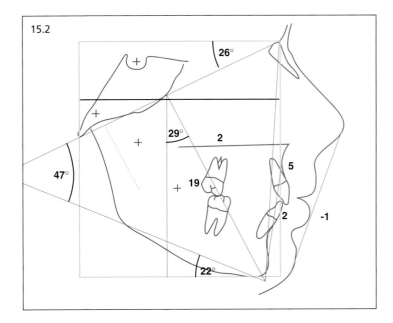

15.2

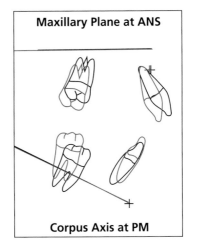

Maxillary Plane at ANS

Corpus Axis at PM

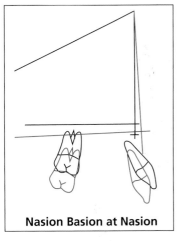

Nasion Basion at Nasion

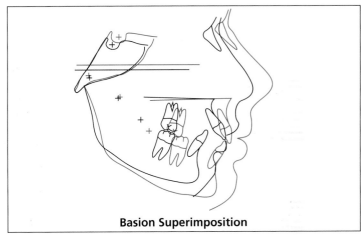

Basion Superimposition

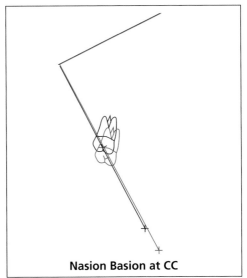

Nasion Basion at CC

E.F.	Age	12.3	15.2
Cranial Base Angle		26	26
Facial Axis Angle		28	29
F/M Plane Angle		22	22
Craniomandibular Angle		47	47
Maxillary Plane		1	2
Convexity		5	5
U/Incisor to Vertical		32	19
L/Incisor to Vertical		39	34
Interincisal Angle		109	127
6 to Pterygoid Vertical		18	19
L/Incisor to A/Po		0	2
L/Lip to Aesthetic Plane		0	−1

67

CASE REPORT: W.L. AGED 10 YEARS 3 MONTHS

This girl presents a severe Class II skeletal pattern with 8 mm convexity, due to severe mandibular retrusion. The 24° facial axis angle indicates a dolichofacial tendency with vertical growth of the chin, which is less favourable for correction. As a result the response to treatment may be slower and the period of treatment is longer (Fig. 6.11).

The screw is operated to expand the maxilla for 3 months.

The overjet reduces from 9 mm to 3 mm in 4 months, and the distal occlusion is corrected by the initial activation of the Twin Blocks. Correction is achieved mainly by mandibular advancement with slight maxillary retraction.

Twin Blocks: 11 months
Support phase: 6 months
Retention: 6 months
Treatment time: 23 months.

CASE REPORT: W.L.

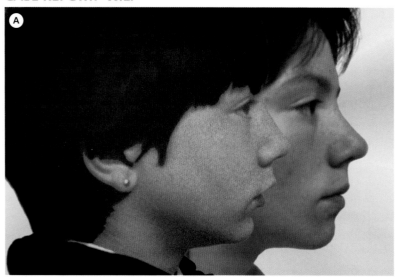

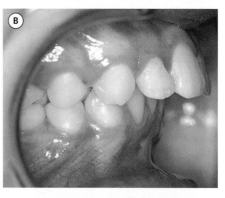
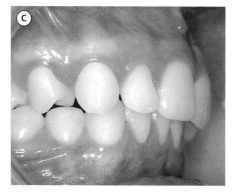
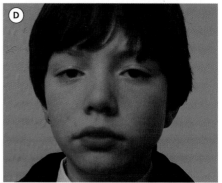
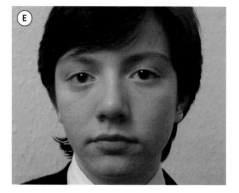

Fig. 6.11 Treatment:
A Profiles at age 10 years 3 months (before treatment) and 11 years 6 months (after treatment).
B Occlusion before treatment.
C Occlusion after treatment.
D Appearance before treatment.
E Appearance after treatment.

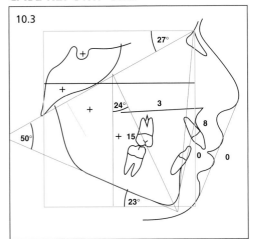

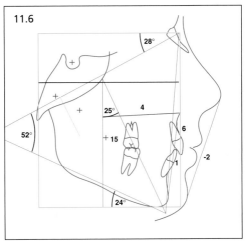

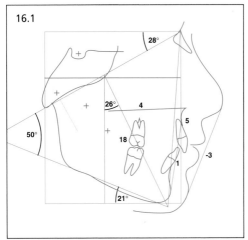

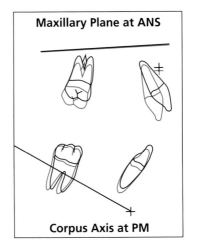

Maxillary Plane at ANS

Corpus Axis at PM

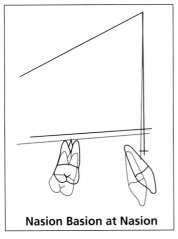

Nasion Basion at Nasion

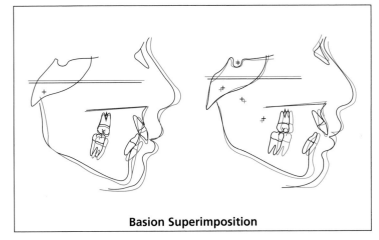

Basion Superimposition

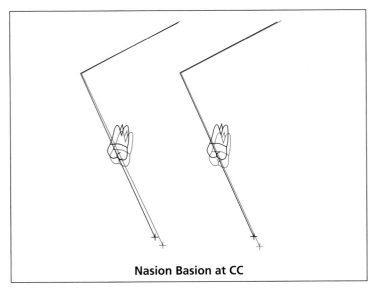

Nasion Basion at CC

W.L.	Age	10.3	11.6	16.1
Cranial Base Angle		27	28	28
Facial Axis Angle		24	25	26
F/M Plane Angle		23	24	21
Craniomandibular Angle		50	52	49
Maxillary Plane		3	4	4
Convexity		8	6	5
U/Incisor to Vertical		31	21	14
L/Incisor to Vertical		34	42	36
Interincisal Angle		115	117	140
6 to Pterygoid Vertical		15	15	18
L/Incisor to A/Po		0	1	1
L/Lip to Aesthetic Plane		0	–2	–3

CASE REPORT: A.F. AGED 11 YEARS

The cephalometric analysis in this case shows a dolichofacial tendency with mandibular retrusion and a facial axis angle of 25°. The convexity is 7 mm and the overjet 9 mm with an increased but incomplete overbite. There was mild upper and lower incisor crowding and disto-labial rotation of 1|1. Brackets were fitted on the upper six anterior teeth to correct the rotation of the incisors during the Twin Block phase, progressing to a simple upper fixed appliance to complete treatment. This was followed by pericision on 1|1 to stabilise their position after treatment. Extraction of all second molars was carried out to reduce the risk of recurrent crowding, and to avert potential impaction of third molars (Fig. 6.12).

Twin Blocks: 6 months
Fixed appliance: 3 months
Retention: 12 months
Treatment time: 21 months.

CASE REPORT: A.F.

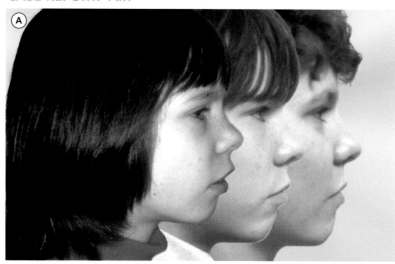

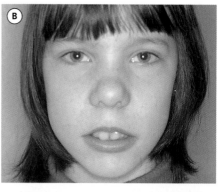

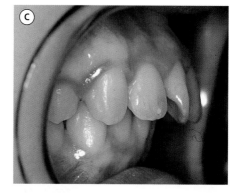

Fig. 6.12 Treatment:
A Profiles at ages 11 years (before treatment) and 17 years 5 months (out of retention).
B Appearance before treatment.
C Occlusion before treatment.
D Appearance 4 years out of retention.
E Occlusion out of retention.

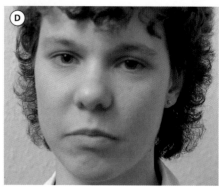

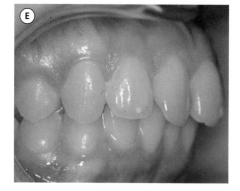

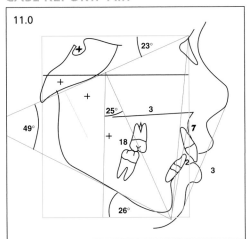

11.0

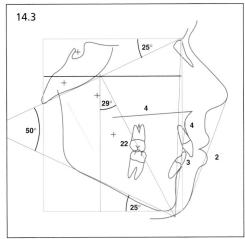

14.3

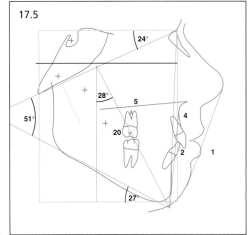

17.5

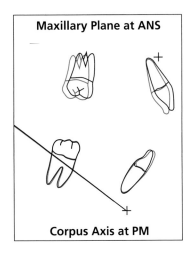

Maxillary Plane at ANS

Corpus Axis at PM

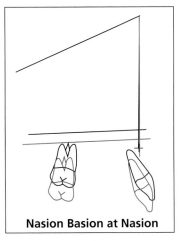

Nasion Basion at Nasion

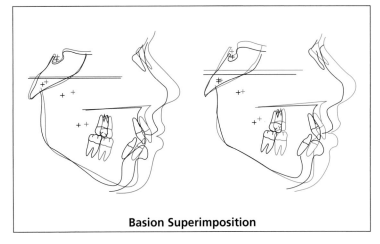

Basion Superimposition

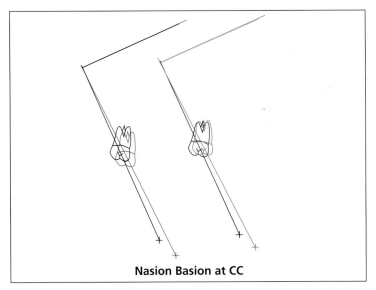

Nasion Basion at CC

A.F.	Age	11.0	14.3	17.5
Cranial Base Angle		23	25	24
Facial Axis Angle		25	29	28
F/M Plane Angle		26	25	27
Craniomandibular Angle		49	50	51
Maxillary Plane		3	4	5
Convexity		7	4	4
U/Incisor to Vertical		27	23	23
L/Incisor to Vertical		37	32	30
Interincisal Angle		116	125	127
6 to Pterygoid Vertical		18	22	20
L/Incisor to A/Po		2	3	2
L/Lip to Aesthetic Plane		3	2	1

CASE REPORT: L.C. AGED 9 YEARS

This girl presents a dolichofacial pattern with a facial axis angle of 22°, indicating severe vertical growth. The face is retrognathic in both the maxilla and mandible, although the mandibular retrusion is more severe. Convexity is 6 mm and the overjet is 14 mm, with excessive overbite.

The response during Twin Block treatment in this case was relatively slow due to the vertical growth pattern. This patient required a second Twin Block appliance to reinforce correction to a Class I dental relationship. Vertical growth is associated with weak musculature and is related to a slower response to treatment because the corrective functional forces are reduced (Fig. 6.13).

Twin Blocks: 16 months
Support and retention: 12 months
Treatment time: 28 months.

CASE REPORT: L.C.

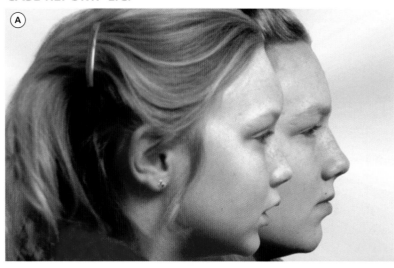

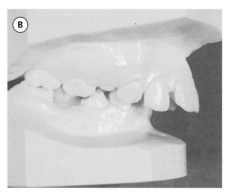

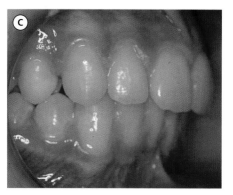

Fig. 6.13 Treatment:
A Profiles at ages 9 years (before treatment) and 14 years 11 months (out of retention).
B Occlusion before treatment.
C Occlusion out of retention.

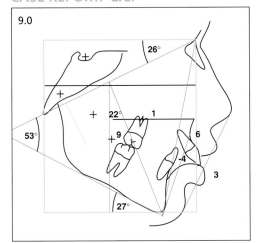

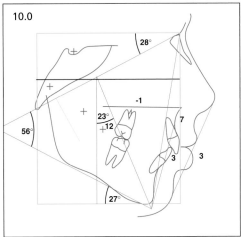

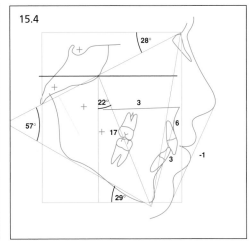

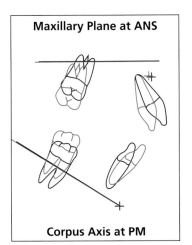

Maxillary Plane at ANS

Corpus Axis at PM

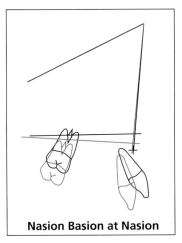

Nasion Basion at Nasion

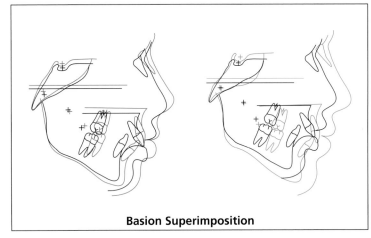

Basion Superimposition

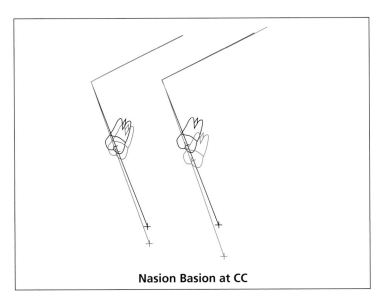

Nasion Basion at CC

L.C.	Age	9.0	10.0	15.4
Cranial Base Angle		26	28	28
Facial Axis Angle		22	23	22
F/M Plane Angle		27	27	29
Craniomandibular Angle		53	56	57
Maxillary Plane		1	−1	3
Convexity		6	7	6
U/Incisor to Vertical		32	15	13
L/Incisor to Vertical		30	42	40
Interincisal Angle		118	123	127
6 to Pterygoid Vertical		9	12	17
L/Incisor to A/Po		−4	3	3
L/Lip to Aesthetic Plane		3	3	−1

Natural head position

It is fully realised that the selection of a single horizontal skeletal plane for the purpose of head orientation in the living subject is a compromise, because the vertical location of landmarks varies among individuals. This limitation was accepted when the Frankfort horizontal was defined after much debate in Germany (1884) to approximate to a standardised head position of the living, in order to orient skulls for craniometric research. In orientating the head relative to the true vertical, therefore, there is good reason to consider alternative skeletal planes for registration, to compensate for individual variation in the position of skeletal landmarks.

Determination of natural head position in relation to the true vertical is a starting point in the aesthetic examination of the facial profile. This method has been used for the purpose of serial cephalometric radiography, as described by other authors in previous studies. The classic natural head position is a reproducible, standardised position of the head, whereby the individual looks at a point in the distance at eye level. The visual axis is horizontal.

This concept cannot always be achieved in a clinical setting, and alternatively the patient may be positioned standing or seated in an upright position opposite a vertical mirror, mounted 150 cm in front of the ear rods, so that the patient can observe his/her eyes in the mirror (Fig. 6.14). The patient is positioned carefully in the cephalostat with the head tilted neither forwards nor backwards, and the true vertical is registered as a plumb line suspended over the cassette holder in the occipital region. Investigation has established a method error of 2.3° for variability of head posture recorded by auxilliaries for head position to the true vertical. (Solow & Tallgren, 1971; Siersbaek-Neilsen & Solow, 1982).

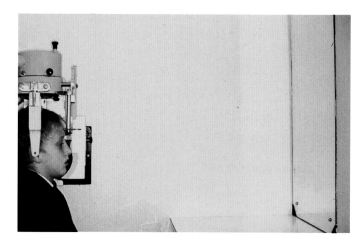

Fig. 6.14 Patient positioned in the cephalostat in natural head position. Note the vertically mounted mirror.

REFERENCES

Bimler, H.P. (1957). A roentgenoscopic method of quantifying the facial proportions. *Trans. Eur. Orthod. Soc.*, 1957: 241–53.

Bimler, H.P. (1977). In *Removable Orthodontic Appliances*, ed. T.M. Graber & B. Neumann. Philadelphia, W.B. Saunders.

Broadbent, B.H. (1937). The face of the normal child. *Angle Orthod.*, **76:** 183–208.

Broadbent, B.H. (1948). *Practical Orthodontics*, ed. G.H. Anderson, 7th edn. St Louis, C.V. Mosby, p. 208.

Brodie, A.G. (1940). Some recent observations on growth of the face and their implications to the orthodontist. *Am. J. Orthod. Oral Surg.*, **26:** 741–57.

Brodie, A.G. (1941). On the growth pattern of the human head from the third month to the eighth year of life. *Am. J. Anatomy*, **68:** 209–62.

Brodie, A.G. (1946). Facial patterns: a theme and variations. *Angle Orthod.*, **16:** 75–87.

Coben, S.E. (1955). The integration of facial skeleton variants. *Am. J. Orthod.*, **41:** 407–34.

Coben, S.E. (1961). Growth concepts. *Angle Orthod.*, **31:** 194–201.

Coben, S.E. (1979). Basion coordinate tracing film. *J. Clin. Orthod.*, 194–201.

Frankel, R. & Frankel, Ch. (1989). *Orthofacial Orthopedics with the Function Regulator*. Basle, Karger.

McNamara, Jr, J.A. (1984). A method of cephalometric evaluation. *Am. J. Orthod.*, **86:** 449–69.

Ricketts, R.M. (1960). A foundation for cephalometric communication. *Am. J. Orthod.*, **46:** 330–57.

Siersbaek-Neilson, S. & Solow, B. (1982). Intra and inter-examiner variability in head posture recorded by dental auxilliaries. *Am. J. Orthod.*, **82:** 50–7.

Solow, B. & Tallgren, A. (1971). Natural head position in standing subjects. *Acta Odont. Scand.*, **29:** 591–607.

Witzig, J.W. & Spahl, T.J. (1989). *The Clinical Management of Basic Maxillofacial Orthopedic Appliances*, Vol. 2, *Diagnostics*. Massachusetts, PSG Publishing Co., pp. 130–1.

FURTHER READING

Ricketts, R.M., Roth, R.H., Chaconas, S.J., Schulhof, R.J. & Engel, G.A. (1982). *Orthodontic Diagnosis and Planning*. Denver, Rocky Mountain Orthodontics.

CHAPTER 7

Appliance Design and Construction

Comfort and aesthetics are the two most important factors in appliance design. It is important to design appliances that are 'patient friendly' to remove any obstacles to compliance and to motivate the patient to cooperate in treatment.

Twin Blocks have the advantage of versatility of design. They meet a wide range of requirements for correction of different types of malocclusion for patients throughout the age range from childhood to adulthood. Because the upper and lower appliances are separate components, the design can be adapted to resolve problems in both arches independently.

The component parts of Twin Block appliances are common to conventional removable appliances with the addition of occlusal inclined planes. Appliance design is modified by the addition of screws and springs or bows to move individual teeth. Arch development can proceed simultaneously with correction of arch relationships in the horizontal and vertical dimensions.

EVOLUTION OF APPLIANCE DESIGN

The earliest Twin Blocks were designed with the following basic components:

- A midline screw to expand the upper arch.
- Occlusal bite blocks.
- Clasps on upper molars and premolars.
- Clasps on lower premolars and incisors.
- A labial bow to retract the upper incisors.
- Springs to move individual teeth and to improve the archform as required.
- Provision for extraoral traction in some cases.

Twin Block appliances are tooth and tissue borne. The appliances are designed to link teeth together as anchor units to limit individual tooth movement, and to maximise the orthopaedic response to treatment. In the lower arch, peripheral clasping combined with occlusal cover exerts three-dimensional control on anchor teeth, and limits tipping and displacement of individual teeth. When indicated, additional clasps may be placed on lower incisors but, in practice, it is found that clasps mesial to the lower canines are equally effective in controlling the lower labial segment. An example of an early design with a labial bow, lower incisor clasps and provision for extraoral traction, which is no longer used to reinforce anchorage, is shown in Fig. 7.1.

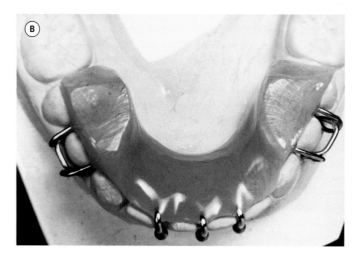

Fig. 7.1 A, B Example of an early Twin Block with a labial bow, lower incisor clasps and provision for extraoral traction, which is no longer used to reinforce anchorage.

A common modification to appliance design preferred by some orthodontists is the addition of incisal capping over the lower incisors. The reasoning is to prevent proclination of the lower incisors, but this concern is usually unfounded, as growth studies by the author and other investigators show that, although the lower incisors procline by up to 5° during the Twin Block stage, they upright during the support stage. After treatment no significant proclination of lower incisors occurs. The author used lower incisal capping during the early stages of development of Twin Blocks, and observed decalcification of the tips of the lower incisors in a few cases where the oral hygiene was poor. One important difference compared to the bionator, for example, is that the Twin Block is worn for eating. Oral hygiene is therefore an important factor during treatment, and because of the risk of decalcification the author abandoned incisal capping.

STANDARD TWIN BLOCKS

Standard Twin Blocks are essentially for treatment of an uncrowded Class II division 1 malocclusion with good archform and an overjet large enough to allow unrestricted forward translation of the mandible to allow full correction of distal occlusion.

Labial bow

In the early stages of development, the upper Twin Block invariably incorporated a labial bow. It was observed that if the labial bow engaged the upper incisors during functional correction it tended to overcorrect incisor angulation. It was, therefore, routinely adjusted out of contact with the upper incisors. Retracting upper incisors prematurely limits the scope for functional correction by mandibular advancement. This led to the conclusion that a labial bow is not always required unless it is necessary to upright severely proclined incisors, and even then it must not be activated until full functional correction is complete and a Class I buccal segment relationship is achieved. If a labial bow is included in the appliance design, and it is activated prematurely to

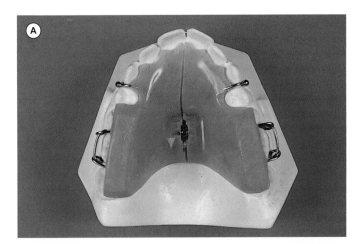
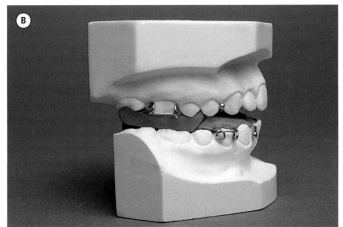
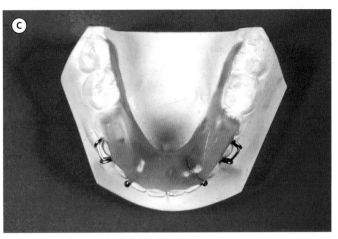
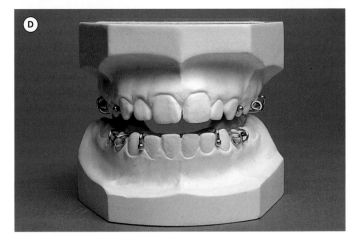

Fig. 7.2 A–D Standard Twin Blocks.

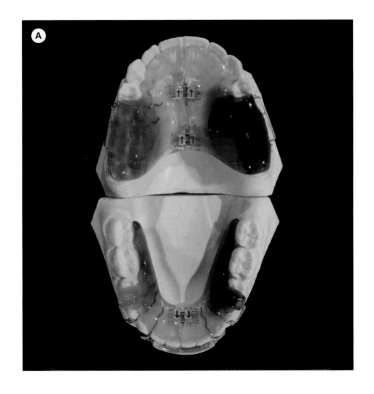

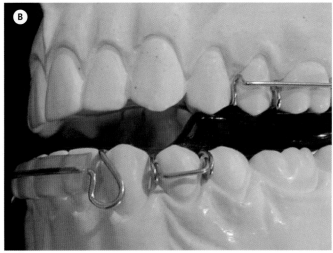

Fig. 7.3 Modified design of the Twin Block lower appliance used by McNamara & Mills.

retract upper incisors, this will act as a brake to limit the functional correction by mandibular advancement. In many cases, the appliance is more effective for functional correction without a labial bow.

In Twin Block treatment a good lip seal is achieved naturally without additional lip exercises, as the appliance is worn for eating and drinking, making it necessary to form a good anterior seal. The lips act like a labial bow and lip pressure is effective in uprighting upper incisors, making a labial bow superfluous. In many cases, the absence of a labial bow improves aesthetics without reducing the effectiveness of the appliance (Fig. 7.2).

An alternative design that has gained some popularity places an acrylic pad labial to the lower incisors as an additional means of retention and control. This procedure has been used in some cases by McNamara and Mills, whose work is referred to in the text of other chapters. An illustration of this modified design of the lower appliance is shown in Fig. 7.3.

TWIN BLOCK CONSTRUCTION

The appliance prescription includes all the details required for correction of the individual malocclusion, with specific instructions on appliance design including springs and screws to correct individual teeth, or segmental correction by transverse and/or sagittal correction to improve archform. A vague request for 'Twin Blocks' does not give sufficient detail for proper construction of the appliance.

The laboratory requires a good set of impressions and an accurate construction bite to record the activation to be built into the appliance. The construction bite should be taken in modelling wax that retains its dimensional stability after it is removed from the mouth. Any excess wax extending over the buccal surfaces of the teeth should be removed to allow the models to seat correctly into the construction bite. In the laboratory the models are mounted on an articulator to register the construction bite before the occlusal bite blocks are constructed. A plasterless articulator may be used, with adjustable screws to position the models in the correct relationship.

THE DELTA CLASP

The delta clasp was designed by the author to improve the fixation of Twin Blocks. The delta clasp is similar to the Adams clasp (Adams, 1970) in principle, but incorporates new features to improve retention, reduce metal fatigue and minimise the need for adjustment. The retentive loops were originally triangular in shape (from which the name 'delta' is derived), or alternatively the loops may be circular or ovoid, both types having similar retentive properties.

The delta clasp retains the basic elements of the Adams clasp, that is, interdental tags, retentive loops and a buccal bridge. The crucial difference is that the retentive loops are shaped as a closed triangle, or a circle or ovoid as opposed to an open U-shaped arrowhead as in the Adams clasp. The

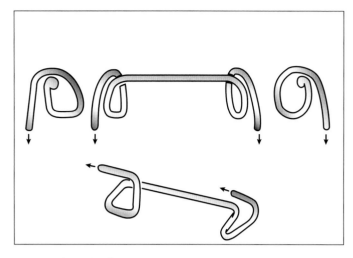

Fig. 7.4 The Delta clasp.

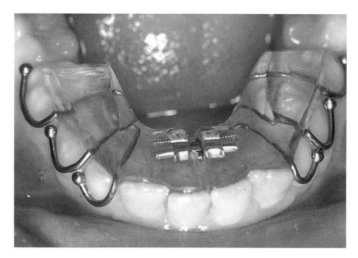

Fig. 7.5 Clasps on deciduous molars and canines.

advantage of the closed loop is that the clasp does not open with repeated insertion and removal and, therefore, maintains its shape better and requires less adjustment, and is less subject to breakage. A further advantage is that the clasp gives excellent retention on lower premolars, and is suitable for use on most posterior teeth (Fig. 7.4).

A comparison of the failure rate of the delta and Adams clasp was made by statistical analysis of two groups of 69 and 72 patients treated consecutively in the author's practice with Twin Blocks between 1979 and 1993 (Clark & Stirrups, pers. comm.).

Results indicated that the incidence of breakage of delta clasps was significantly reduced compared with appliances retained with the modified arrowhead clasp. The percentage of breakages was 10% for the modified arrowhead (Adams) clasp and 1% for the delta clasp.

According to the area of best retention there are two possible methods of construction for the delta clasp. The first is similar to the Adams clasp, with the retentive loop angled to follow the curvature of the tooth into mesial and distal undercuts. This design is appropriate if the tooth is favourably shaped, with good undercuts mesially and distally.

If the individual teeth are not favourably shaped, the loop of the clasp may be directed interdentally. The loop is then constructed at right angles to the bridge of the clasp, so that it passes into the interdental undercut to gain retention from adjacent teeth.

In the permanent dentition, delta clasps are placed routinely on upper first molars and on lower first premolars. They may also be used on deciduous molars. Additional interdental ball-ended clasps, finger clasps or C-shaped clasps may be placed to improve retention and provide resistance to anteroposterior tipping.

Ball-ended clasps are routinely employed mesial to lower canines and in the upper premolar or deciduous molar region to gain interdental retention from adjacent teeth. C-clasps are useful in mixed dentition where they can be used for peripheral clasping on deciduous molars and canines (Fig. 7.5).

ADJUSTMENT OF THE DELTA CLASP

The delta clasp may be adjusted gingivally into an interdental undercut by placing pliers on the wire as it emerges from the acrylic interdentally. Bird beak or 139 pliers have a short round beak that is placed under the wire and the square beak is placed on top. A slight adjustment extends the retentive loop of the clasp into the gingival or interdental undercut.

The other method of adjustment is to grasp the arrowhead from the buccal aspect and twist the retentive loop inwards towards the tooth to adjust into a mesial or distal undercut.

THE BASE PLATE

Appliances may either be made with heat cure or cold cure acrylic. Heat cure acrylic has the advantage of additional strength and accuracy. Making the appliances in wax first allows the blocks to be formed with greater precision.

Cold cure acrylic has the advantage of speed and convenience, but sacrifices something in strength and accuracy. It is essential to use a top-quality cold cure acrylic to avoid problems with breakage, especially in the later stages of treatment, after trimming the blocks to allow eruption in treatment of deep overbite. The inclined planes can lose their definition as a result of wear if a soft acrylic is used.

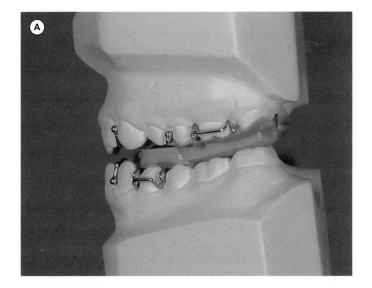

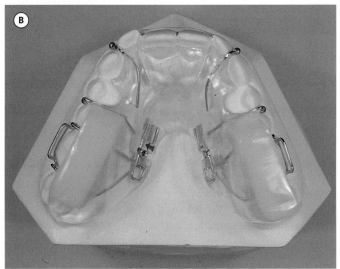

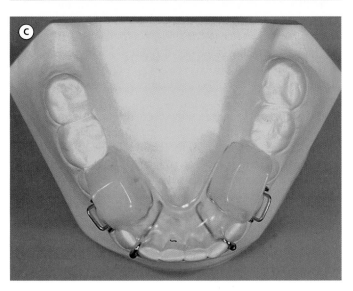

The disadvantages of cold cure acrylic can be overcome by using preformed blocks made from a good-quality heat cured acrylic. This has the important advantage of making construction easier and increasing the accuracy of the inclined planes by providing a consistent angle for occlusion of the blocks (Fig. 7.6).

The author has observed that laboratory construction of Twin Block appliances in cold cure acrylic is time consuming, especially in forming the occlusal bite blocks, and subsequently in trimming and finishing the appliances. This is the most common method of appliance construction and there is scope to improve the process and to simplify this stage in construction of the appliances. After recent research new preformed patterns have been designed to facilitate laboratory construction of the bite blocks by producing preformed modules which greatly simplify appliance construction and finishing.

TWIN BLOCKS FOR ARCH DEVELOPMENT

It is important to realise that when crowding or irregularity is present in the dental arches provision must be made for this in the appliance design, and the Twin Blocks must be modified by the addition of springs or screws to correct the irregularity.

Transverse development

Upper and lower Schwarz appliances (Schwarz & Gratzinger, 1966) were commonly used in the past for transverse development in mixed dentition. It is now possible to combine transverse arch development simultaneously with sagittal and vertical correction of arch relationships by combining Twin Block and Schwarz appliances (Fig. 7.8).

Screws may be incorporated in the upper and lower Twin Blocks to develop the archform in mixed dentition. This allows independent control of arch width in both arches to improve anterior crowding or correct posterior crossbite. An upper transpalatal arch or lower Jackson design (Jackson, 1887) may be used as an alternative to screws for arch development (Fig. 7.9).

The Twin Block Crozat appliance (Crozat, 1920) provides a useful alternative that is suitable for adult treatment with minimum palatal and lingual coverage. This appliance requires careful adjustment to maintain symmetry (Fig. 7.10).

The palate-free Twin Block is an excellent alternative for added comfort and to improve speech. This is illustrated in Chapter 10 in the section on 'Concurrent Straightwire and Twin Block Therapy'.

Fig. 7.6 A–C Appliances with preformed heat-cured blocks.

OCCLUSAL INCLINED PLANES

The position and angulation of the occlusal inclined planes is crucial to efficiency in correcting arch relationships. In most cases, the inclined planes are angled at 70° to the occlusal plane, although the angulation may be reduced to 45° if the patient fails to posture forwards consistently and thereby to occlude the blocks correctly.

The position of the inclined plane is determined by the lower block and is critical in the treatment of deep overbite. It is important that the inclined plane is clear of mesial surface contact with the lower molar, which must be free to erupt unobstructed in order to reduce the overbite. The inclined plane on the lower bite block is angled from the mesial surface of the second premolar or deciduous molar at 70° to the occlusal plane. The lower block should extend distally to the buccal cusp of the lower second premolar or deciduous molar, stopping short of the distal marginal ridge. This allows the leading edge of the inclined plane on the upper appliance to be positioned mesial to the lower first molar so as not to obstruct eruption. The position of the inclined plane is especially important in correction of deep overbite, where the upper block is trimmed to allow eruption of lower molars. If the inclined plane extends too far distally, subsequent trimming of the upper block weakens the upper inclined plane and leads to breakage.

Buccolingually the lower block covers the occlusal surfaces of the lower premolars or deciduous molars to occlude with the inclined plane on the upper Twin Block (Fig. 7.7). The flat occlusal bite block passes forwards over the first premolar to become thinner buccolingually in the lower canine region. The full thickness of the blocks need not be maintained in the canine region. Reducing the bulk in this area is important, as speech is improved by allowing the tongue freedom of movement in the phonetic area.

As this can be the most vulnerable part of the appliance, the lingual flange of the lower appliance in the midline should be sufficiently thick to give adequate strength to avoid breakage.

The upper inclined plane is angled from the mesial surface of the upper second premolar to the mesial surface of the upper first molar. The flat occlusal portion then passes distally over the remaining upper posterior teeth in a wedge shape, reducing in thickness as it extends distally.

Because the upper arch is wider than the lower, it is only necessary to cover the lingual cusps of the upper posterior teeth, rather than the full occlusal surface. This has the advantage of making the clasps more flexible and allows access to the interdental wires of the clasps for adjustment.

In constructing the blocks a decision must be made concerning the angulation of the blocks in relation to the line of the arch. There are two alternatives, both of which are effective in practice.

First, the blocks may be aligned in each quadrant at right angles to the line of the arch in the same pattern as the teeth are aligned. Alternatively, the lower blocks may be aligned at right angles to the midline bisecting the arch. The upper blocks would be constructed to match this angulation. This second method has the advantage that the blocks maintain the same angulation relative to each other even if the midline screws are turned to widen the archform.

Appliance design has been progressively simplified over the years and additional designs have been developed to treat different types of malocclusion.

The position of the inclined plane

Angle stressed the importance of the first permanent molars and described the development of the key ridge in the first molar region in response to functional forces applied to the molars. The permanent molars are designed to resist the forces of occlusion and the muscles of mastication apply the optimum forces in this region. It is logical that the inclined plane should be placed mesial to the upper first molars in order to optimise the functional forces to achieve the best response to treatment.

The author tested the response to moving the inclined plane mesially to the first premolar region 20 years ago, during the early stages of development of the technique. This change appeared to reduce both the efficiency of the appliance and the response to mandibular advancement. Mesial movement of the inclined plane is therefore not recommended, as reduction in the functional forces applied results in a corresponding reduction in the response to treatment.

Mahoney and Witzig (1999) proposed moving the inclined plane forward to coincide with the distal of the lower canine in order to free the posterior teeth to erupt. In addition to reducing efficiency, this approach removes posterior occlusal support, and may result in overloading of the condyle and lack of occlusal support can damage the articular disc.

The same article suggests that there is less need for a support phase, but in the author's experience, it is important to realise that insufficient support and retention following functional correction can lead to relapse. While recognising that any improvements in the design of Twin Blocks are to be encouraged, these proposals are more likely to reduce the efficiency of the technique, and lack of support and retention may produce unstable results.

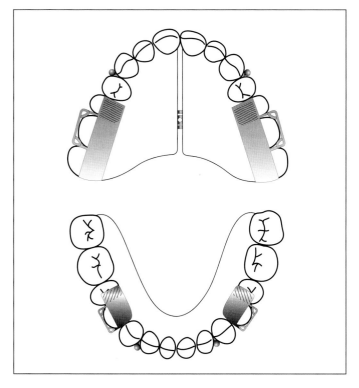

Fig. 7.7 Occlusal view of standard Twin Blocks. Two upper midline screws may be used to improve stability.

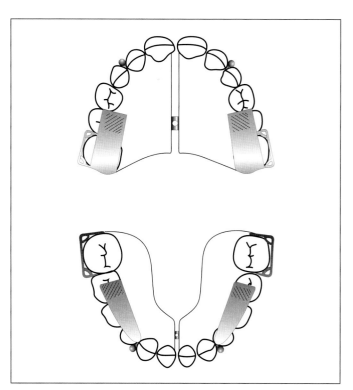

Fig. 7.8 Twin Block Schwarz appliances.

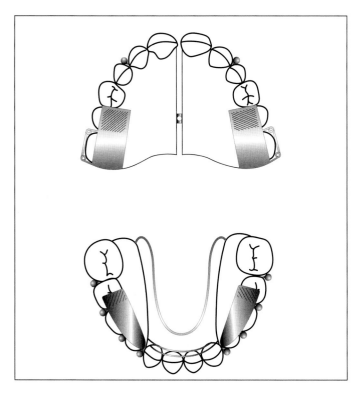

Fig. 7.9 Upper Schwarz/Lower Jackson Twin Block.

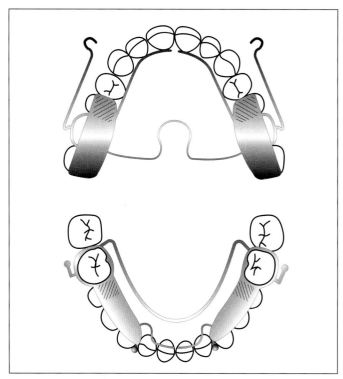

Fig. 7.10 Twin Block Crozat appliances.

SAGITTAL DEVELOPMENT

Twin Block sagittal appliance

Sagittal arch development is required when upper or lower incisors are retroclined with deep overbite. As the name implies, the Twin Block sagittal appliance is designed primarily for anteroposterior arch development by positioning two screws which are aligned anteroposteriorly in the palate. Some oblique movement is also possible by offsetting the angulation of the screws to achieve an additional component of buccal expansion. Normally, the palatal screws are angled to drive the upper posterior segments distally along the line of the arch.

The anteroposterior positioning of the screws and the location of the cuts determines whether the appliance acts mainly to move upper anterior teeth labially or to distalise upper posterior teeth. The position of the anterior cut determines how many teeth are included in the anterior segment. If only the central incisors are retroclined, a cut distal to the central incisors will move only these teeth labially or, alternatively, the lateral incisors may also be advanced by placing the cut distal to the lateral incisors. The incisor teeth are then pitted against the posterior teeth to advance the labial segment (Fig. 7.11).

In cases with asymmetrical arch development, if more distal movement is required unilaterally the screw on one side may be activated more than the other. If the cut is positioned distal to the canines or premolars the distalisation of posterior teeth increases in proportion to the number of teeth included as anchorage in the anterior segment.

In placing the screws in the palate it is important that they are set in the horizontal plane, and not inclined downwards anteriorly, which would cause the appliance to ride down the anterior teeth, reducing its effectiveness.

The lower Twin Block sagittal appliance applies similar principles in the lower arch. To advance the lower labial segment, curved screws are placed in the lower canine region, or to open premolar spaces, straight screws are placed in the second premolar region.

Transverse and sagittal development

Many cases require a combination of transverse and sagittal development. A three-way screw incorporates two screws in a single housing and allows independent activation for transverse and sagittal expansion, although it is fairly bulky in the anterior part of the palate and therefore interferes with speech (Fig. 7.12).

The three-screw sagittal appliance achieves this objective with an additional midline screw, which can be positioned anteriorly or posteriorly in the palate to achieve a similar objective (Fig. 7.13).

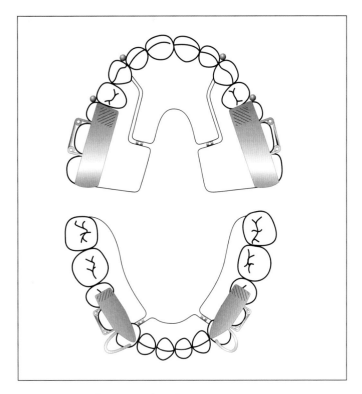

Fig. 7.11 Twin Block sagittal appliance.

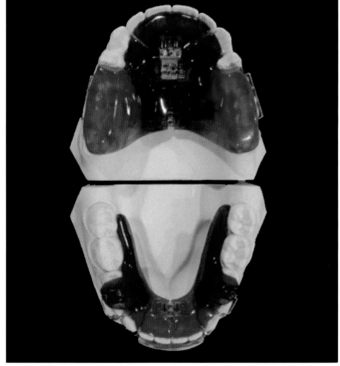

Fig. 7.12 Three-way screw for upper arch development.

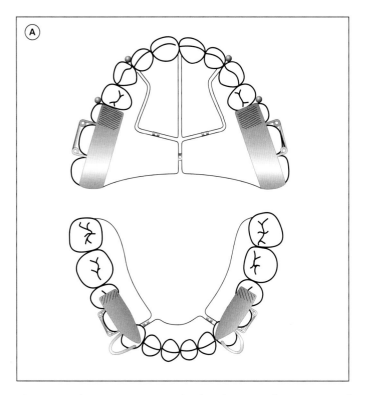

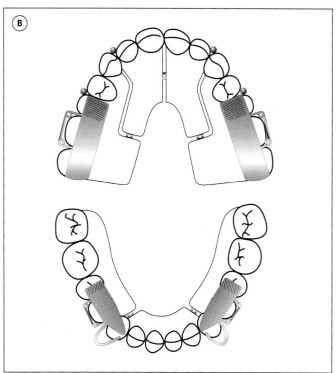

Fig. 7.13 A Three-screw upper sagittal appliance, with posterior midline screw.
B Three-screw upper sagittal appliance, with anterior midline screw.

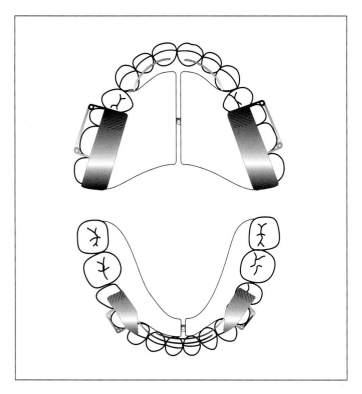

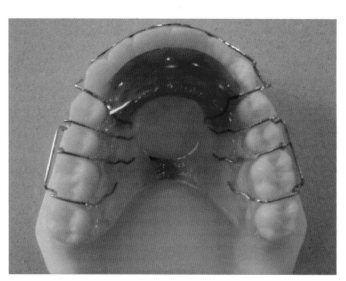

Fig. 7.15 Modified anterior inclined plane with palate-free area to control tongue thrust.

Fig. 7.14 Twin Blocks to open the bite and advance anterior teeth; springs advance upper and lower incisors.

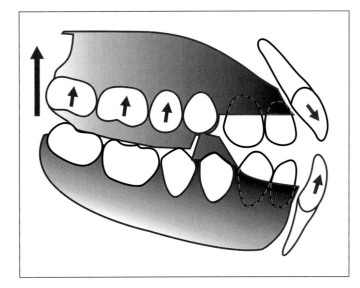

Fig. 7.16 Vertical extraoral traction force to intrude upper posterior teeth. The appliance is relieved lingual to upper and lower incisors to allow them to erupt.

Alternatively, a midline screw may be combined with lingual wires to advance and align upper and lower incisors. This design of appliance may be used in both arches to advance retroclined upper and lower incisors and to open the bite in treatment of bimaxillary retrusion (Fig. 7.14).

Twin Blocks to close anterior open bite

Twin Blocks are designed to close an anterior open bite by applying an intrusive force to the posterior teeth. Occlusal contact of the bite blocks on all the posterior teeth is essential to prevent eruption, which would open the bite. Similar principles apply in designing both upper and lower appliances to achieve these objectives (Fig. 7.15).

The upper appliance must extend distally to cover all the upper posterior teeth including second molars to prevent overeruption. Occlusal rests should extend distally to control second molars if they are about to erupt. Prevention is better than cure, as failure to control second molars will increase the open bite and cause treatment to fail.

The design of the lower appliance is modified for anterior open bite to prevent eruption of posterior teeth by placing clasps on lower molars and first premolars or deciduous molars to give good stability to the appliance. There is no need to add additional clasps in the lower labial segment.

The appliances should be designed to allow the upper and

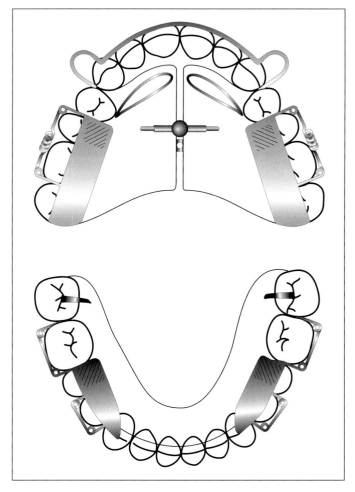

Fig. 7.17 Spinner to control tongue thrust – Clasps on lower first molars; occlusal rests to prevent eruption of second molars – E.O.T. tubes.

lower incisors to erupt in order to reduce the anterior open bite. The acrylic base plate may be extended over the cingulum of the upper and lower incisors before trimming the acrylic slightly to relieve contact with the incisors. This method has the advantage that the lingual flange serves to shield the incisors from the tongue, thus allowing the incisors to erupt to reduce the anterior open bite (Fig. 7.16). A labial bow may be added to upright proclined upper incisors and help reduce the anterior open bite. Tongue thrust may be controlled by the addition of a spinner or tongue guard. In some cases, both may be indicated (Fig. 7.17).

Provision can be made in the support appliance to control tongue thrust by using a modified anterior inclined plane with a palate-free target area for the tongue thrust (Fig. 7.15).

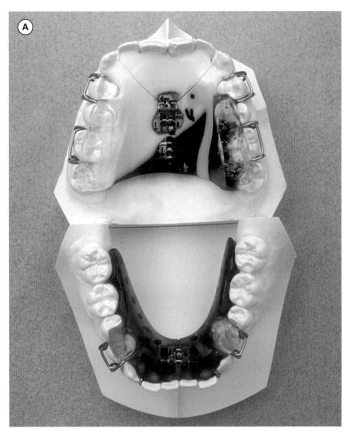

Designer Twin Blocks

Attention to detail is important in designing Twin Block appliances and the design should be selected to suit the individual patient. Young patients like to be involved in choosing the colour and design of their appliances. Orthodontic laboratories have the skill and expertise to individualise appliances to meet many different styles. Figure 7.18 illustrates examples of 'Designer Twin Blocks'. The range is unlimited, depending on the imagination of the designer. A list of recommended orthodontic laboratories is included on page 359.

Fig. 7.18 Designer Twin Blocks:
A The flamingo and the water melon. The upper appliance gives 3-way expansion.
B The Hole in One Twin Block and the Zebra. An alternative design for 3-way expansion in the upper arch.
C The dinner-suit appliance for stage 2.
These appliances were made by Ortholab, Melbourne, Australia, and are reproduced by kind permission of Graham Manley. They are representative of the high standard of work observed in specialist orthodontic laboratories.

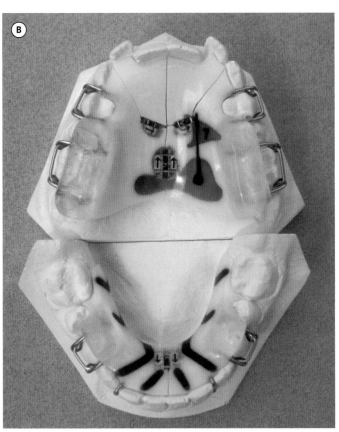

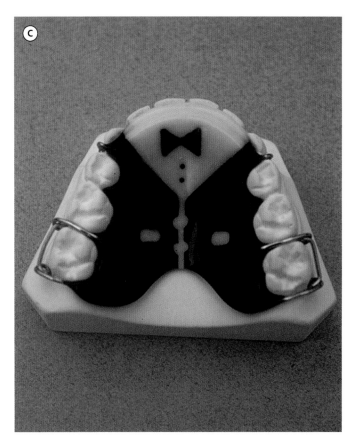

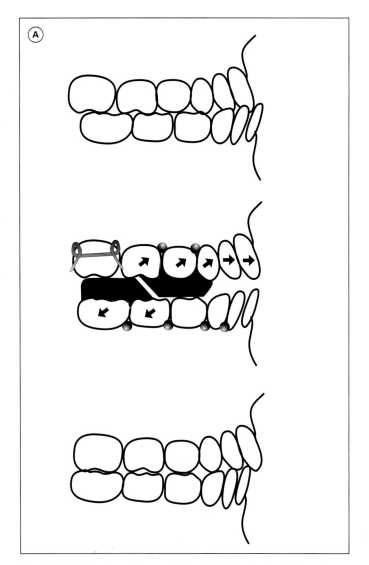

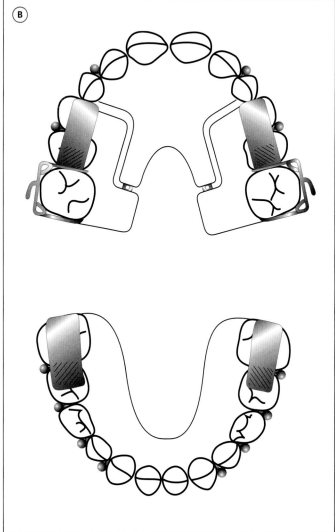

Fig. 7.19 A Side view of reverse Twin Blocks. **B** Occlusal view of reverse Twin Blocks.

TREATMENT: CLASS III MALOCCLUSION

Reverse Twin Blocks

The position of the bite blocks is reversed compared with that of Twin Blocks for the treatment of Class II malocclusion. The occlusal blocks on the upper appliance are positioned over the deciduous molars to occlude distally with blocks placed over the lower first permanent molars.

The addition of two sagittal screws in the palate provides a means of activation to advance the upper incisors, and the reciprocal force on the inclined planes uses anchorage in the lower arch to drive the upper arch labially. Apart from the reverse position of the blocks and inclined planes, the design of the upper appliance is similar in principle to the sagittal design used in the treatment of Class II division 2 malocclusion and the same principles apply in relation to positioning the screws.

A contracted maxilla frequently requires three-way expansion. This is achieved by a three-screw sagittal design or the three-way screw to combine transverse and sagittal arch development (Figs 7.19, 7.20).

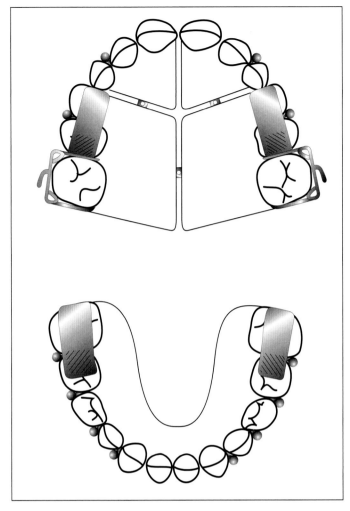

Fig. 7.20 Reverse Twin Block with three-way expansion in the upper arch.

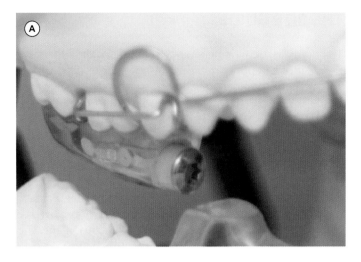

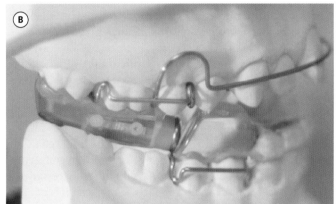

Fig. 7.21 A, B Screw Advancement mechanism

SCREW ADVANCEMENT MECHANISM FOR PROGRESSIVE ACTIVATION OF TWIN BLOCKS

A recent modification has been described (Carmichael, Banks & Chadwick, 1999) to enable controlled progressive advancement of the Twin Block. The activating mechanism uses a conical screw installed in a housing incorporated in the upper block. A laboratory kit includes components for installation and alignment and is supported by a chairside kit with cylindrical co-polymer spacers of different sizes for progressive advancement. In treatment of deep overbite the placement of an occlusal screw does not permit trimming of the upper block to allow eruption of lower molars. This is an advantage. The following are indications for use:

- Stepwise advancement may be used to facilitate reactivation in the treatment of large overjets.
- Unilateral activation may be used to correct asymmetrical mandibular development.
- Patients with vertical growth patterns tend to have weak musculature and are not able to tolerate large mandibular advancements. In such cases gradual mandibular advancement may be more effective.
- Smaller adjustments are possible to improve patient tolerance.
- More gradual advancement may be more physiological, at cellular level, and may produce an improved mandibular response.
- The system may also be used for progressive activation of Reverse Twin Blocks in correction of Class III malocclusion.

THE BITE GUIDE

Technological developments are playing an increasing role in the evolution of orthodontic and orthopaedic techniques. The recent development of a lingual attachment, the Bite Guide is a significant factor, not only related to Twin Block Technique, but also relevant in many clinical situations where vertical control of increased overbite is an important aspect of treatment.

The specific application in Twin Block treatment relates to the support phase, when vertical control is necessary during the transition to the support phase in order to maintain the corrected overjet and overbite. The bite guide acts as a fixed retainer to maintain the corrected vertical dimension after the molars have erupted into occlusion, and during the transitional period when the premolars and canines (or the deciduous teeth in mixed dentition) are erupting to establish the buccal segment occlusion. The inclined plane provided by the Bite Guide is specifically designed to engage the lower incisors when the overjet is up to 3 mm. If the overjet is more than 3 mm the lower incisors would then bite lingual to the Bite Guide, therefore it is necessary for the overjet to be fully corrected before the Bite Guide is fitted.

The Bite Guide provides an elegant solution to this phase of treatment, also when Twin Blocks are to be followed by a second phase of fixed appliances. By bonding bite guides on the lingual of the central incisors, it is no longer necessary to fit a removable appliance to support the corrected overjet and overbite until the posterior teeth have erupted into occlusion. Correction of the Class II relationship may be reinforced by the attachment of Class II inter-maxillary elastics to encourage the lower incisors to engage correctly on the Bite Guide until the posterior teeth have erupted fully, and the posterior occlusion has settled into a Class I relationship.

It is possible to invert the lingual attachment to form a Bite Ramp, as a horizontal platform to engage the lower incisors. While this is an effective method of controlling deep overbite by encouraging eruption of the posterior teeth in treatment of Class I occlusion, the inclined plane provided by the Bite Guide is better suited to act as a fixed support mechanism after Twin Block treatment after correction of a Class II malocclusion.

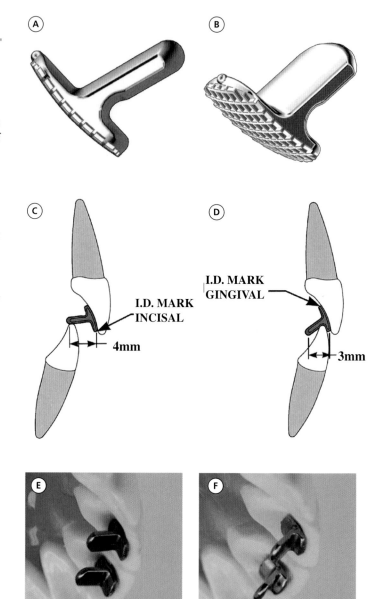

Fig. 7.22 Bite Guide and Bite Ramp appliances. Courtesy of Ortho Organizers.

REFERENCES

Adams, C.P. (1970). *The Design and Construction of Removable Orthodontic Appliances*, 4th edn. Bristol, John Wright & Sons Ltd.

Carmichael, G.J., Banks P.A., Chadwick S.M. (1999). A modification to enable controlled progressive advancement of the Twin Block Appliance. *Br. J. Orthodon.*, **26**: 9–14.

Crozat, G.B. (1920). Possibilities and use of removable labio-lingual spring appliances. *Int. J. Oral Surg.*, **6**: 1–7.

Jackson, V.H. (1887). Some methods of regulating. *Dent. Cosmos*, **29**: 373–87.

Mahoney, D.R. & Witzig, J. (1999). A modification of the Twin Block technique for patients with a deep bite. *The Functional Orthodontist*, **16**: 2, 4–10.

Schwarz, A.M. & Gratzinger, M. (1966). *Removable Orthodontic Appliances*. Philadelphia, W.B. Saunders.

CHAPTER 8

Treatment of Class II Division 1 Malocclusion Deep Overbite

CLINICAL MANAGEMENT OF TWIN BLOCKS

After a century of development of functional techniques it is surprising that the forces of occlusion have not been used to any significant extent as a functional mechanism to correct malocclusion. Twin Blocks adapt the functional mechanism of the natural dentition, the occlusal inclined plane, to harness the forces of occlusion to correct the malocclusion.

The Twin Block is a natural progression in the evolution of functional appliance therapy. It represents a fundamental transition from a one-piece appliance that restricts normal function to twin appliances that promote normal function.

Twin Blocks are designed on aesthetic principles to free the patient of the restrictions imposed by a one-piece appliance made to fit the teeth in both jaws. With Twin Blocks the patient can function quite normally. Eating and speaking can be accomplished without overly restricting normal movements of the tongue, lips and mandible. This means that the patient eats with the appliances in the mouth and the forces of mastication are harnessed to maximise the functional response to treatment.

Bite registration

The procedure of bite registration for construction of Twin Blocks for a Class II division 1 malocclusion with deep overbite is described in greater detail.

The Exactobite or Projet Bite Gauge is designed to record a protrusive bite for construction of Twin Blocks. The blue bite gauge registers 2 mm vertical clearance between the incisal edges of the upper and lower incisors, which is an appropriate interincisal clearance for bite registration in most Class II division 1 malocclusions with increased overbite.

The incisal portion of the bite gauge has three incisal grooves on one side that are designed to be positioned on the incisal edge of the upper incisor and a single groove on the opposing side that engages the incisal edge of the lower incisor. The appropriate groove in the bite gauge for bite registration is selected depending on the ease with which the patient can posture the mandible forwards.

In Class II division 1 malocclusion a protrusive bite is registered to reduce the overjet and the distal occlusion on average by 5–10 mm on initial activation, depending on the freedom of movement in protrusive function. The length of the patient's protrusive path is determined by recording the overjet in centric occlusion and fully protrusive occlusion. The activation should not exceed 70% of the protrusive path.

In the growing child with an overjet of up to 10 mm, provided the patient can posture forwards comfortably, the bite may be activated edge-to-edge on the incisors with a 2 mm interincisal clearance. This allows an overjet of up to 10 mm to be corrected on the first activation, without further activation of the Twin Blocks. Larger overjets invariably require partial correction, followed by reactivation after the initial correction is complete.

It is best first to rehearse the procedure of bite registration, with the patient using a mirror. The patient is instructed to close correctly into the bite gauge before applying the wax. When the patient understands what is required, softened wax is applied to the bite gauge from a hot water bath. The clinician then places the bite gauge in the patient's mouth to register the bite. After removing the registration bite from the mouth, the wax is chilled in cold water and should now be firm and dimensionally stable.

In registering the bite the wax is kept clear of the incisors, so that the operator has an unobstructed view of the anterior teeth. This helps the laboratory to position the models correctly in the squash bite (Fig. 8.1). Silicone putty may be used as an alternative to wax to register the bite, but the elasticity of the material can make it more difficult to locate the models correctly in the construction bite.

Centre lines should be coincident provided no dental asymmetry is present. To reduce the overjet when the lower incisors close into the incisal guidance groove on the

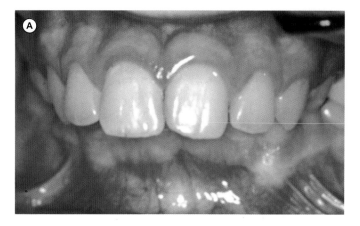

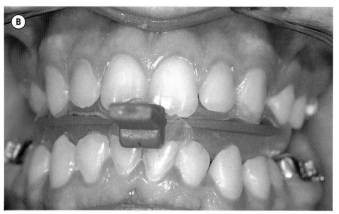

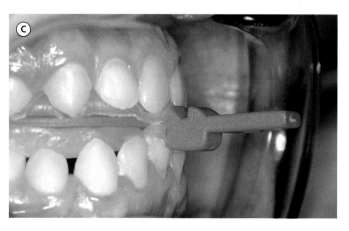

Fig. 8.1 A–C Construction bite for deep overbite with the projet.

underside of the bite gauge, the bite gauge is positioned with the upper incisors occluding in the appropriate groove. It is essential that the patient bites 'fully home' into the bite gauge to register the correct vertical opening for the occlusion.

In the vertical dimension a 2 mm interincisal clearance is equivalent to an approximately 5- or 6 mm clearance in the first premolar region. This usually leaves 3 mm clearance distally in the molar region, and ensures that space is available for vertical development of posterior teeth to reduce the overbite.

It is very important to open the bite slightly beyond the clearance of the free-way space to encourage the patient to close into the appliance rather than allow the mandible to drop out of contact into rest position, which is one of the disadvantages of making the blocks too thin.

APPLIANCE DESIGN: TWIN BLOCKS TO OPEN THE BITE

In designing Twin Blocks to open the bite the inclined planes must be positioned carefully to achieve vertical control by selective eruption of posterior teeth. The inclined planes must be clear of the lower molars so that they can erupt without obstruction (Fig. 8.2).

Fitting Twin Blocks Instructions to the patient

Patient motivation is an important aspect of all removable appliance therapy. The process of patient education and motivation continues when the patient attends to have Twin Blocks fitted. It is often helpful to the patient if the clinician demonstrates Twin Blocks on models to confirm that it is a simple appliance system and is easy to wear, with no visible anterior wires.

Simply biting the blocks together guides the lower jaw forwards to correct the bite. The appliance system is easily understood even by young patients, who can see that biting the blocks together corrects the jaw position. It is important to emphasise positive factors and to motivate the patient before treatment.

The patient is shown how to insert the Twin Blocks with the help of a mirror, pointing out the immediate improvement in facial appearance when the Twin Block is fitted and explaining that the appliances will produce this change in a few months, provided they are worn full time.

A removable appliance only corrects the teeth when it is in the mouth, not in the pocket. Both appliances must be worn full time, especially during eating, and removed only for cleaning. Exceptions may be made for swimming and contact sports.

At first the appliance will feel large in the mouth, but within a few days it will be very comfortable and easy to wear. Twin Blocks cause much less interference to speech than a one-piece functional appliance. For the first few days speech will be affected, but will steadily improve and should return to normal within a week.

When the patient has learned to insert and remove the appliance, instruction is given on operating the expansion screw, one quarter turn per week, explaining the necessity to widen the upper arch as the lower arch is advanced to correct the bite. The screw should be turned for the first time after a few days, when the appliances have settled in comfortably.

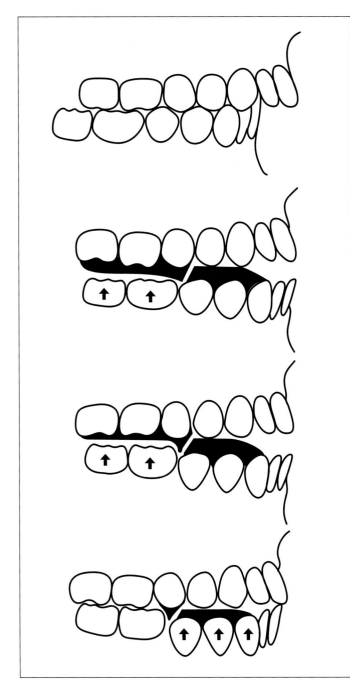

Fig. 8.2 Twin Blocks to open the bite – side view.

As with any new appliance it is normal to expect a little initial discomfort. But it is important to encourage the patient to persevere and keep the appliance in the mouth at all times except for hygiene purposes. The patient should also be instructed not to hesitate to contact the office if it is not comfortable within a few days.

The patient may be advised to remove the appliance for eating for the first few days. Then it is important to learn to eat with the appliance in the mouth. The force of biting on the appliance corrects the jaw position, and learning to eat with the appliance in is important to accelerate treatment. In a few days, patients should be eating with the Twin Blocks and, within a week, should be more comfortable with the appliance in the mouth than they are without it.

It is necessary to check the initial activation and confirm that the patient closes consistently on the inclined planes with the mandible protruded in its new position. The overjet is measured with the mandible fully retruded and this measurement should be recorded in the patient's notes and checked at every visit to monitor progress.

FULL-TIME APPLIANCE WEAR

Temporary fixation of Twin Blocks

The most crucial time to establish good cooperation with the patient is in the first few days after fitting the Twin Blocks, when he or she is learning to adjust to the new appliance. Twin Blocks have the unique advantage compared to other functional appliances in that they can be fixed to the teeth. Such temporary fixation guarantees full-time wear, 24 hours per day, and excellent cooperation is established at the start of treatment.

The technique for fixing the appliances in place is simple. The teeth should first be fissure sealed and treated with topical fluoride as a preventive measure prior to fixation. There are two alternative methods of fixation of Twin Blocks:

* The appliances may be fixed to the teeth by spreading cement on the tooth-bearing areas of the appliance but not on the gingival areas. The appliance is then inserted and secured in place with cement adhering to the teeth. Zinc phosphate or zinc oxide cement is suitable for temporary fixation. Alternatively, a small quantity of glass ionomer cement may be used, taking care to ensure that the appliance can be freed easily from the teeth (Fig. 8.3).

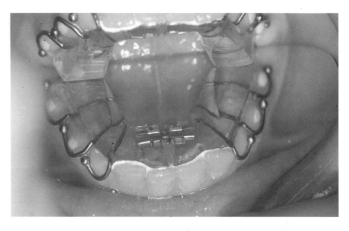

Fig. 8.3 Twin Blocks cemented in position.

- Twin Blocks may also be bonded directly to the teeth by applying composite around the clasps. This is a useful approach in mixed dentition when ball clasps may be bonded directly to deciduous molars to improve fixation.

After 10–14 days, when the patient has adapted to the Twin Block and is wearing it comfortably, the appliance can be removed by freeing the clasps with a sickle scaler. Sharp edges of composite can be smoothed over, leaving some composite attached to the teeth. The altered contour of the deciduous teeth will improve the retention of the appliance.

If cooperation is doubtful at any stage of treatment, the operator should not hesitate to fix the appliance in for 10 days to regain control and restore full-time wear. After 10 days full-time wear the patient is more comfortable with the appliance in the mouth than without it.

MANAGEMENT OF DEEP OVERBITE

Overbite reduction is achieved by trimming the occlusal blocks on the upper appliance, so as to encourage eruption of the lower molars. A progressive sequence of trimming aims to encourage selective eruption of posterior teeth to increase the vertical dimension. The objective is to increase lower facial height and improve facial balance by controlling the vertical

dimension (Fig. 8.4). Provided the correct sequence of trimming is carried out to control eruption, closure of a posterior open bite is accelerated in Twin Block treatment compared with a one-piece functional appliance, which is removed for eating, and allows the tongue to spread between the teeth and prevent eruption of the posterior teeth. Posterior support is established as the molars erupt into occlusion before relieving the appliance over the premolars until they also are free to erupt into occlusion.

The management of deep overbite begins even before the appliance is fitted – by placing elastic separators in the molar region. When the appliance is fitted, the separators are removed and the appliance is adjusted to encourage the molars to erupt.

In the treatment of deep overbite, it is important to encourage vertical development of the lower molars from the start of treatment, by trimming the upper bite block occlusodistally to allow the lower molars to erupt.

The upper bite block is progressively trimmed at each visit over several months, leaving only a small vertical clearance of 1 or 2 mm over the lower molars to allow them to erupt into occlusion. The clearance between the upper appliance and the lower molars is checked by inserting a probe (or explorer) between the posterior teeth to establish that the lower molars are free to erupt. At each subsequent visit for appliance adjustment the occlusion is cleared by sequentially trimming the upper block occlusodistally to allow further eruption of the lower molars, again checking that the clearance is correct.

This sequence of adjustment does not allow the tongue to spread laterally between the teeth to prevent eruption of lower molars, and results in a more rapid development of the vertical dimension. The molars will erupt into occlusion normally within 6–9 months.

It is important that the mandible continues to be supported in a protruded position throughout the sequence of trimming the blocks. The leading edge of the inclined plane on the upper bite block remains intact, leaving a triangular wedge in contact with the lower bite block.

When the molars have erupted into occlusion, a lateral open bite is present in the premolar region because the lower bite block is still intact. The final adjustment at the end of the Twin Block stage aims to reduce the lateral open bite by trimming the upper occlusal surface of the lower bite block over the premolars by 2 mm. To maintain adequate inclined planes to support the corrected arch relationships, the lower bite block is shaped into a triangular wedge distally in contact with the upper block.

Relieved of occlusal contact, the lower premolars erupt, carrying the lower appliance up into occlusion. The occlusal height of the upper premolars is maintained by interdental clasps that effectively prevent their eruption. The lateral open bite in the premolar region now reduces and the occlusal plane begins to level.

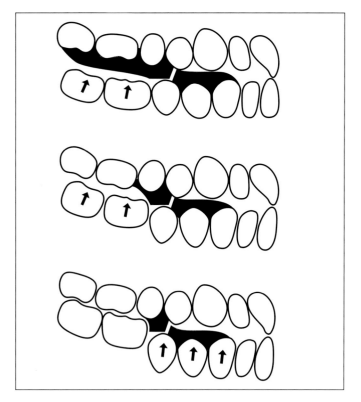

Fig. 8.4 Sequence of trimming blocks to reduce overbite.

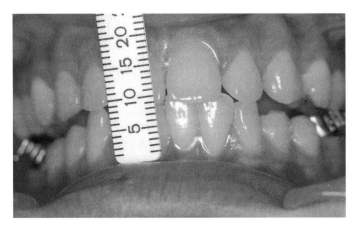

Fig. 8.5 Measuring the intergingival height.

ESTABLISHING VERTICAL DIMENSION

The Intergingival Height

A simple guideline is used to establish the correct vertical dimension during the Twin Block phase of treatment. The intergingival height is measured from the gingival margin of the upper incisor to the gingival margin of the lower incisor when the teeth are in occlusion (Fig. 8.5).

This measurement has proved to be beneficial for temporomandibular joint practitioners who use the intergingival height to establish the vertical dimension in a restorative approach to rebuild the occlusion in treatment of patients with temporomandibular joint dysfunction.

The 'comfort zone' for intergingival height for adult patients is generally found to be 17–19 mm. This is equivalent to the combined heights of the upper and lower incisors minus an overbite within the range of normal. Patients whose intergingival height varies significantly from the 'comfort zone' are at greater risk of developing temporomandibular joint dysfunction. This applies both to patients with a deep overbite, whose intergingival height is significantly reduced, and to patients with an anterior open bite who have an increased intergingival height.

The intergingival height is a useful guideline to check progress and to establish the correct vertical dimension during treatment. Measurement of intergingival height is made by using a millimetre ruler or dividers with a vernier scale to measure the distance between the upper and lower gingival margins. To keep track of progress in opening or closing the bite, this measurement should be noted on the record card at every visit.

In Twin Block treatment the correct intergingival height is achieved with great consistency. Deep overbite may be overcorrected to an intergingival height of 20 mm to allow for a slight 'settling in' with a resultant increase in overbite after treatment. Overcorrection of deep overbite is advisable as a precaution against any tendency to relapse.

The intergingival height varies according to the patient's age and stage of development, and the height of the incisor crowns. It is smaller in a young patient whose incisors have recently erupted, and larger in an older patient with gingival recession. In the younger patient a range of 15–17 mm is normal and allowance should be made for the diminutive height of the clinical crowns.

SOFT TISSUE RESPONSE

Rapid changes occur in the craniofacial musculature in response to the altered muscle function that results from treatment of malocclusion by a full-time functional appliance. As a result of altered muscle balance, significant changes in facial appearance are seen within 2 or 3 weeks of starting treatment with Twin Blocks. The rapid improvement in muscle balance is very consistent and is observed on photographs as a more relaxed posture within minutes, hours or days of starting treatment.

The Twin Block appliance positions the mandible downwards and forwards, increasing the intermaxillary space. As a result it is difficult to form an anterior oral seal by contact between the tongue and the lower lip, and patients adopt a natural lip seal without instruction. As the appliance is worn full time, even during eating, rapid soft-tissue adaptation occurs to assist the primary functions of mastication and swallowing that necessitate an effective anterior oral seal. The patient adopts a lip seal when the overjet is eliminated in the most natural way possible, by eating and drinking with the appliance in the mouth. This encourages a good lip seal as a functional necessity to prevent food and liquid escaping from the mouth. A good lip seal is always achieved by normal function with Twin Blocks, without the need for lip exercises.

CASE REPORT: L.J. AGED 10 YEARS 9 MONTHS

This is an example of treatment of an uncrowded Class II division 1 malocclusion with good archform, deep overbite, a full unit distal occlusion and an 11 mm overjet. The Class II skeletal discrepancy is measured by a convexity of 7 mm, due to a combination of maxillary protrusion and mandibular retrusion. The maxilla is narrow, typical of a distal occlusion, and the patient shows only four upper incisors when she smiles. The upper intercanine distance is reduced due to lack of support from the lower labial segment. This is a major aetiological factor causing the mandible to be locked in distal occlusion. Maxillary expansion is required together with functional mandibular advancement in order to unlock the malocclusion.

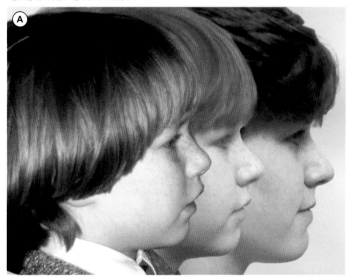

Fig. 8.6 Treatment:
A Profiles at ages 10 years 9 months (before treatment), 11 years 3 months (after treatment) and 16 years 11 months.
B–D Occlusion before treatment: a narrow upper arch with a 10 mm overjet and lower incisors biting into the palate.
E After 6 months the overjet is corrected and a posterior open bite is present in the early stages of treatment. The upper block is trimmed to encourage lower molar eruption.
F After the lower molars have erupted into occlusion, the lower occlusal block is trimmed to allow the lateral open bite in the premolar region to reduce. The lower occlusal plane now begins to level, while the upper premolar height is maintained by the upper appliance. After 9 months of treatment the patient is ready to proceed to the support stage.
G An anterior inclined plane is fitted to support the corrected incisor relationship. The lower appliance is left out and the lower premolars and canines are free to erupt into occlusion.

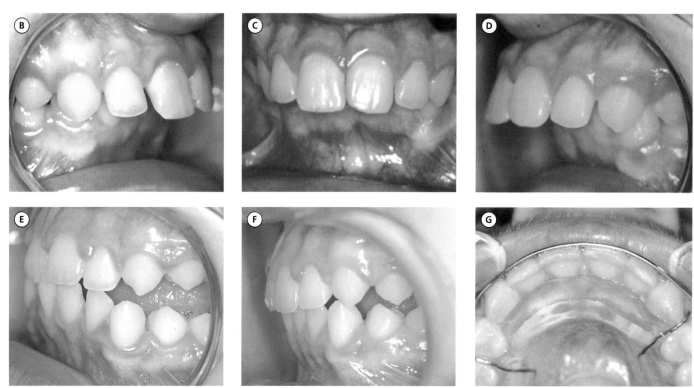

The facial type is mild brachyfacial, and there is normally a good prognosis for correction of this type of malocclusion provided the unfavourable occlusal factors are eliminated to allow the mandible to develop forward into a normal relationship with the maxilla. Clinical examination confirms that the profile improves when the patient postures the mandible downwards and forwards to a normal overjet with the lips closed (Fig. 8.6).

Bite registration

A construction bite with a blue Exactobite registers an edge-to-edge occlusion with 2 mm interincisal clearance. This results in a vertical clearance in the first premolar region of 6 mm.

Adjustment:

• When the appliance is fitted at the insertion appointment, the patient is instructed to turn the midline screw one

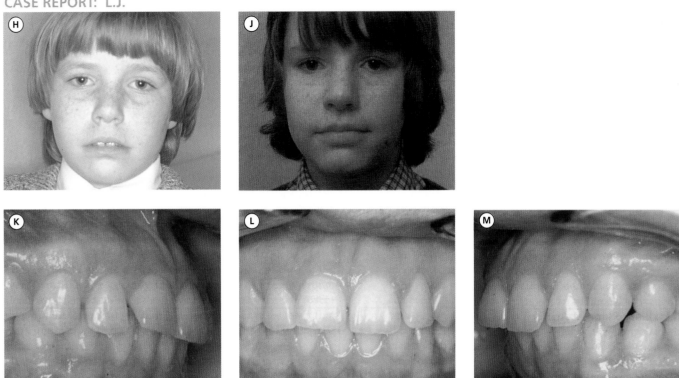

Fig. 8.6 Treatment (cont.):
H Appearance before treatment at age 10 years 9 months.
J Appearance after treatment.
K–M The occlusion 5 years out of retention.

quarter turn per week, expanding the upper arch to assist in unlocking the mandible from distal occlusion.

- Correction of deep overbite is initiated at the start of treatment by trimming the upper bite block clear of the lower molars, thereby stimulating molar eruption. It is important to leave only 1 or 2 mm occlusal clearance to encourage eruption, so that the tongue cannot spread between the teeth and delay vertical development. The leading edge of the inclined plane of the upper bite block remains intact to provide contact with the lower bite block. This contact is the key mechanism which provides the functional stimulus to growth by occlusion with the inclined plane on the lower appliance.
- To avoid gingival irritation in the initial stages of adaptation to the appliance, the fitting surface of the lower appliance is trimmed slightly in the area of the sulcus lingual to the lower incisors and canines.

After 3 months of treatment the overjet is reduced from 10 mm to 3 mm. The posterior teeth are still out of occlusion at this stage. Over the next 3 months the occlusal surface of the upper bite block is trimmed in a sequential fashion at each visit, still maintaining the leading edge of the inclined

plane intact. This will eventually result in the removal of all the acrylic covering the upper molars. This allows the lower molars freedom to erupt fully into occlusion. The biting surface of the lower Twin Block is then trimmed slightly in the premolar region to allow eruption of the premolars carrying the lower appliance vertically with them as they erupt. This will then reduce the lateral open bite in the premolar region.

The open bite quickly resolves and after 6 weeks an upper support appliance is fitted with an anterior inclined plane and the lower Twin Block is left out. The occlusion settles without further adjustment. Full-time appliance wear continues for 4 months, followed by 4 months of night-time wear to retain the corrected occlusion.

Duration of treatment:

- Active phase: 7 months with Twin Blocks.
- Support phase: 4 months full time with an anterior inclined plane.
- Retention: 4 months anterior inclined plane at night only.
- Total treatment time: 15 months, including retention.
- Final records: 5 years out of retention.

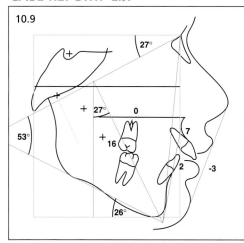

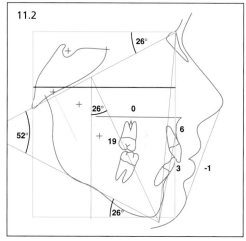

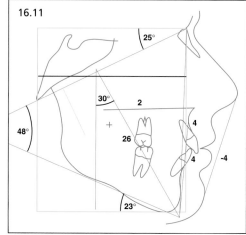

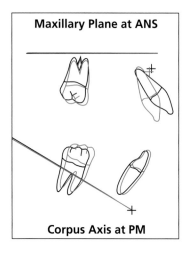

Maxillary Plane at ANS

Corpus Axis at PM

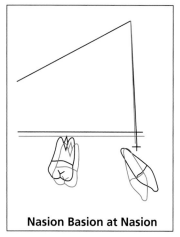

Nasion Basion at Nasion

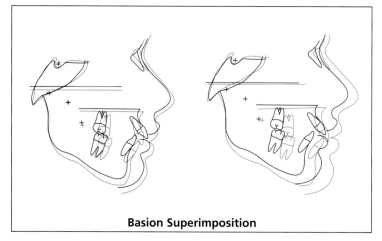

Basion Superimposition

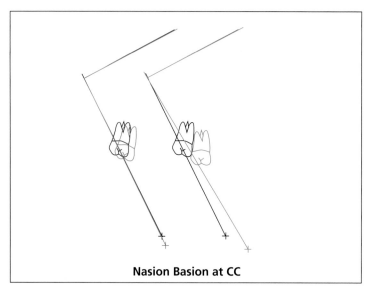

Nasion Basion at CC

L.J.	Age	10.9	11.2	16.11
Cranial Base Angle		27	26	25
Facial Axis Angle		27	26	30
F/M Plane Angle		26	26	23
Craniomandibular Angle		53	52	48
Maxillary Plane		0	0	2
Convexity		7	6	4
U/Incisor to Vertical		41	19	29
L/Incisor to Vertical		37	36	36
Interincisal Angle		102	125	115
6 to Pterygoid Vertical		16	19	26
L/Incisor to A/Po		2	3	4
L/Lip to Aesthetic Plane		−3	−1	−4

REACTIVATION OF TWIN BLOCKS

As indicated previously, an overjet of up to 10 mm in a patient who is growing well and has free protrusive movement may be corrected without reactivation of the Twin Blocks during treatment. If growth is less favourable, or in treatment of larger overjets, or when the protrusive path of the mandible is restricted, it is necessary to reactivate the inclined planes more gradually in progressive increments during treatment.

Reactivation is a simple procedure that is achieved by extending the anterior incline of the upper Twin Block mesially to increase the forward posture. Cold cure acrylic may be added at the chairside, inserting the appliance to record a new protrusive bite before the acrylic is fully set. Even in cases with an excessive overjet, a single reactivation of Twin Blocks is normally sufficient to correct most malocclusions (Fig. 8.7).

It is important that no acrylic is added to the distal incline of the lower Twin Block, especially in the treatment of deep overbite. Extending occlusal acrylic of the lower block distally would prevent eruption of the lower first molar. It is necessary to leave the lower first molars free to erupt so that the overbite is reduced by increasing the vertical dimension.

If the patient's rate of growth is slow or the direction of growth is vertical rather than horizontal, it is advisable to advance the mandible more gradually over a longer period of time to allow compensatory mandibular growth to occur. This can be taken into account by reactivating Twin Blocks progressively to extend the inclined plane of the upper bite block mesially (Petrovic & Stutzmann, 1977).

After extending the upper block forwards, the contact of the upper block on the lower molar should be checked to make any necessary adjustment to clear the occlusion with the lower molar for correction of deep overbite.

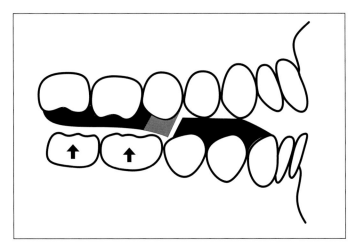

Fig. 8.7 Addition of acrylic to the anterior incline of the upper inclined plane to reactivate Twin Blocks. It is incorrect to reactivate by addition to the lower Twin Block.

PROGRESSIVE ACTIVATION OF TWIN BLOCKS

Progressive activation of the inclined planes is indicated as follows:

- If the overjet is greater than 10 mm it is advisable to step the mandible forwards, usually in two stages. The first activation is in the range of 7–10 mm. The second activation brings the incisors to an edge-to-edge occlusion.
- In any case where full correction of arch relationships is not achieved after the initial activation, an additional activation is necessary.
- If the direction of growth is vertical rather than horizontal, the mandible may be advanced more gradually to allow adequate time for compensatory mandibular growth to occur.
- Phased activation is recommended in adult treatment, where the muscles and ligaments are less responsive to a sudden large displacement of the mandible (see Chapter 20).
- In the treatment of temporomandibular joint dysfunction, care must be exercised so as not to introduce activation that is beyond the level of tolerance of injured tissue. It is best to be conservative and advance the mandible slowly to a position that is comfortable and will allow the patient to rest and function without discomfort (see Chapter 21).

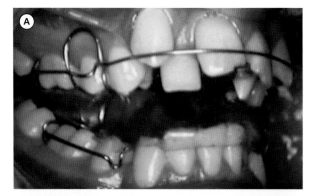
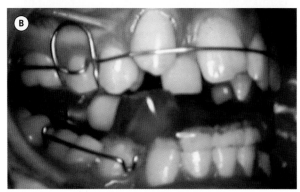

Fig. 8.8 A, B Screw advancement mechanism described in Chapter 7.

FUNCTIONAL ORTHOPAEDIC THERAPY

CASE REPORT: P.K. AGED 11 YEARS 4 MONTHS

This young girl presents a disfiguring Class II division 1 malocclusion with an overjet of 17 mm and an excessive overbite. A combination of maxillary protrusion and mandibular retrusion has resulted in a severe distal occlusion and an equally severe transverse discrepancy with buccal occlusion of the upper premolars and a traumatic occlusion of the lower incisors in the palate. The malocclusion is further complicated by the congenital absence of the second lower premolar on the left side, resulting in displacement of the lower centre line to the left. The dramatic facial and dental changes in this case illustrate the benefits of a functional orthopaedic approach to treatment compared to a conventional orthodontic approach.

Before treatment this patient has the typical listless appearance of many severe Class II division 1 malocclusions. This has been described as 'adenoidal facies' and is evident in the dull appearance of the eyes and poor skin tone. A large overjet with a distal occlusion is frequently associated with a backward tongue position, and a restricted airway. These patients cannot breathe properly and, as a result, are subject to allergies, and upper respiratory problems due to inefficient respiratory function.

After only 3 months of treatment the patient undergoes a dramatic change in facial appearance, which exceeds the parameters of orthodontic treatment in this time scale. The patient appears more alert and there is a marked improvement in the eyes and the complexion. This is a fundamental physiological change, extending beyond the limited objective of correcting a malocclusion. The upper pharyngeal space increased from 5 mm before treatment to 20 mm after treatment. Increasing the airway achieves the crucially important benefit of improving respiratory function and may influence basal metabolism as a secondary effect. Increase in the pharyngeal airway is a consistent feature of mandibular advancement with a full-time functional appliance. This is the most significant functional benefit of advancing the mandible, as opposed to retracting the maxilla in the treatment of Class II malocclusion.

Conventional fixed appliances with brackets cannot produce equivalent physiological changes in the treatment of patients with severe malocclusions. A functional approach achieves a rapid improvement in the facial appearance and can be followed by a simplified orthodontic phase of treatment to detail the occlusion (Fig. 8.9).

Treatment plan:

To retract the maxilla and advance the mandible. The dental asymmetry would be difficult to eliminate in view of the absence of ⌐5. An orthodontic phase of treatment was planned to complete the treatment.

Appliances:

- Standard Twin Blocks.
- Support phase with an anterior inclined plane.
- Fixed appliances to complete the treatment.

Adjustment:

The registration bite reduced the overjet from 17 mm to 8 mm on the initial activation. This correction was achieved in 8 weeks, when the inclined planes were reactivated to an edge-to-edge incisor occlusion by adding cold cure acrylic to the mesial of the upper inclined plane. The normal adjustments were made to reduce the overbite by trimming the occlusal surface of the upper bite blocks to allow eruption of the lower molars.

Twin Blocks were effective in quickly reducing the overjet from 17 mm to 2 mm in 6 months. After 7 months of treatment the lower appliance was left out and an anterior inclined plane was fitted to retain the position as the remaining posterior open bite resolved and the buccal teeth settled into occlusion. The space was closed with a simple fixed appliance, and the slight displacement of the centre line was accepted. This was followed by an orthodontic phase to complete treatment.

Duration of treatment:

- Active phase: Twin Blocks for 7 months.
- Support phase: 6 months full-time wear.
- Orthodontic phase: 12 months.

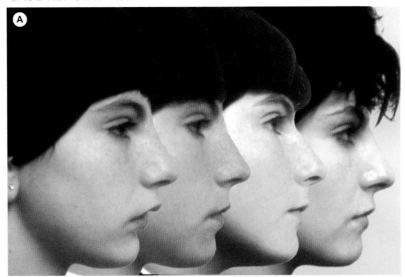

Fig. 8.9 Treatment:
A Profiles at ages 11 years 4 months (before treatment), 11 years 7 months (3 months after treatment), 12 years 3 months and 18 years 4 months.
B–D Occlusion before treatment: overjet = 17 mm.
E–G Occlusal change after 11 months.
H Facial appearance before treatment at age 11 years 4 months.
J Facial change after 3 months of treatment, showing marked physiological improvement.
K Facial change after 11 months of treatment.

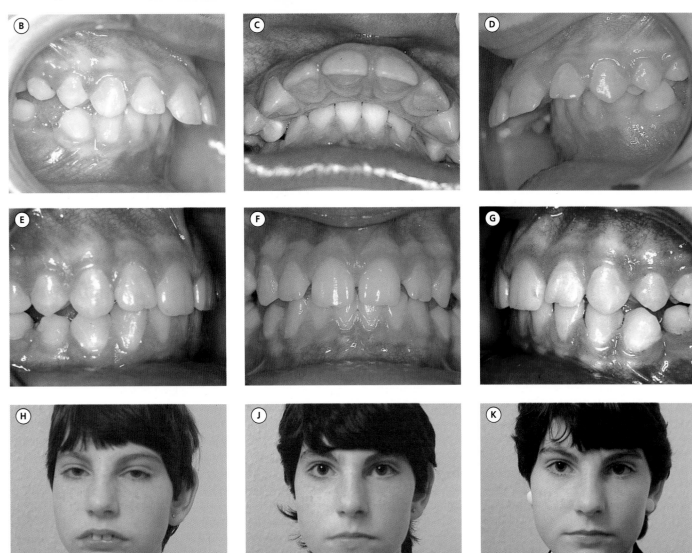

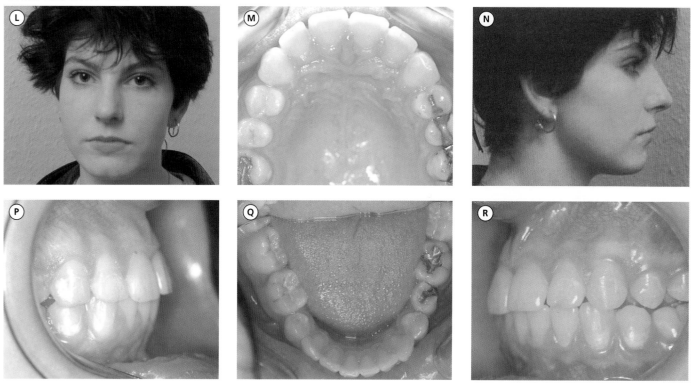

Fig. 8.9 Treatment (cont.):
L, N Facial appearance at 18 years 4 months.
M Upper occlusal view after treatment.
P, R Occlusion at age 18 years 7 months.
Q Lower occlusal view after treatment, note congenital absence of ⌈5.

SUMMARY: ADJUSTMENT AND CLINICAL MANAGEMENT

Stage 1: active phase

Appliance fitting

It is first necessary to check that the patient bites comfortably in a protrusive bite with the inclined planes occluding correctly. To avoid irritation as the appliance is driven home by the occlusion during the first few days of wear, it is important to relieve the lower appliance slightly over the gingivae lingual to the lower incisors. The clasps are adjusted to hold the appliance securely in position without impinging on the gingival margin. If a labial bow is present, it should be out of contact with the upper incisors.

Initial adjustment – after 10 days

The patient should now be wearing the appliances comfortably and eating with them in position. The initial discomfort of a new appliance should have resolved and the patient should be biting consistently in the protrusive bite.

Patient motivation is reinforced by offering encouragement for their success on becoming accustomed to the appliance so quickly, and reassurance on any difficulties.

The patient should now be turning the upper midline screw one quarter turn per week. In the treatment of deep overbite the upper bite block should be trimmed clear of the lower molars leaving a clearance of 1–2 mm to allow these to erupt.

At this stage, it is important to detect if the patient is failing to posture forwards consistently to occlude correctly on the inclined planes. This would indicate that the appliance has been activated beyond the level of tolerance of the patient's musculature. It would then be appropriate to reduce the activation by trimming the inclined planes, to reduce the forward mandibular displacement until the patient closes comfortably on the appliances. The angulation of the inclined planes may be reduced to 45° if the patient is failing to posture consistently forwards to occlude the blocks correctly.

This may be an early sign that progress will be slower than normal, due to weakness in the patient's musculature reducing the functional response. This response is more likely in the patient who has a vertical growth pattern. Mandibular advancement will then be more gradual, usually requiring incremental activation of the occlusal inclined planes.

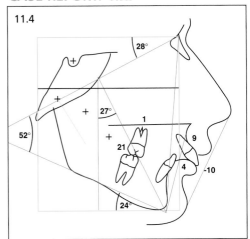

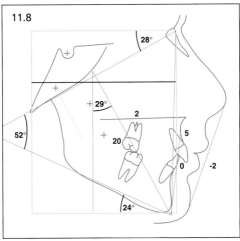

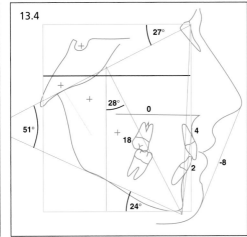

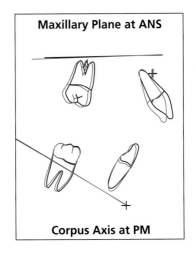

Maxillary Plane at ANS

Corpus Axis at PM

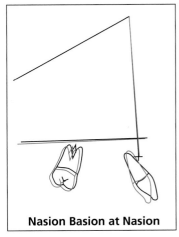

Nasion Basion at Nasion

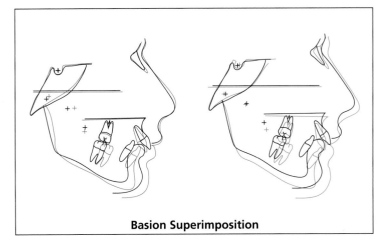

Basion Superimposition

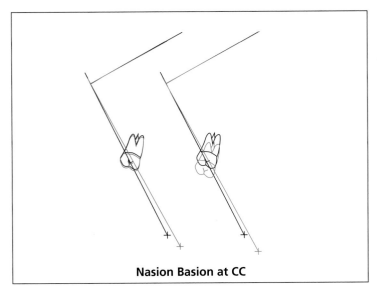

Nasion Basion at CC

P.K.	Age	11.4	11.8	13.4
Cranial Base Angle		28	28	27
Facial Axis Angle		27	29	28
F/M Plane Angle		24	24	24
Craniomandibular Angle		52	52	51
Maxillary Plane		1	2	0
Convexity		9	5	4
U/Incisor to Vertical		35	27	19
L/Incisor to Vertical		33	24	25
Interincisal Angle		112	129	136
6 to Pterygoid Vertical		21	20	18
L/Incisor to A/Po		−4	0	2
L/Lip to Aesthetic Plane		−10	−2	−8

Adjustment visit – after 4 weeks

At the first monthly visit positive progress should already be evident with respect to better facial balance. Photographs demonstrate this very clearly, and may be repeated at this stage to record progress.

Progress can be confirmed also by noting the amount of reduction in overjet, as measured intraorally with the mandible fully retracted. To monitor progress, the overjet should be measured and noted on the record card at each visit. This allows any lapse in progress or cooperation to be detected readily. There should be a steady and consistent reduction of overjet and correction of distal occlusion. If cooperation is suspect it is advisable to fix the appliance in place in the mouth to exert immediate control and restore full-time appliance wear.

Apart from monitoring progress, only minor adjustment is required at this stage. Check that the screw is operating correctly, and adjust the clasps if necessary to improve retention. If the appliance includes a labial bow, adjust it so as to be out of contact with the upper incisors.

In the treatment of deep overbite ensure that the lower molars are not in contact with the upper block. The upper block is trimmed occluso-distally to clear the occlusion, using a probe (explorer) to confirm that the lower molars do not contact the upper block.

Routine adjustment – time interval 6 weeks

A similar pattern of adjustment continues with steady correction of distal occlusion and reduction of overjet. The upper arch width is checked at each visit, until the expansion is sufficient to accommodate the lower arch in its corrected position and no further turns of the screw are required.

Trimming of the upper block continues until all the occlusal cover is removed from the upper molars to allow the lower molars to erupt completely into occlusion.

The overjet, overbite and distal occlusion should be fully corrected by the end of the Twin Block phase. A slight open bite in the buccal segments should be limited to the premolar region. It is now appropriate to proceed to the support phase.

Stage 2: support phase

Antero-posterior and vertical control remain equally important in the support phase to maintain the correction achieved in the active phase.

The purpose of the support phase is to maintain the corrected incisor relationship until the buccal segment occlusion is fully established. To achieve this objective, an upper removable appliance is fitted with an anterior inclined plane to engage the lower incisors and canines.

The lower appliance is left out at this stage and removal of the posterior bite blocks allows the posterior teeth to erupt into occlusion. The anterior inclined plane extends distally to engage all six lower anterior teeth and the patient must not be able to occlude lingual to the inclined plane. It must be adequate to retain the incisor relationship effectively, but at the same time should be neat and unobtrusive so as not to interfere with speech.

Many anterior inclined planes are mistakenly made too large and bulky which causes discomfort for the patient, who may then be discouraged from wearing such an appliance. There is no necessity for the anterior inclined plane to extend much beyond the level of the incisal tips of the upper incisors, provided it also extends far enough distally to engage the canines.

The patient must understand the importance of wearing the support appliance full time to prevent relapse at this critical stage of treatment. An appliance that is comfortable and carefully designed is more readily accepted by the patient.

Vertical control is essential during the support phase after reduction of overbite. To maintain the corrected vertical dimension, a flat occlusal stop of acrylic extends forwards from the inclined plane to engage the lower incisors. The occlusal stop is an important addition to maintain the corrected intergingival height as the posterior teeth erupt into occlusion. The upper and lower buccal teeth should normally settle into occlusion within 2–6 months, depending on the depth of the overbite.

Retention

Treatment is followed by a normal period of retention. As the buccal segments settle in fully, full-time wear of the support appliance allows time for internal bony remodelling to support the corrected occlusion. A good buccal segment occlusion is the cornerstone of stability after correction of arch-to-arch relationships. Appliance wear is reduced to night-time only when the occlusion is fully established.

If treatment is carried out in the mixed dentition, retention may continue with an anterior inclined plane to support the occlusion during the transition to the permanent dentition. In early treatment of severe skeletal discrepancies a night-time functional appliance of the monobloc type may be used as a retainer. This gives additional functional support and may be activated to enhance the orthopaedic response to treatment during the transitional dentition. An excellent alternative is the occluso-guide, which is a preformed appliance resembling a mini-positioner. It is available in a range of sizes and is designed to retain the corrected incisor relationship with a functional component to retain the correction to a Class I occlusion. The management of this appliance is described in Chapter 9 on mixed dentition treatment.

Advantages of Twin Blocks

The Twin Block is the most comfortable, the most aesthetic and the most efficient of all the functional appliances. Twin Blocks have many advantages compared to other functional appliances:

- **Comfort.** Patients wear Twin Blocks 24 hours per day and can eat comfortably with the appliances in place.
- **Aesthetics.** Twin Blocks can be designed with no visible anterior wires without losing efficiency in correction of arch relationships.
- **Function.** The occlusal inclined plane is the most natural of all the functional mechanisms. There is less interference with normal function because the mandible can move freely in anterior and lateral excursion without being restricted by a bulky one-piece appliance.
- **Patient compliance.** Twin Blocks may be fixed to the teeth temporarily or permanently to guarantee patient compliance. Removable Twin Blocks can be fixed in the mouth for the first week or 10 days of treatment to ensure that the patient adapts fully to wearing them 24 hours per day.
- **Facial appearance.** From the moment Twin Blocks are fitted the appearance is noticeably improved. The absence of lip, cheek or tongue pads, as used in some other appliances, places no restriction on normal function, and does not distort the patient's facial appearance during treatment. Improvements in facial balance are seen progressively in the first 3 months of treatment.
- **Speech.** Patients can learn to speak normally with Twin Blocks. In comparison with other functional appliances, Twin Blocks do not distort speech by restricting movement of the tongue, lips or mandible.
- **Clinical management.** Adjustment and activation is simple. The appliances are robust and not prone to breakage. Chairside time is reduced in achieving major orthopaedic correction.
- **Arch development.** Twin Blocks allow independent control of upper and lower arch width. Appliance design is easily modified for transverse and sagittal arch development.

- **Mandibular repositioning.** Full-time appliance wear consistently achieves rapid mandibular repositioning that remains stable out of retention.
- **Vertical control.** Twin Blocks achieve excellent control of the vertical dimension in treatment of deep overbite and anterior open bite. Vertical control is significantly improved by full-time wear.
- **Facial asymmetry.** Asymmetrical activation corrects facial and dental asymmetry in the growing child.
- **Safety.** Twin Blocks can be worn during sports activies with the exception of swimming and violent contact sports, when they may be removed for safety.
- **Efficiency.** Twin Blocks achieve more rapid correction of malocclusion compared to one-piece functional appliances because they are worn full time. This benefits patients in all age groups.
- **Age of treatment.** Arch relationships can be corrected from early childhood to adulthood. However, treatment is slower in adults and the response is less predictable.
- **Integration with fixed appliances.** Integration with conventional fixed appliances is simpler than with any other functional appliance. In combined techniques, Twin Blocks can be used to maximise the skeletal correction while fixed appliances are used to detail the occlusion. Because Twin Blocks do not need to have anterior wires, brackets can be placed on the anterior teeth to correct tooth alignment simultaneously with correction of arch relationships during the orthopaedic phase. During the support phase an easy transition can be made to fixed appliances.
- **Treatment of temporomandibular joint dysfunction.** The Twin Block may at times also be used as an effective splint in the treatment of patients who present temporomandibular joint dysfunction due to displacement of the condyle distal to the articular disc. Full-time wear allows the disc to be recaptured, when disc reduction is possible in early stage temporomandibular joint problems, and at the same time sagittal, vertical and transverse arch development proceeds to eliminate unfavourable occlusal contacts (see Chapter 21).

REFERENCE

Petrovic, A. & Stutzmann, J. (1977). Further investigations into the functioning of the 'comparator' of the servosystem (respective positions of the upper and lower dental arches) in the control of the condylar cartilage growth rate and of the lengthening of the jaw. In *The Biology of Occlusal Development*, ed. J.A. McNamara Jr, Monograph No. 6, Craniofacial Growth series. Center for Human Growth & Development, University of Michigan, pp. 225–91.

CHAPTER 9

Treatment in Mixed Dentition

Treatment of skeletal discrepancies should not be delayed until the permanent dentition has been established. Interceptive treatment is frequently indicated in the mixed dentition to restore normal function and correct arch relationships by means of functional appliance therapy.

Not all orthodontists favour early treatment, and indeed some are actively opposed to the concept. As a result treatment may be delayed until the permanent canines and premolars have erupted. The straightwire pre-adjusted appliance is the most popular fixed appliance system of the present day. It is designed for treatment in the permanent dentition and lends itself to a highly organised practice environment. While this is undoubtedly an excellent finishing appliance for detailing the occlusion, it can not deal effectively with severe skeletal problems. Straightwire technique must therefore be used in combination with surgery, or functional correction. Many such problems can be dealt with more efficiently by early treatment and it is important to offer an effective functional orthopaedic technique as a viable alternative to surgery.

Prominent upper incisors are vulnerable to accidental trauma and breakage, and early treatment is advisable to avoid fracture or damage by placing the incisors within the protection of the lips. Early treatment of crowded dentitions can combine arch development with correction of arch relationships.

The principles of treatment are unchanged in the mixed dentition, although the response to treatment may prove to be slower depending on the patient's rate of growth. Bite registration follows the same procedures as described for treatment in the permanent dentition.

APPLIANCE DESIGN

Appliance design may be modified to meet the requirements of the mixed dentition, when retention may be limited by deciduous teeth that are unfavourably shaped with respect to adequately accepting retention clasps of removable appliances.

Twin Block appliance design for Class II division 1 malocclusion in the mixed dentition is similar to appliance design for the permanent dentition. Delta clasps may be fitted on lower first or second deciduous molars if they are suitably shaped for retention.

Alternatively, C-clasps may be used for retention on deciduous molars. The C-clasp is well suited to this stage of development of the dentition and there are several ways to improve retention even if the teeth are unfavourably shaped (Fig. 9.1).

The simplest method of improving retention on deciduous teeth is to bond composite on to the buccal surfaces of these teeth to create an additional undercut. Both cooperation and retention can be improved by bonding C-clasps directly to deciduous molars for the first week or 10 days before freeing the clasps and rounding the edges of the composite that remains attached to the teeth to improve retention.

It is also possible to grind retention grooves into the buccal surfaces of deciduous teeth to improve undercuts; for example, gingival to the line of a C-clasp. Alternatively, a round bur may be used to grind a concavity to accommodate a ball clasp. Sealant can then be applied to protect the tooth and a ready-made undercut has been created.

Synthetic crown contours (Truax) are preformed plastic pads, which may be bonded to the buccal surfaces of deciduous cuspids and molars to reshape these teeth with additional undercuts, in order to improve the retention of clasps (Fig. 9.2).

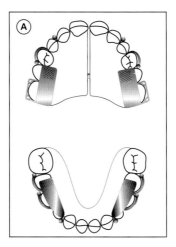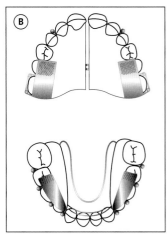

Fig. 9.1 A, B Typical appliance design for mixed dentition.

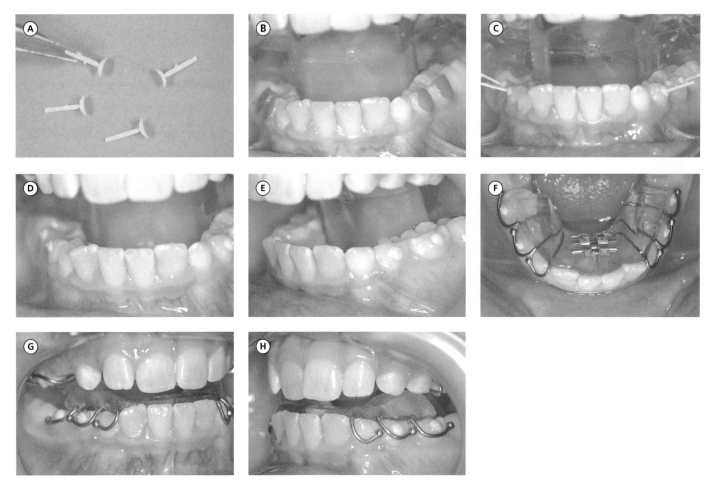

Fig. 9.2 The appliance with crown contours to improve fixation in mixed dentition:
A Crown contours.
B Etching deciduous molars with paper pads soaked in etching fluid.

C The crown contours bonded to the teeth.
D, E After cutting off the sprues, the impression is taken to make the appliance.
F–H The C-clasps are shaped to gain retention from the crown contours.

CASE REPORT: F.D. AGED 9 YEARS 7 MONTHS

This is a typical example of a young boy in mixed dentition who has a severe Class II dental relationship with the lower lip trapped under a large overjet of 12 mm. Early treatment is indicated for many reasons, not least of which is to protect the upper incisors from injury by placing them inside the protective envelope of the lips. There is a severe Class II skeletal base with 9 mm convexity, mainly due to maxillary protrusion with proclination of upper incisors and lower incisors which are slightly retroclined. On clinical examination the profile improves when the mandible postures forwards with the lips closed together. The upper pharyngeal airway is restricted before treatment to 8 mm and increased to 11 mm during the Twin Block stage of treatment, as a result of mandibular advancement.

Twin Blocks: 1 year
Support phase: 6 months of full-time wear with an anterior inclined plane
Retention: continued for 2 years of night-time wear with an occluso-guide appliance until the occlusion is fully established in the permanent dentition
Final records: 5 years out of retention at age 18 years, when the occlusion has settled satisfactorily without further treatment (Fig. 9.3).

After treatment in the mixed dentition there is diminished occlusal support during the transition to the permanent dentition. A night-time functional appliance may be selected as a retention appliance to provide a positive functional stimulus to growth during the transitional stage of dental development.

CASE REPORT: F.D.

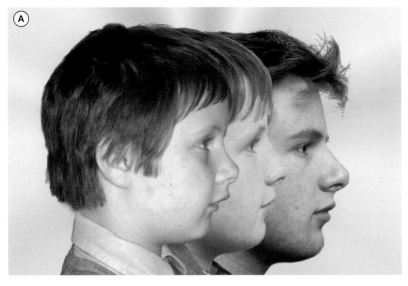

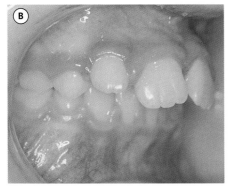

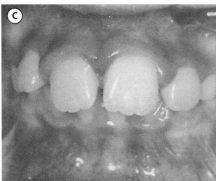

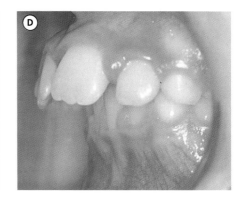

Fig. 9.3 Treatment:
A Profiles at ages 9 years 7 months (before treatment), 11 years 4 months (after retention) and 18 years 7 months.
B–D The patient has a 12 mm overjet and a four-tooth smile before treatment due to the constricted maxillary arch.

CASE REPORT: F.D.

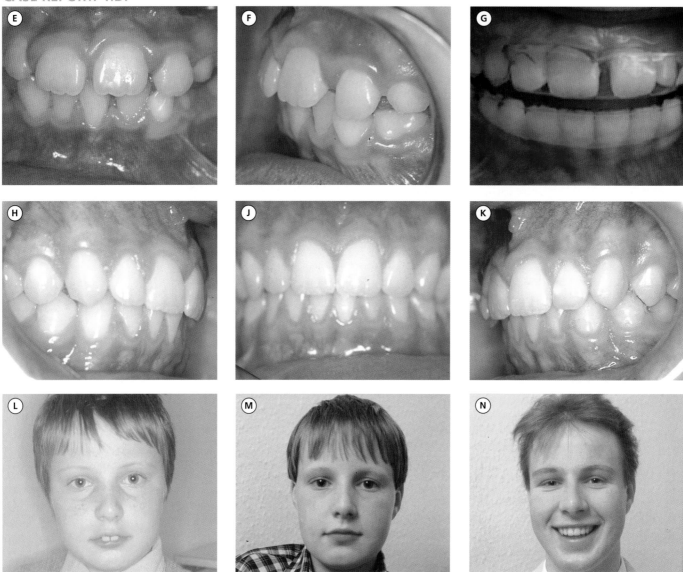

Fig. 9.3 Treatment (cont.):
E, F The overjet is corrected after 8 months and the overbite is reduced.
G Occluso-guide appliance for retention.
H–K Occlusion at age 18 years. No further treatment was required after support and retention.
L Appearance before treatment at age 9 years 7 months.
M Appearance at age 11 years 4 months after retention.
N Appearance at age 16 years 7 months.

The occluso-guide is an excellent functional retainer during the transition from mixed to permanent dentition (see also p.114). It is a simple preformed appliance, resembling a mini-positioner, which can be worn at night to retain the incisor and molar relationship, while maintaining space for eruption of premolars and canines. The occluso-guide should be worn for 1 or 2 hours during the day and the patient is instructed to actively bite into the appliance. This is effective in maintaining the vertical dimension after correction of deep overbite. The material is sufficiently flexible to allow correction of minor tooth irregularities, in addition to acting as a retainer to reinforce the sagittal and vertical correction. One version of the appliance is specifically designed to engage the upper and lower incisors in an edge-to-edge occlusion with troughs in the buccal segments to guide the eruption of premolars and canines.

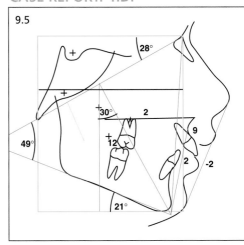

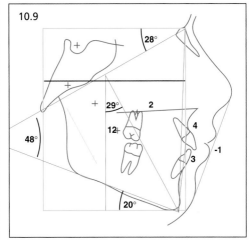

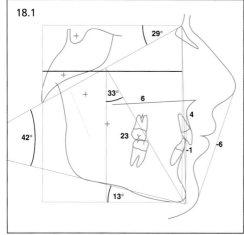

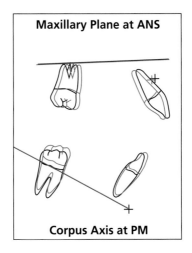

Maxillary Plane at ANS

Corpus Axis at PM

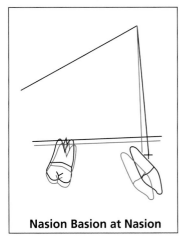

Nasion Basion at Nasion

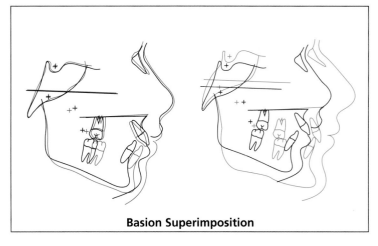

Basion Superimposition

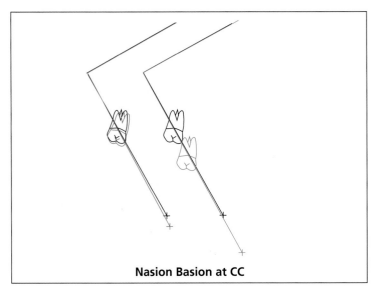

Nasion Basion at CC

F.D.	Age	9.5	10.9	18.1
Cranial Base Angle		28	28	29
Facial Axis Angle		30	29	33
F/M Plane Angle		21	20	13
Craniomandibular Angle		49	48	42
Maxillary Plane		2	2	6
Convexity		9	4	4
U/Incisor to Vertical		35	35	24
L/Incisor to Vertical		35	34	24
Interincisal Angle		110	111	132
6 to Pterygoid Vertical		12	12	23
L/Incisor to A/Po		−2	3	−1
L/Lip to Aesthetic Plane		−2	−1	−6

TRANSVERSE DEVELOPMENT

Twin blocks for arch development

CASE REPORT: A.G. AGED 9 YEARS 6 MONTHS

This boy has a mild Class II division 1 malocclusion in the mixed dentition but a convexity of 1 mm indicates a normal skeletal base relationship with a brachyfacial growth pattern. The maxilla is narrow and crowding in the lower labial segment is related to the restricted maxillary width. The lower lip is trapped in the overjet, causing proclination of the upper incisors, while the lower incisors are retroclined, at –3 mm to the A–Po line.

The straight profile dictates non-extraction therapy and expansion is indicated in both arches. The orthopaedic phase of treatment was initiated before the growth spurt during a period of slow growth, to minimise the skeletal change. No labial bow is used in order to maintain the labial position of the upper incisors. This case illustrates the use of upper and lower Schwarz Twin Blocks for expansion in both arches in mixed dentition, followed by a lower fixed appliance during support phase (Figs 9.4, 9.6).

Twin Blocks: 8 months
Support appliance: continued while premolars and canines erupted
Lower fixed appliance: 6 months
Retention: 1 year.

CASE REPORT: A.G.

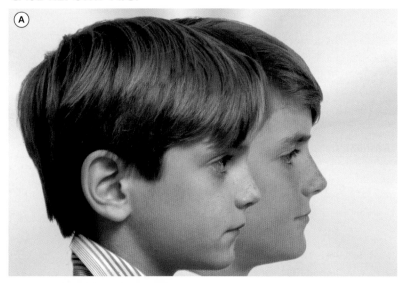

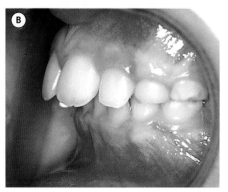

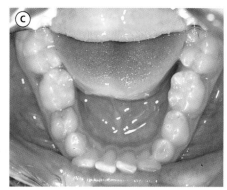

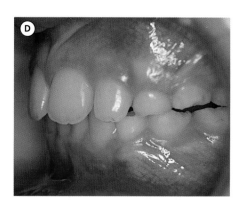

Fig. 9.4 Treatment:
A Profiles at ages 9 years 6 months (before treatment) and 13 years 6 months.
B, D Overjet correction after 4 months of treatment.
C Lower arch before treatment.

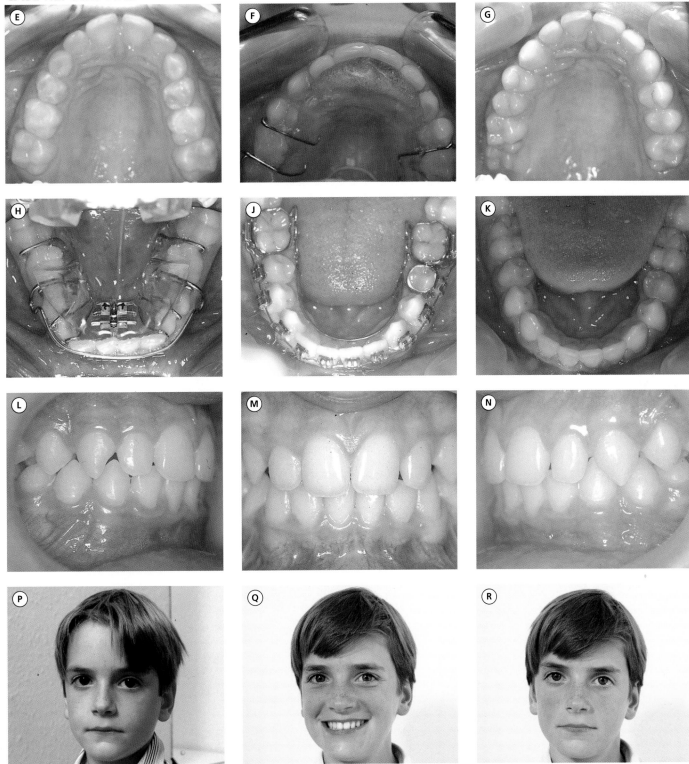

Fig. 9.4 Treatment (cont.):

E, G Expansion achieved in the upper arch.

F The anterior inclined plane with occlusal stops to control the vertical dimension.

H The lower Twin Block has a midline screw for expansion.

J, K Because of the lower arch crowding a lower fixed appliance with three-dimensional control is necessary to correct the labial segment.

L–N Occlusion at age 13 years 6 months.

P Facial appearance at age 9 years 6 months.

Q, R Appearance at age 13 years 6 months.

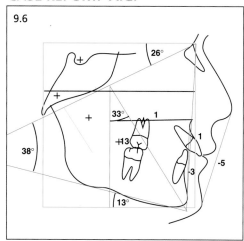

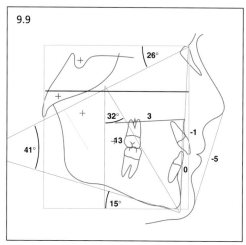

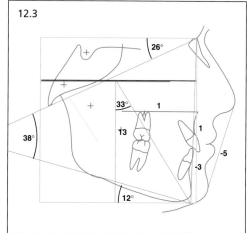

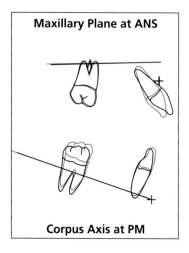

Maxillary Plane at ANS

Corpus Axis at PM

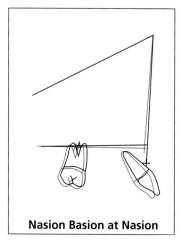

Nasion Basion at Nasion

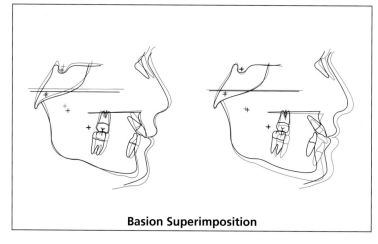

Basion Superimposition

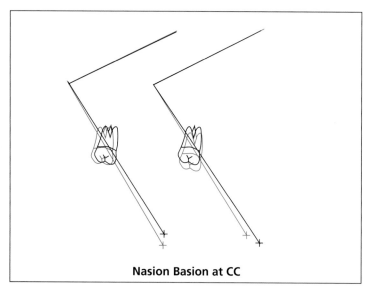

Nasion Basion at CC

A.G.	Age	9.6	9.9	12.3
Cranial Base Angle		26	26	26
Facial Axis Angle		33	32	33
F/M Plane Angle		13	15	12
Craniomandibular Angle		38	41	38
Maxillary Plane		1	3	1
Convexity		1	–1	1
U/Incisor to Vertical		42	32	31
L/Incisor to Vertical		18	22	21
Interincisal Angle		120	126	128
6 to Pterygoid Vertical		13	13	13
L/Incisor to A/Po		–3	0	–3
L/Lip to Aesthetic Plane		–5	–5	–5

OCCLUSO-GUIDE APPLIANCE

The occluso-guide is a preformed mini-positioner appliance designed to fit the upper and lower anterior teeth and to act as a functional retainer by engaging the teeth in an edge-to-edge relationship in a slightly open position with an inter-incisal distance of 3 mm. There is therefore a slight forward positioning of the mandible to maintain the corrected overjet after Twin Block treatment. This type of appliance may be used as a retainer during the transition from mixed to permanent dentition, after correction of arch relationships in mixed dentition with Twin Blocks.

The occluso-guide is manufactured in a range of sizes and the correct size is selected using a flexible ruler to measure the width of the six upper anterior teeth. A pointer is placed between the upper left cuspid and bicuspid and the ruler is bent along the incisal edge of the incisors to the interproximal area between the right cuspid and bicuspid, where the size is registered on a scale for measurement.

The occluso-guide is designed to fit the anterior teeth in well aligned arches. In common with the positioner, it can accommodate only slight irregularity in the anterior teeth; neither is it sufficiently active to correct significant distal occlusion or increased overjet. The construction is sufficiently robust to permit the appliance to be worn comfortably as a long-term retainer. It is important that the patient is motivated to wear the appliance consistently as instructed. The patient and parents should be advised that failure to wear the retainer correctly may result in set-back if the inherent growth pattern is allowed reassert itself.

The occluso-guide should be worn for one or two hours during the day and the patient is instructed to actively bite into the appliance. This is effective in maintaining the vertical dimension after correction of deep overbite. The material is sufficiently flexible to allow correction of minor tooth irregularities, in addition to acting as a retainer to reinforce the sagittal and vertical correction. One version of the appliance is specifically designed to engage the upper and lower incisors in an edge-to-edge occlusion with troughs in the buccal segments to guide the eruption of premolars and canines.

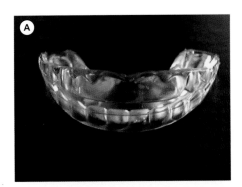
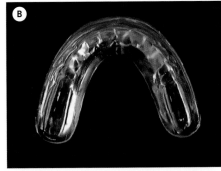
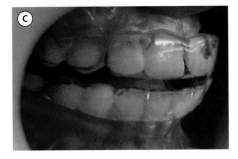
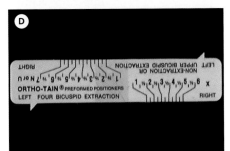

Fig. 9.5
A, B The occluso-guide appliance.
C Upper and lower incisors are engaged in an edge-to-edge occlusion.
D A flexible ruler is used to select the correct size. Courtesy of Ortho-Tain® Preformed Positioners.

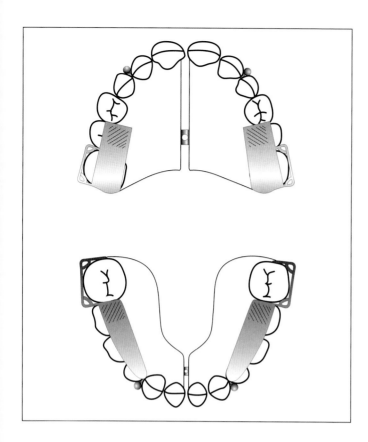

Fig. 9.6 The use of upper and lower Schwarz Twin Blocks for expansion in both arches in mixed dentition.

TWO-PHASE TREATMENT IN MIXED AND PERMANENT DENTITION

CASE REPORT: J.C. AGED 8 YEARS 9 MONTHS

This boy presents a disfiguring malocclusion in the early mixed dentition with the upper incisors extremely vulnerable to trauma, resting completely outside the lower lip. The lower lip is trapped under an overjet of 15 mm. The lower incisors are biting into the soft tissue of the palate 5 mm lingual to the upper incisors. Early treatment is essential in this type of malocclusion to place the upper incisors safely under lip control.

Mandibular retrusion accounts for a convexity of 9 mm, and this is evident in the profile. There is a vertical growth tendency with a facial axis angle of 25° and a Frankfort mandibular plane angle of 29°. The maxilla is typically narrow with a full unit distal occlusion. The upper pharyngeal airway is severely restricted at 7 mm, due to the mandibular retrusion (Fig. 9.7).

Functional correction is planned in two steps to reduce the excessive overjet of 15 mm. The Twin Blocks are constructed to a registration bite that reduces the overjet initially by 8 mm, planning to reactivate the blocks during treatment to complete reduction of the overjet.

After 4 months, the occlusion has corrected by 8 mm to

the position of initial activation of the occlusal inclined planes and the Twin Block is now reactivated by the addition of acrylic to the mesial incline of the upper appliance. This adjustment is made at the chairside to bring the mandible forwards to an edge-to-edge incisor relationship to complete correction of the overjet.

A 'gummy' smile necessitates intrusion of the upper incisors during treatment to improve the position of the upper lip relative to the incisors. This improves to some extent when the patient develops a lip seal during the Twin Block phase, but a further stage is necessary to intrude the upper incisors and detail the occlusion.

Orthopaedic correction to a Class I occlusion by Twin Blocks was followed in the permanent dentition by a short period of orthodontic treatment during which time fixed appliances were worn for a year to detail the occlusion. A utility arch was used to intrude the upper incisors to improve the 'gummy' smile.

Response to treatment

The upper pharyngeal space increased from 7 to 11 mm after 1 year of treatment, then to 14 mm 2 years later and, finally, to 21 mm after 6 years. Radiographic examination of the temporomandibular joints confirms that the condyles are in good position in the articular fossa at the age of 11 years 11 months, 3 years after the start of treatment.

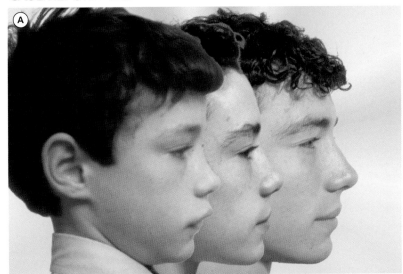

Fig. 9.7 Treatment:
A Profiles at ages 8 years 9 months (before treatment), 10 years 1 month and 14 years 11 months.
B–D Occlusion before treatment.
E–G Twin Blocks were worn for 14 months. Occlusion after 8 months of treatment.
H, J Appearance before treatment at age 8 years 9 months. Note the 'gummy' smile.
K After treatment at age 10 years 1 month.

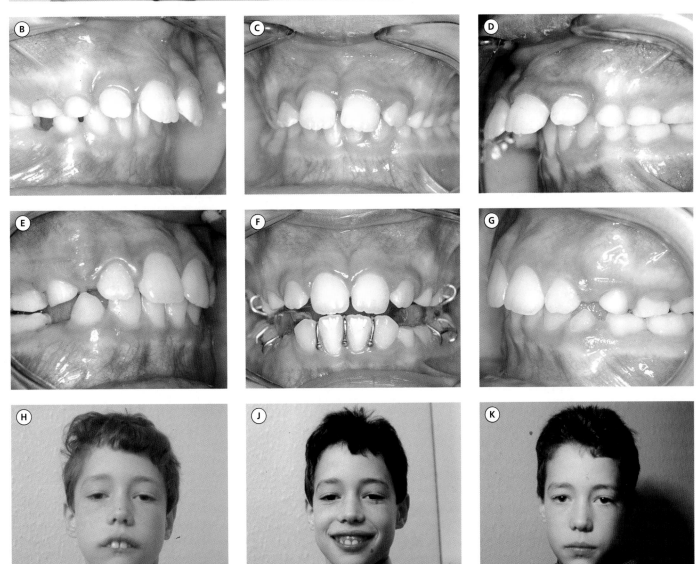

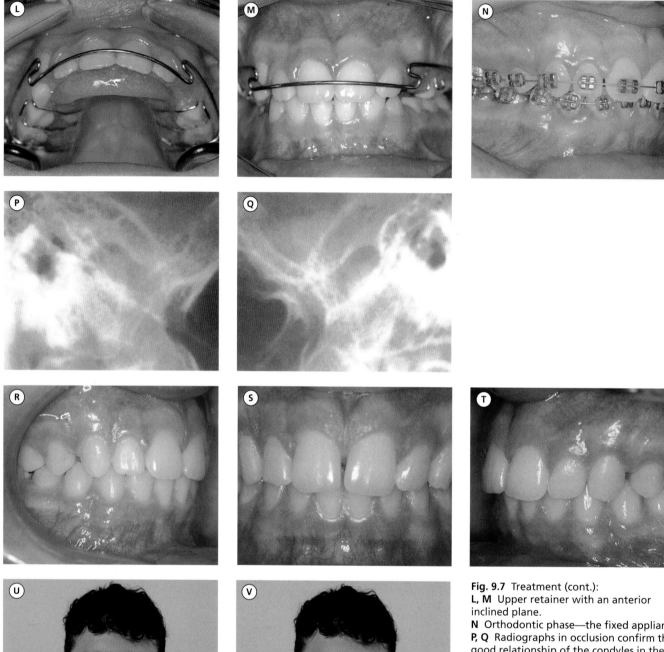

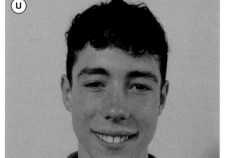

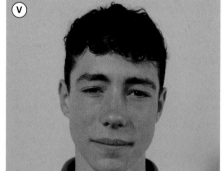

Fig. 9.7 Treatment (cont.):
L, M Upper retainer with an anterior inclined plane.
N Orthodontic phase—the fixed appliances.
P, Q Radiographs in occlusion confirm the good relationship of the condyles in the glenoid fossae at age 13 years 6 months.
R–T Occlusion 1 year out of retention at age 14 years 11 months.
U, V Facial views 1 year out of retention at age 14 years 11 months.

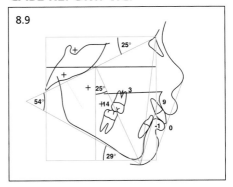

8.9

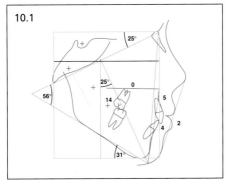

10.1

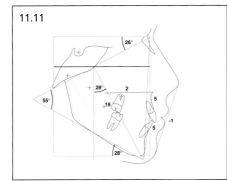

11.11

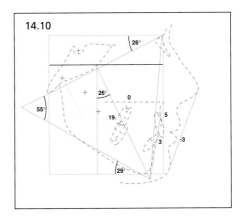

14.10

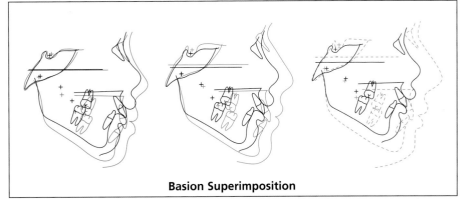

Basion Superimposition

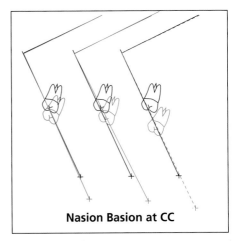

Nasion Basion at CC

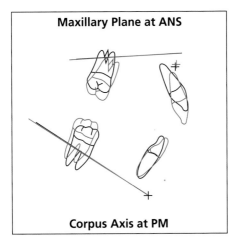

Maxillary Plane at ANS

Corpus Axis at PM

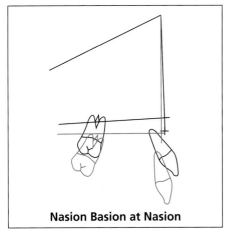

Nasion Basion at Nasion

J.C.	Age	8.9	10.1	11.11	14.10
Cranial Base Angle		25	25	26	26
Facial Axis Angle		25	25	28	26
F/M Plane Angle		29	31	28	29
Craniomandibular Angle		54	56	55	55
Maxillary Plane		3	0	2	0
Convexity		9	5	5	5
U/Incisor to Vertical		30	12	23	14
L/Incisor to Vertical		32	41	40	41
Interincisal Angle		118	127	117	125
6 to Pterygoid Vertical		14	14	19	19
L/Incisor to A/Po		−1	4	5	3
L/Lip to Aesthetic Plane		0	2	−1	−3

CASE REPORT: J.B. AGED 9 YEARS 11 MONTHS

This girl presents a Class II division 1 malocclusion with a maxillary protrusion contributing to prognathic facial profile in late mixed dentition. The skeletal discrepancy is mild, with a 5 mm convexity and the overjet is 7 mm. A tongue thrust is associated with an incomplete overbite and incompetent lip behaviour. The profile improves when the mandible postures forwards, indicating that functional therapy will improve the facial appearance in spite of the prognathic growth pattern. Clinical assessment takes precedence over cephalometric norms in predicting the response to functional treatment.

During the support phase an upper appliance was fitted with a tongue guard formed from heavy gauge wire, which also served as an anterior inclined plane to retain the corrected incisor relationship. After 18 months of treatment with functional appliances, upper and lower fixed appliances were fitted to complete the treatment.

Growth during support and retention resulted in a slight return of convexity in the profile. Twin Blocks were integrated with fixed appliances for 3 months to improve the facial result before detailing the occlusion with fixed appliances. The additional short orthopaedic phase was successful in improving the profile.

In this case, a two-phase approach combined the advantages of orthopaedic and orthodontic treatment to achieve a satisfactory dental occlusion and a pleasing improvement in facial balance. Treatment was initiated in late mixed dentition and completed in permanent dentition (Fig. 9.8).

Mixed dentition:
Twin Blocks: 3 months
Support and retention: 18 months.

Permanent dentition:
Twin Blocks: 3 months
Fixed appliances: 12 months.

CASE REPORT: J.B.

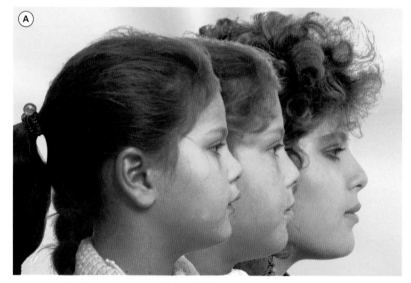

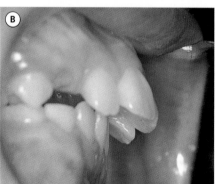
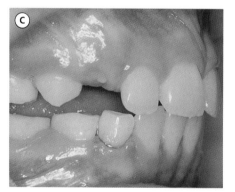
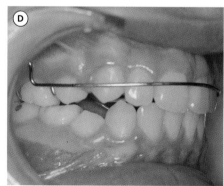

Fig. 9.8 Treatment:
A Profiles at ages 9 years 11 months (before treatment), 10 years 8 months and 18 years 6 months.
B–D Occlusion before treatment, after 6 weeks and after 1 year.

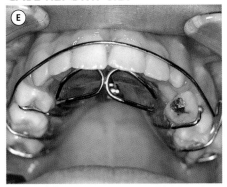

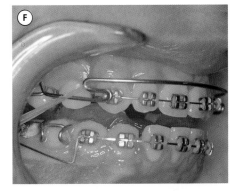

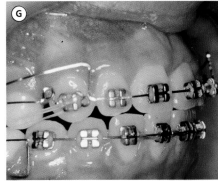

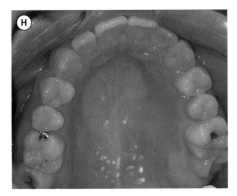

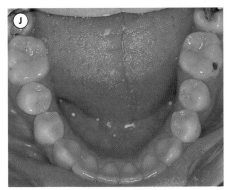

Fig. 9.8 Treatment (cont.):
E The recurved lingual tongue guard acts as an inclined plane.
F Phase 2: Twin Blocks combined with fixed appliance.
G Fixed appliance to finish.
H, J Occlusal views after treatment.
K, L Facial appearance at ages 9 years 11 months and 15 years 8 months.
M–P Occlusion at age 18 years 6 months.

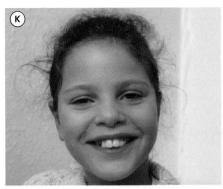

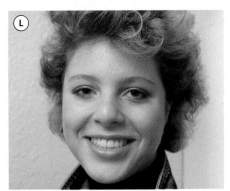

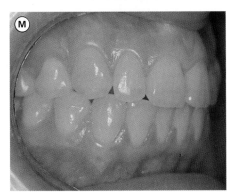

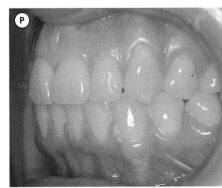

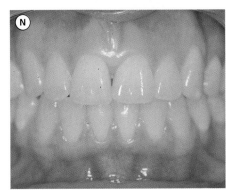

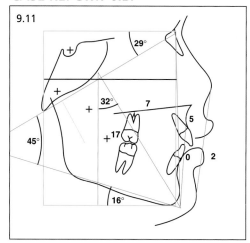

9.11

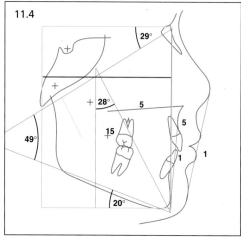

11.4

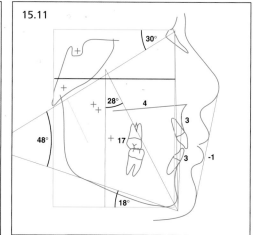

15.11

Maxillary Plane at ANS

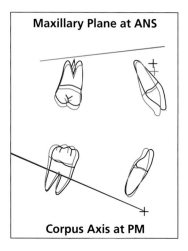

Corpus Axis at PM

Nasion Basion at Nasion

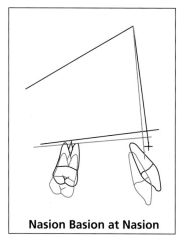

Basion Superimposition

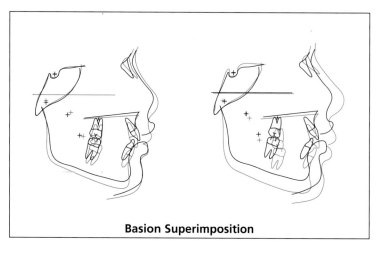

Nasion Basion at CC

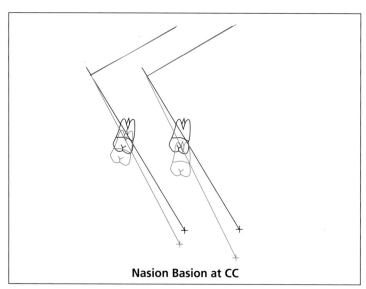

J.B.	Age	9.11	11.4	15.11
Cranial Base Angle		29	29	30
Facial Axis Angle		32	28	28
F/M Plane Angle		16	20	18
Craniomandibular Angle		45	49	48
Maxillary Plane		7	5	4
Convexity		5	5	3
U/Incisor to Vertical		33	20	27
L/Incisor to Vertical		30	28	31
Interincisal Angle		117	132	122
6 to Pterygoid Vertical		17	15	17
L/Incisor to A/Po		0	1	3
L/Lip to Aesthetic Plane		2	1	−1

CASE REPORT: C.M.

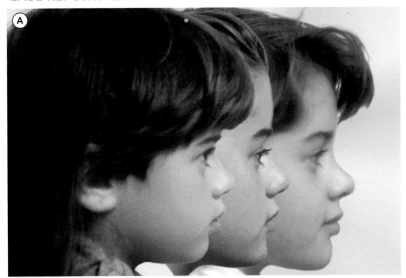

Fig. 9.9 Treatment:
A Profiles at ages 7 years 10 months (before treatment), 8 years 7 months and 11 years 7 months.
B–D Occlusion before treatment.
E Twin Block appliances.
F, G Occlusion after 11 months of treatment at age 8 years 7 months.

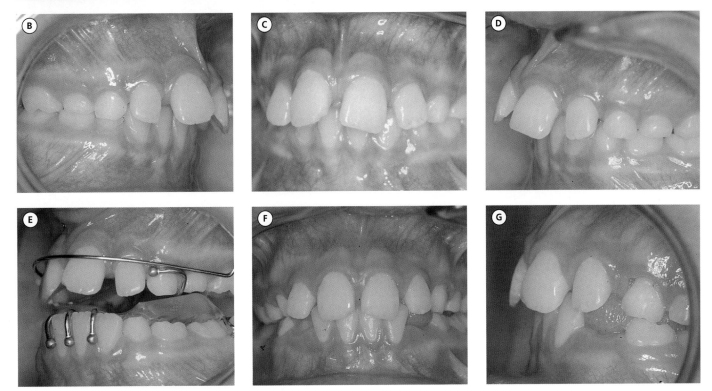

CASE REPORT: C.M. AGED 7 YEARS 10 MONTHS

This patient presents a prognathic profile with upper incisors proclined and flared in the early mixed dentition. The patient also exhibits a reduced anterior facial height and deep overbite, associated with a brachyfacial growth pattern. In spite of the prognathic appearance, the profile improves when the mandible postures downwards and forwards. Treatment is accomplished in two stages: first with interceptive functional treatment to correct to Class I occlusion in the mixed dentition and, second, with a finishing stage of straightwire technique in the permanent dentition (Fig. 9.9).

Mixed dentition:
Twin Blocks: 6 months
Support phase: 7 months
Retention: 15 months, awaiting eruption followed by a period without appliances.

Permanent dentition:
Fixed appliances: 7 months, followed by retention.

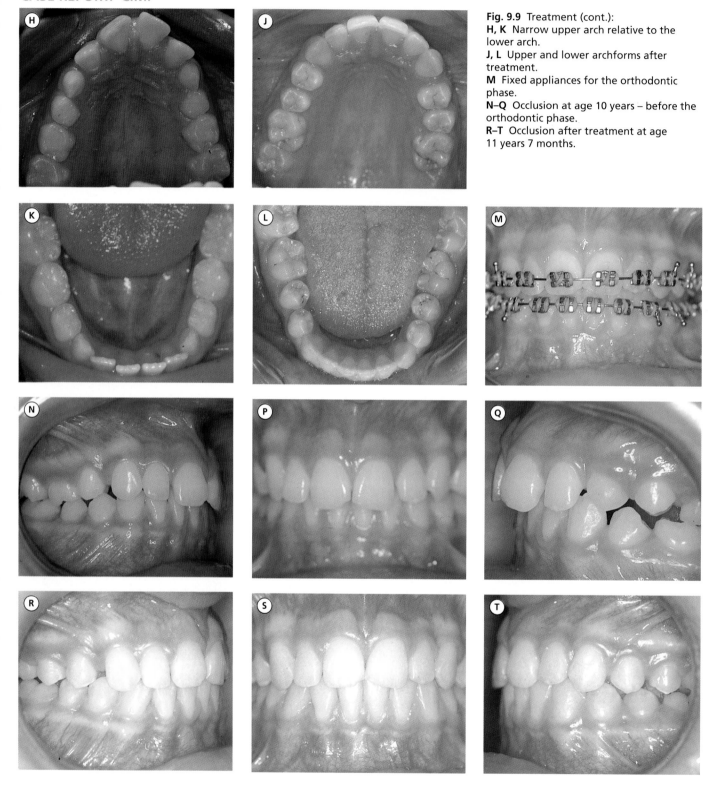

Fig. 9.9 Treatment (cont.):
H, K Narrow upper arch relative to the lower arch.
J, L Upper and lower archforms after treatment.
M Fixed appliances for the orthodontic phase.
N–Q Occlusion at age 10 years – before the orthodontic phase.
R–T Occlusion after treatment at age 11 years 7 months.

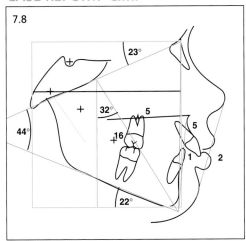

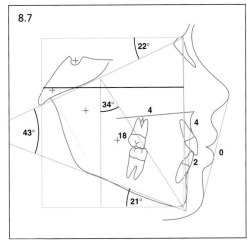

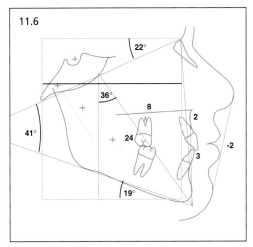

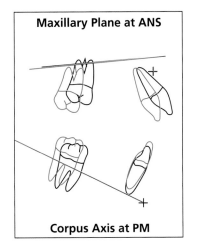

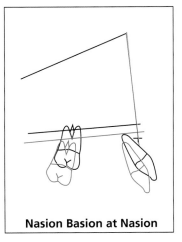

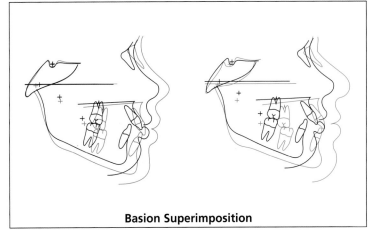

Maxillary Plane at ANS

Corpus Axis at PM

Nasion Basion at Nasion

Basion Superimposition

Nasion Basion at CC

C.M.	Age	7.8	8.7	11.6
Cranial Base Angle		23	22	22
Facial Axis Angle		32	34	36
F/M Plane Angle		22	21	19
Craniomandibular Angle		44	43	41
Maxillary Plane		5	4	8
Convexity		5	4	2
U/Incisor to Vertical		37	25	24
L/Incisor to Vertical		24	27	24
Interincisal Angle		119	128	124
6 to Pterygoid Vertical		16	18	24
L/Incisor to A/Po		1	2	3
L/Lip to Aesthetic Plane		2	0	−2

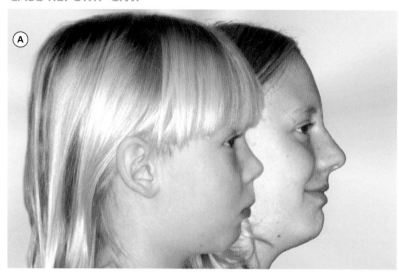

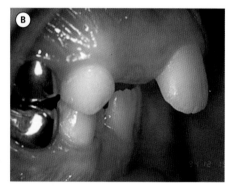
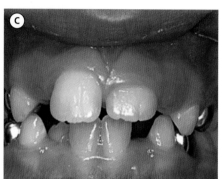

Fig. 9.10 Treatment:
A Profiles at ages 7 years 6 months (before treatment) and 13 years (after treatment).
B, C Occlusion before treatment.

PAEDODONTIC PRACTICE

Paedodontic practice is geared to early correction and the following patients are examples of interceptive treatment in mixed dentition carried out by Dr Gordon Kluzak in his paedodontic practice in Calgary. In suitable cases no additional treatment may be required.

CASE REPORT: C.W. AGED 7 YEARS 6 MONTHS

by Gordon Kluzak

This patient presented a disfiguring malocclusion and was successfully treated in the early mixed dentition stage when the permanent incisors were erupting. A thumb sucking habit was associated with upward tipping of the palatal plane and anterior open bite. An anterior open bite in mixed dentition responded well to a short period of treatment with Twin Blocks. An occluso-guide appliance was used to retain the position pending eruption of premolars and canines. This appliance was worn every night and for 2 hours in the day time. Finally a fixed lingual retainer was fitted to retain the lower labial segment. The occlusion is settling well 3 years out of retention when permanent teeth have erupted. Extraction of all second molars is planned to relieve potential impaction of third molars, which may otherwise contribute to recurrent late crowding in the lower arch (Fig. 9.10).

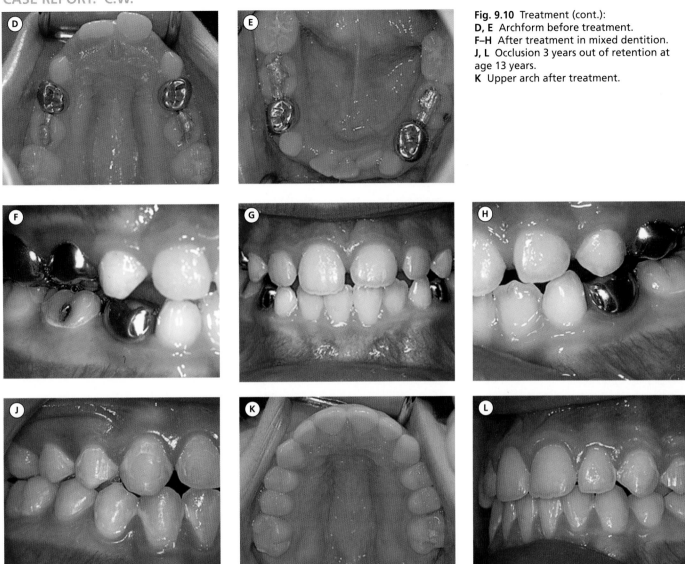

Fig. 9.10 Treatment (cont.):
D, E Archform before treatment.
F–H After treatment in mixed dentition.
J, L Occlusion 3 years out of retention at age 13 years.
K Upper arch after treatment.

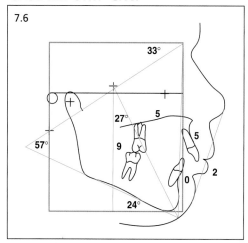

7.6

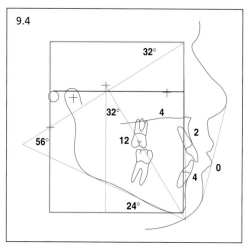

9.4

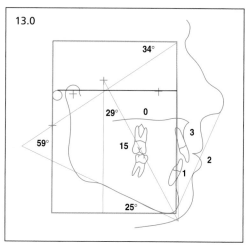

13.0

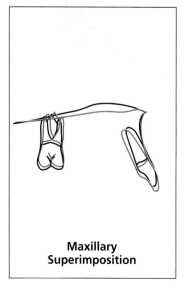

Maxillary Superimposition

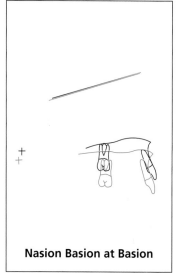

Nasion Basion at Basion

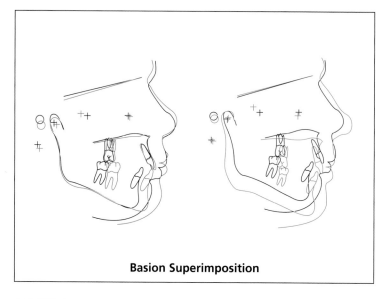

Basion Superimposition

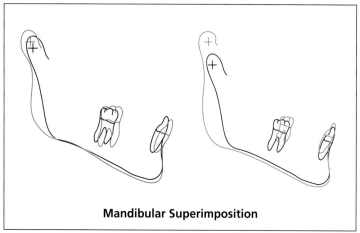

Mandibular Superimposition

CW Age	7.6	9.4	13.0
Cranial Base Angle	33	32	34
Facial Axis Angle	27	32	29
F/M Plane Angle	24	24	25
Craniomandibular Angle	57	56	59
Maxillary Plane	5	4	0
Convexity	5	2	3
U/Incisor to Vertical	23	28	18
L/Incisor to Vertical	27	28	23
L/Incisor to A/Po	0	4	1
L/Lip to Aesthetic Plane	2	0	2
6 to Pterygoid vertical	9	12	15

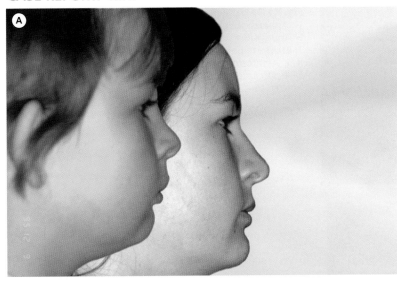

Fig. 9.11 Treatment:
A Profiles at ages 8 years 9 months (before treatment) and 13 years 9 months (after treatment).
B–D Occlusion before treatment.
E, F Anterior occlusion before treatment.

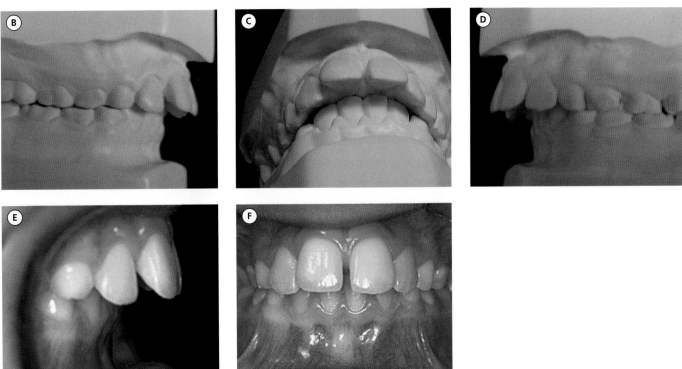

CASE REPORT: K.H. AGED 8 YEARS 9 MONTHS

by Gordon Kluzak

This case is an example of interceptive treatment in mixed dentition for a patient with a favourable growth pattern, who responded well to early treatment. This patient had Twin Blocks for 6 months, followed by an occluso-guide retainer. During the first 5 months of retention the occluso-guide was worn for 2 hours during the day and at nights. The patient was then given the option of wearing the occluso-guide at nights only, or for 1 hour during the day. During the transition to permanent dentition when deciduous teeth are shed the occluso-guide is a useful functional retainer. Retention was discontinued after 1 year. No further treatment was necessary and the occlusion is stable 4 years out of retention (Fig. 9.11).

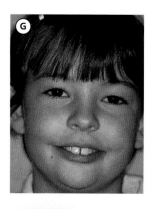

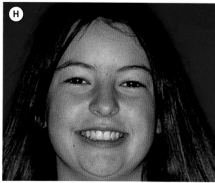

Fig. 9.11 Treatment (cont.):
G Appearance before treatment.
H Appearance after treatment.
J Archform before treatment.
K, L Archform after treatment.
M–P Occlusion out of retention at age 13 years 9 months.

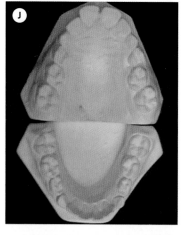

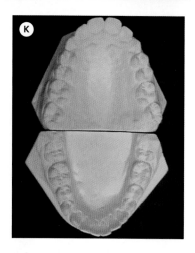

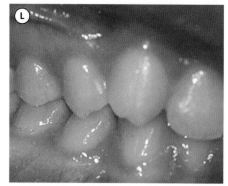

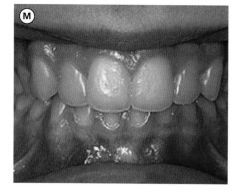

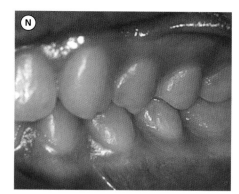

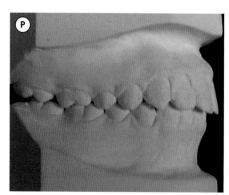

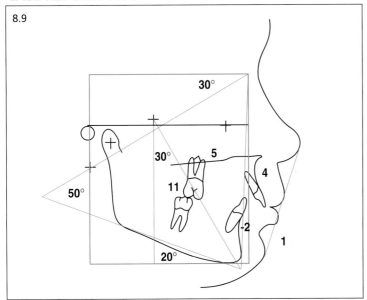

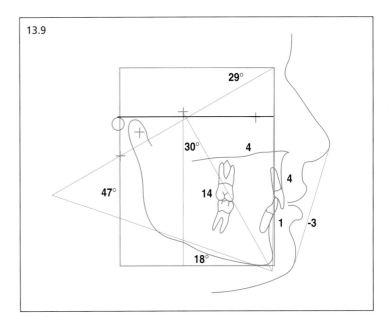

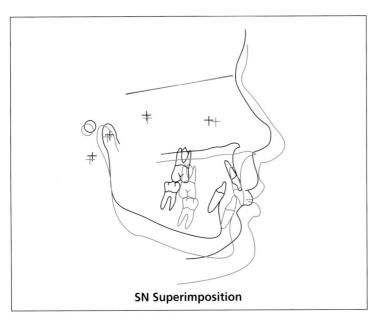

SN Superimposition

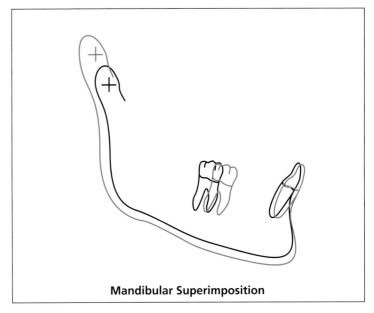

Mandibular Superimposition

KH Age	8.9	13.9
Cranial Base Angle	30	29
Facial Axis Angle	30	30
F/M Plane Angle	20	18
Craniomandibular Angle	50	47
Maxillary Plane	5	4
Convexity	6	4
U/Incisor to Vertical	28	14
L/Incisor to Vertical	30	25
L/Incisor to A/Po	−2	1
L/Lip to Aesthetic Plane	1	−3
6 to Pterygoid vertical	11	14

REFERENCES

Bergason, E.O. (1981). The preformed orthodontic positioner and eruption guidance appliance. *North Western Univ. Am. Dent. Assn. Library*, Chicago, Il. USA.

Bergason, E.O. (1985). The eruption guidance myofunctional appliance: case selection timing, motivation, indications and contraindictions in its use. *The Functional Orthodontist*, **2**: 17–13.

FURTHER READING

McNamara, J.A. & Brundon, W.L. (1993) *Orthodontic and orthopedic treatment in the mixed dentition*. Needham Press, Ann Arbor, Michigan.

CHAPTER 10

Combination Therapy
Permanent Dentition

Only the very wise or very foolish marry themselves to but one appliance or method.

Robert E. Moyers

Combination therapy describes the combined use of functional and fixed techniques in the management of malocclusion. In many respects this represents the best of both worlds, where orthopaedic and orthodontic techniques are combined to achieve correction of the skeletal discrepancy and detailing of the occlusion. The timing of treatment is a significant factor in planning combination therapy. By definition this is a one-phase treatment and should be timed to coincide with eruption of the permanent teeth. The optimum timing for this approach is either in late mixed dentition or early permanent dentition. It is then possible to integrate the fixed and functional therapy into a single phase of treatment, and to select either commencement with Twin Blocks or a fixed appliance according to preference or the requirements of the individual case. In some cases Twin Blocks may be adapted for simultaneous use with fixed appliances.

The following examples illustrate alternative approaches to combination therapy.

CASE REPORT: C.D. AGED 11 YEARS 1 MONTH

This is a typical example of treatment of a girl in the early permanent dentition, using Twin Blocks for initial functional correction, followed by fixed appliances to detail the occlusion. Mild mandibular retrusion accounts for 6 mm convexity with an overjet of 9 mm and a full unit distal occlusion (Fig. 10.1).

Facial convexity reduced from 6 mm to 3 mm during treatment by a combination of maxillary retraction and mandibular advancement. This improvement was maintained by good post-treatment growth which further reduced convexity to 2 mm by compensatory mandibular growth after the occlusion had been corrected. The dental and facial improvement was maintained at the age of 18 years 8 months, when third molars erupted into good occlusion.

Twin Blocks: 5 months
Support phase: 3 months
Fixed appliances: 12 months
Retention: 12 months
Final records: 18 years 8 months; 5 years out of retention.
Summary: The integration of Twin Blocks and fixed appliances combines the benefits of fixed and functional therapy. Contrary to many other forms of cosmetic treatment, the benefits of combined dental orthopaedic and orthodontic therapy are not temporary, but permanent. These techniques improve facial development and are of benefit as the patient grows from childhood into maturity. Interceptive treatment in the growing child by an orthopaedic approach to treatment can enhance facial growth. In many cases it helps to avoid surgical correction at a later stage of development. When required, orthopaedic correction is followed by an orthodontic phase of treatment to detail the occlusion.

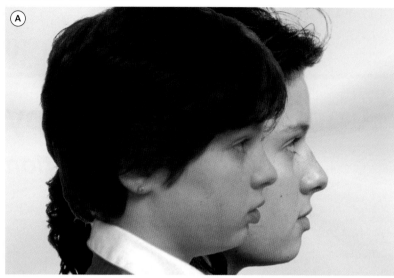

Fig. 10.1 Treatment:
A Profiles at ages 11 years 1 month (before treatment) and 15 years 11 months.
B–D Occlusion before treatment.
E, F Appliances in the orthodontic phase.

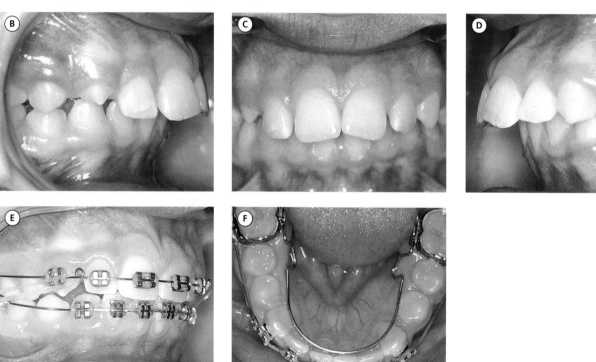

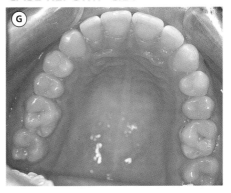

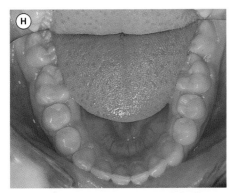

Fig. 10.1 Treatment (cont.):
G, H Upper and lower archforms after treatment at 15 years 11 months.
J–L Occlusion after treatment.
M Appearance before treatment at age 11 years 1 month.
N Appearance at 15 years 11 months.
P Appearance at 18 years 5 months.

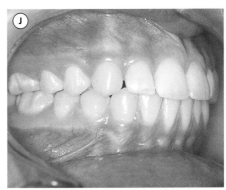

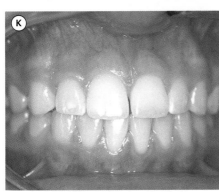

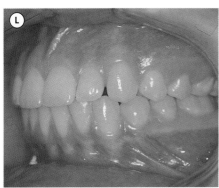

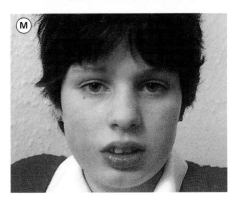

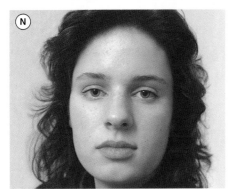

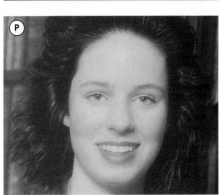

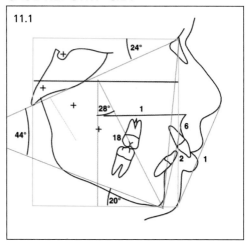

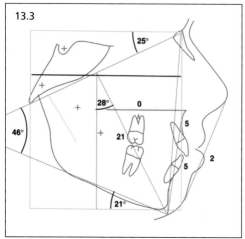

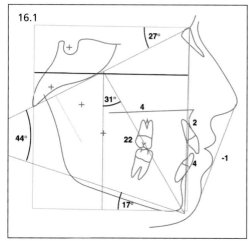

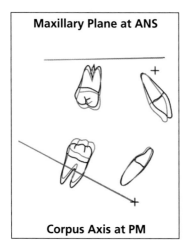

Maxillary Plane at ANS

Corpus Axis at PM

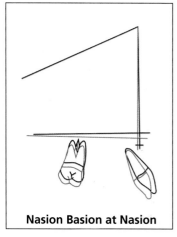

Nasion Basion at Nasion

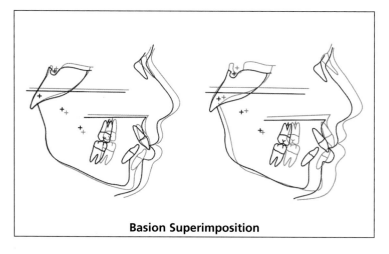

Basion Superimposition

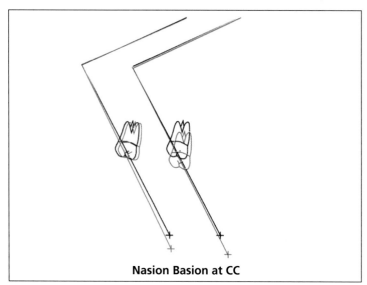

Nasion Basion at CC

C.D.	Age	11.1	13.3	16.1
Cranial Base Angle		24	25	27
Facial Axis Angle		28	28	31
F/M Plane Angle		20	21	17
Craniomandibular Angle		44	46	44
Maxillary Plane		1	0	4
Convexity		6	5	2
U/Incisor to Vertical		35	27	26
L/Incisor to Vertical		41	34	31
Interincisal Angle		104	119	123
6 to Pterygoid Vertical		18	21	22
L/Incisor to A/Po		2	5	4
L/Lip to Aesthetic Plane		1	2	−1

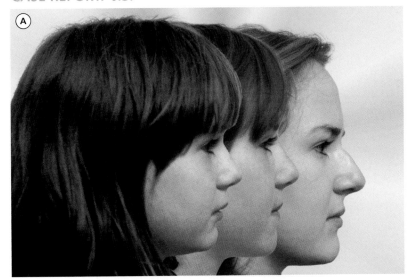

Fig. 10.2 Treatment:
A Profiles at ages 10 years 3 months (before treatment), 11 years 3 months (after the Twin Blocks phase) and 17 years.
B–D Occlusion before treatment; the anterior view shows the tongue thrust.
E–G After 11 months of treatment.

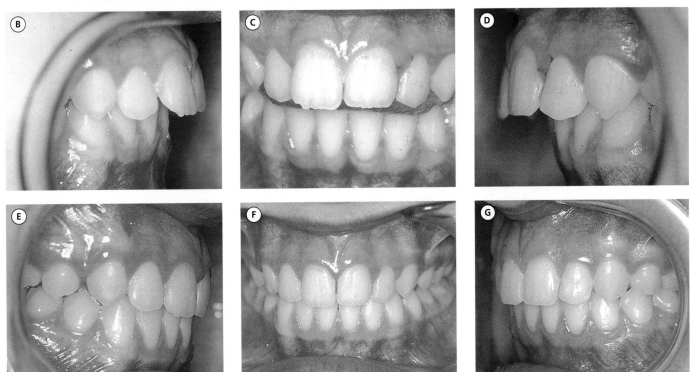

CASE REPORT: J.S. AGED 10 YEARS 3 MONTHS

This case illustrates controlled functional correction of a Class II division 1 malocclusion on a retrognathic Class I skeletal base to improve the profile without excessive mandibular advancement. An overjet of 7 mm with an incomplete overbite is due to tongue thrust and there is a full unit distal occlusion. Although a good occlusion was achieved during the Twin Block phase, this demonstrates the improvement resulting from detailing the occlusion with a finishing stage of straightwire technique (Fig. 10.2).

Twin Blocks: 7 months
Support phase: 4 months
Fixed appliances: 9 months followed by retention.

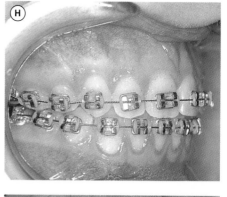

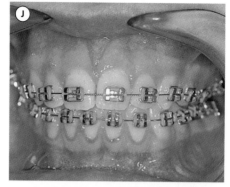

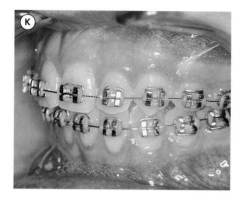

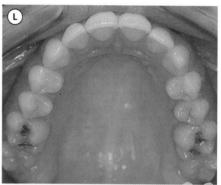

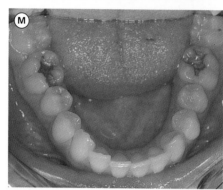

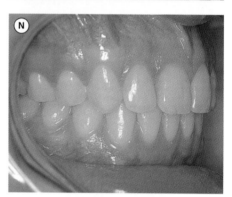

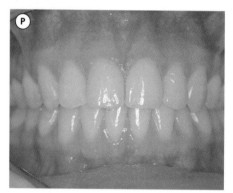

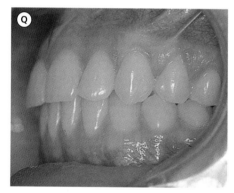

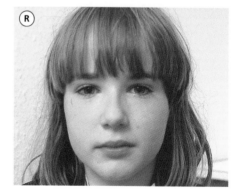

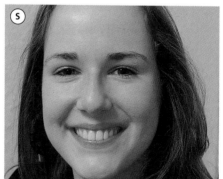

Fig. 10.2 Treatment (cont.):
H–K Fixed appliances phase.
L, M Upper and lower archforms.
N–Q Occlusion at age 17 years.
R Appearance before treatment at age 10 years 3 months.
S Appearance at age 17 years.

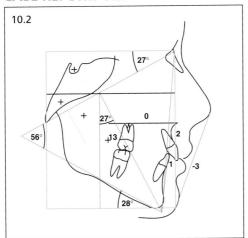

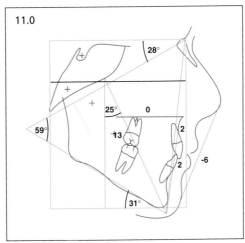

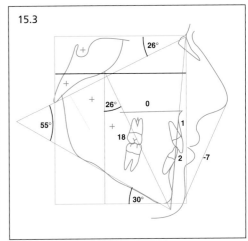

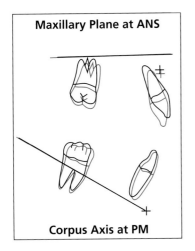

Maxillary Plane at ANS

Corpus Axis at PM

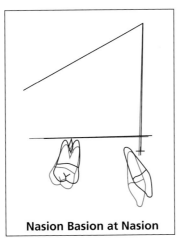

Nasion Basion at Nasion

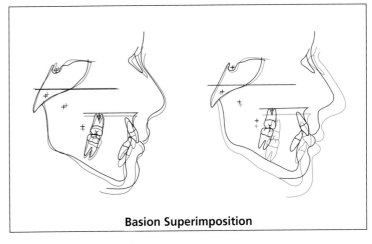

Basion Superimposition

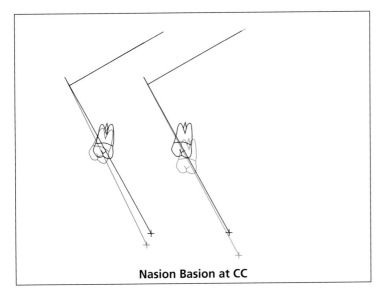

Nasion Basion at CC

J.S.	Age	10.2	11.0	15.3
Cranial Base Angle		27	28	26
Facial Axis Angle		27	25	26
F/M Plane Angle		28	31	30
Craniomandibular Angle		56	59	55
Maxillary Plane		0	0	0
Convexity		2	2	1
U/Incisor to Vertical		20	12	14
L/Incisor to Vertical		31	32	32
Interincisal Angle		129	136	134
6 to Pterygoid Vertical		13	13	18
L/Incisor to A/Po		1	2	2
L/Lip to Aesthetic Plane		-3	-6	-7

CONCURRENT STRAIGHTWIRE AND TWIN BLOCK THERAPY

An alternative approach is to initiate treatment with fixed appliances, correcting archform and applying torque to correct incisor angulation prior to fitting Twin Blocks, which are integrated with straightwire technique. This is a useful modification of technique, and one which many practitioners would appreciate. The following account is based on material provided by Dr Gary Baker and is illustrated by patients treated in his dental practice in Vancouver, Canada.

Timing is everything

by Gary Baker DMD and Beverly Ireland CDA

Classically described, the Twin Block technique corrects skeletal discrepancies first, both in the anteroposterior and vertical dimensions (development of the mandibular posterior segments), followed by alignment of the teeth. Depending on the timing of treatment, the two stages may frequently be separated by many months, resulting in two separate and distinct phases of treatment. The first phase (skeletal correction) may occur in mixed dentition, and the second phase (dental correction) may follow when all, or most of the adult dentition has erupted.

Experience suggests that this approach is more time consuming, and more demanding on patient cooperation than a single continuous phase of treatment. In addition, the delay between the first and second phases of treatment may allow time for the inherent Class II skeletal growth pattern to reassert itself, necessitating a further phase of functional correction. As well, early treatment with only Twin Blocks, especially in cases where the maxillary incisors are retroclined (e.g. Class II/2) may not allow for complete mandibular advancement.

A valid alternative in order to minimise the time required, and therefore improve patient cooperation, is to wait until all or most of the permanent dentition has erupted before commencing with treatment. At this stage in development the straight wire appliances are fitted first to achieve dental correction, followed concurrently by the correction of skeletal deficiencies with Twin Blocks. Initial dental alignment, especially incisor torque to advance the maxillary incisors helps to create optimal 'overjet-power' and thus gain greater control in achieving full mandibular advancement and posterior occlusal development. There is the additional advantage in that this protocol usually coincides with the pubertal mandibular growth spurt, thus enhancing the response to functional mandibular advancement.

Where a deep overbite is present this technique first aligns the maxillary dentition sufficiently to create adequate clearance before placing bands and brackets to align the mandibular teeth. When both arches have progressed to .018 round wires an orthopantomograph is taken to assess proper root tip and carry out any necessary rebracketing. In cases where the maxillary incisors are retroclined, the arch is taken to .020 × .020 straight wire (2–3 months) which widens the arch and torques out the incisors. Finally a .021 × .025 rectangular wire is placed to develop the arch as much as possible prior to the addition of Twin Blocks. This arch wire, by stabilising and anchoring the maxillary teeth, also mitigates the retracting forces of the Twin Block appliances on the upper anterior teeth, thereby facilitating a more complete advancement of the mandibular arch to Class I relationships.

The mandibular arch is taken to a .020 round wire or, less frequently, a .020 × 020 square wire. Anchorage control, to decrease the proclining effect on the mandibular incisors from the mandibular Twin Block, is improved by figure-eighting a .009 metal ligature from second premolar to second premolar. The archwire is then placed on top of this ligation, using conventional elastic ligatures.

The dental phase of treatment requires approximately 8–12 months, at which time the Twin Block appliances are placed. The maxillary appliance is designed with .028 ball clasp wires mesial and distal to the cuspids and mesial to the first molars. An open palate design is used where possible to facilitate increased tongue space and better speech. The mandibular appliance has .028 ball clasps mesial and distal to the cuspids and between the bicuspids in a full dentition case.

To ensure patient cooperation these appliances are fixed in place for a period of 2–3 weeks, using metal ligatures from .024 fixation loops on the appliances to the brackets. After this time the ligatures and fixation loops are removed to free the appliance. A soft .0175 braided wire is placed in the mandibular arch (over the 5 to 5 ligation) extending to the molars to maintain arch control during their eruption. At this appointment, and subsequent monthly appointments, the maxillary pads are relieved. To measure accurately the amount of clearance for eruption of the lower molars a double layer of thick articulating paper (700 microns) is used to mark the posterior maxillary blocks. In order to ensure molar eruption the patient wears short Class II interarch elastics from hooks on the mandibular molars to hooks on the second maxillary premolars.

The molars are generally in occlusion within a further 6–8 months of treatment and the incisors ideally exhibit an open bite of approximately 0–2 mm depending on the amount of overbite initially present. The mandibular 5 to 5 ligation is now removed and clearance is made for lower second premolars to erupt with elastics passing from these teeth to the upper first premolars, at times in conjunction with the original elastic bands. During all of these adjustments the integrity of the inclined planes is maintained to ensure that the mandible is held forward. After 2–3 months of further eruption, adding new braided wires as needed to maintain mandibular arch integrity, the appliances are discontinued and short Class II elastics are continued from the mandibular premolars to the maxillary premolars and canines to bring the mandibular teeth into occlusion. During this phase the mandibular teeth are levelled and aligned back to .018 or .020 round wires, and the 5 to 5 ligation is removed. The maxillary .021 × .025 wire is downsized to an .020 or .018 round arch to allow increased closure. This final interdigitation is generally achieved within 2–3 months without the use of a support appliance, and treatment is concluded usually within a 24- to 30-month period, with the placement of conventional Hawley retainers.

Fig. 10.3 illustrates the approach to this technique and the [following] three case reports refer to patients treated by Gary Baker and Beverly Ireland in Dr Baker's practice in Vancouver, Canada.

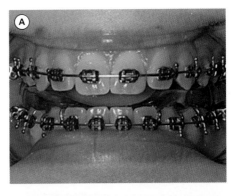

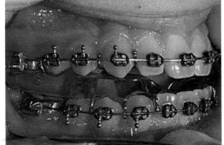

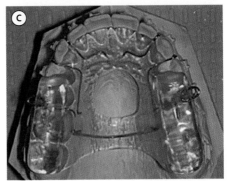

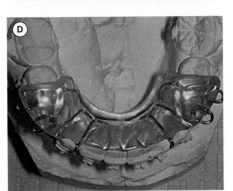

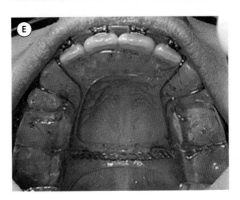

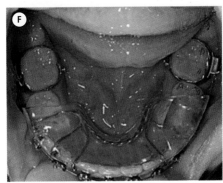

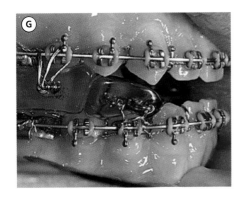

Fig. 10.3 The approach to the concurrent straightwire Twin Block therapy technique:
A Mx aligned to 021 025 and Md to 020 wire at initial insertion of appliances.
B Mx 028 ball clasps mesial to Mx 6s and mesial and distal to Mx 3s. Md 028 ball clasps mesial and distal to Md 3s and Md 4s.

C, D Appliances fixed in place for 2–3 weeks break-in period using 024 loops embedded in acrylic pads.

E Open palate design for ease of wear and to facilitate tongue and freedom of speech.
F Md appliance extends distally 2–3 mm anterior to Md 5/6 contact point.
G Loops are ligated to brackets and wire using 009 metal ligatures.

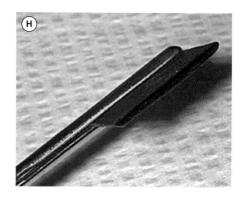

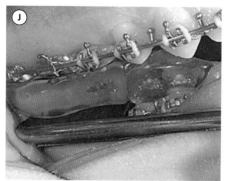

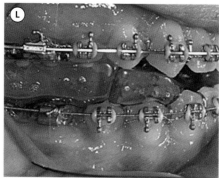

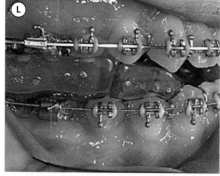

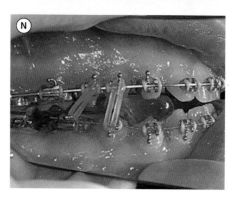

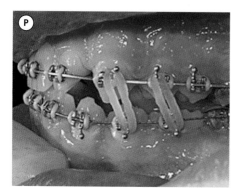

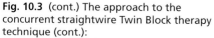

Fig. 10.3 (cont.) The approach to the concurrent straightwire Twin Block therapy technique (cont.):

H, J After the break-in period the Mx pads are relieved monthly using double thickness of thick articulating paper placed distal to the Md pad.

K Mx pads are marked and relieved until paper no longer marks on the pads. Barrel shaped acrylic bur used in slow-speed handpiece.

L Approximately 1–1.5 mm of clearance is created. Note Md 4/4 metal ligation under 0175 braided wire extended to molars.

M Intra-arch rubber bands initially worn from Mx 5s to Md 6s to predictably erupt lower 6s.

N When lower 6s are mostly in contact with Mx 5s and 6s, an additional rubber band is added from Mx 4s to Md 5s. Clear acrylic around Md 5s to allow for this eruption.

P Appliances then discontinued; rubber bands worn from Mx 3s and 4s to Md 4s and 5s to complete dental closure.

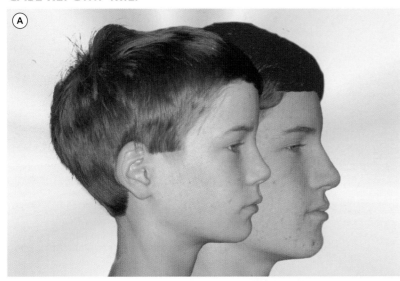

Fig. 10.4 Treatment:
A Profiles at ages 12 years 6 months (before treatment) and 15 years 3 months (after treatment).
B–D Occlusion before treatment.
E, F Archforms before treatment.
G, H Appearance before treatment at age 12 years 6 months.

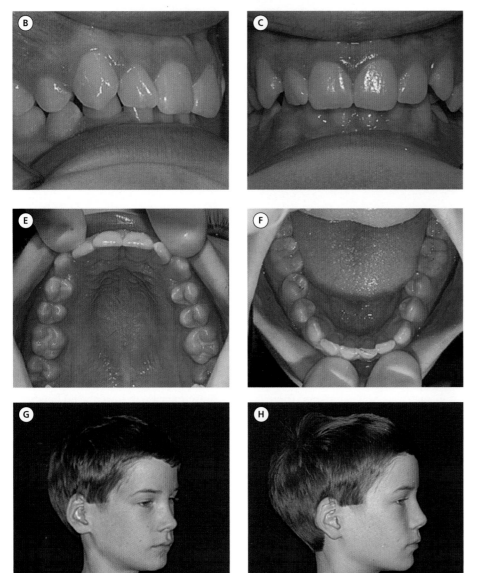

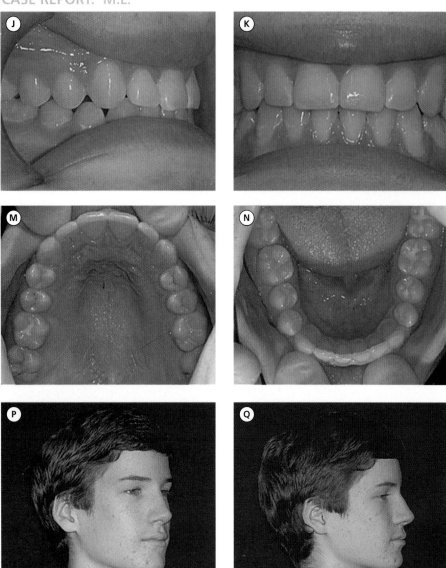

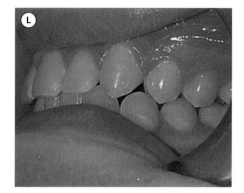

Fig. 10.4 Treatment (cont.):
J–L Occlusion after treatment.
M, N Archforms after treatment.
P, Q Appearance after treatment at age 15 years 3 months.

CASE REPORT: M.L. AGED 12 YEARS 6 MONTHS

This boy is treated in early permanent dentition at an appropriate stage to commence treatment with fixed appliances. The dental relationship is dictated by retroclination of all four upper incisors with deep overbite, causing a distal occlusion by restricting mandibular development. There is mild crowding of the upper canines, and minimal crowding in the lower arch. Cephalometric analysis reveals a retrognathic profile with a Class I skeletal base relationship, and in profile the retrognathic pattern is evident, especially in the mandible. A long anterior cranial base is a factor in the retrognathic appearance. The growth potential is good in view of a brachyfacial pattern with a horizontal growth vector in the mandible.

The facial change after treatment shows a much stronger profile, as a result of a good mandibular growth response made possible by the proper torquing of the maxillary incisors. There is a significant increase in lower facial height brought about by mandibular posterior development, which contributes to improved facial balance and resolution of the deep overbite (Fig. 10.4).

Total active treatment: 27 months
Fixed appliances: upper arch, 22 months; lower arch, 18 months
Twin Blocks: 11 months
Final detailing/Hawley retainers: 5 months.

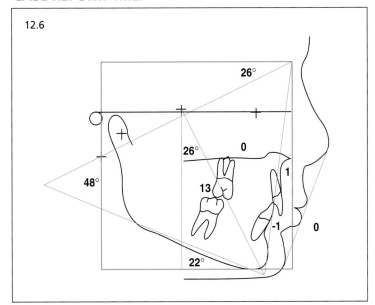

12.6

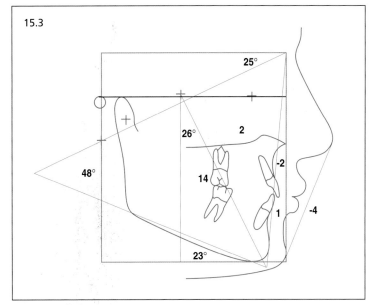

15.3

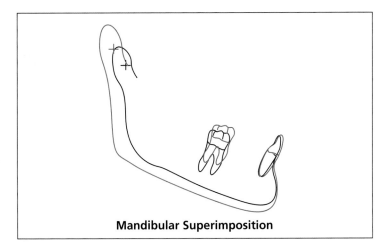

Mandibular Superimposition

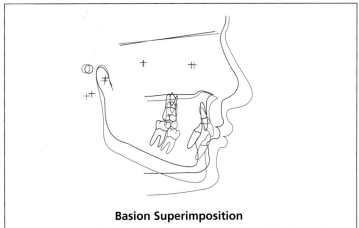

Basion Superimposition

M.L. Age	12.6	15.3
Cranial Base Angle	26	25
Facial Axis Angle	26	26
F/M Plane Angle	22	23
Craniomandibular Angle	48	48
Maxillary Plane	0	2
Convexity	1	−2
U/Incisor to Vertical	9	23
L/Incisor to Vertical	28	27
L/Incisor to A/Po	−1	1
L/Lip to Aesthetic Plane	0	−4
6 to Pterygoid vertical	13	14

CASE REPORT: C.S.

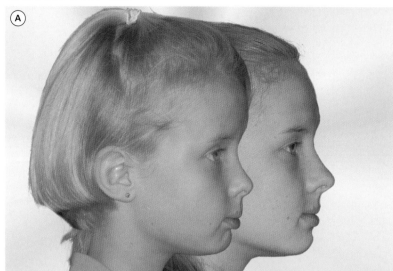

Fig. 10.5 Treatment:
A Profiles at ages 9 years 11 months (before treatment) and 14 years 5 months.
B–D Occlusion before treatment.
E, F Archforms before treatment.
G, H Appearance before treatment.

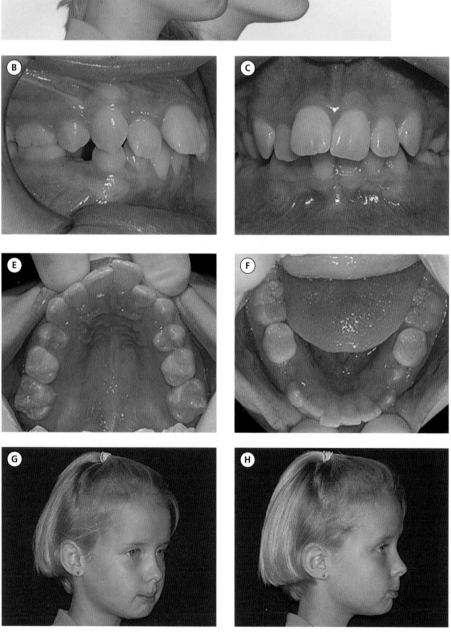

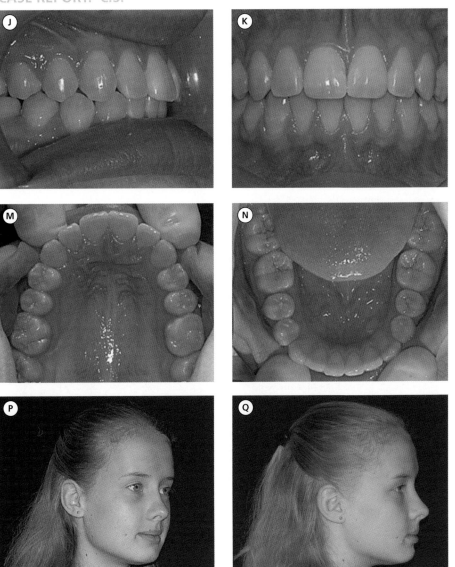

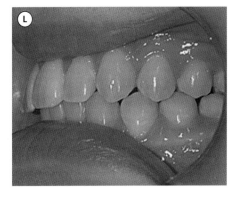

Fig. 10.5 Treatment (cont.):
J–L Occlusion after treatment.
M, N Archforms after treatment.
P, Q Appearance after treatment.

CASE REPORT: C.S. AGED 9 YEARS 11 MONTHS

This young girl presents a Class II division 1 malocclusion in late mixed dentition with crowding in the upper and lower labial segments. The appearance confirms severe mandibular retrusion. This is an appropriate time to initiate treatment for a girl, as it is important to start treatment in good time to allow for arch development to proceed and still be able to take advantage of the pubertal growth spurt. Treatment was initiated with upper fixed appliances, followed 3 months later by lower fixed appliances. When the arches were aligned, with correct maxillary incisor torque, Twin Blocks were fitted to advance the mandible and correct the occlusal relationship to Class I.

There is a pleasing improvement in facial appearance, and occlusal detailing is completed with fixed appliances to an excellent result. The growth response is positive during treatment with a significant increase in mandibular length and a resulting improvement in the mandibular retrusion (Fig. 10.5).

Total active treatment: 27 months
Fixed appliances: upper arch, 23 months; lower arch, 20 months
Twin Blocks: 10 months
Final detailing/Hawley retainers: 4 months.

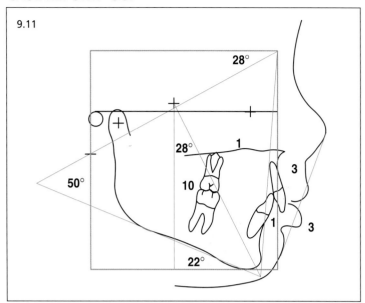

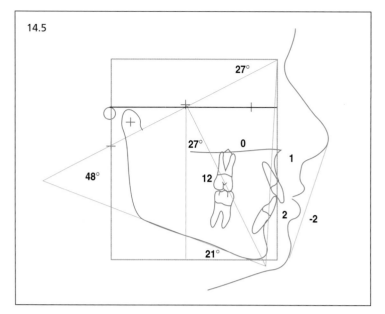

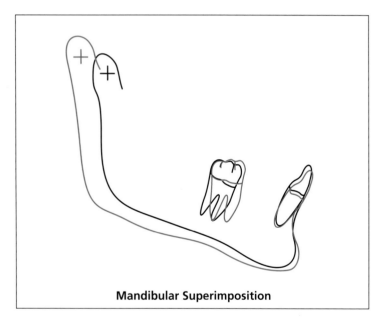

Mandibular Superimposition

C.S. Age	9.11	14.5
Cranial Base Angle	28	27
Facial Axis Angle	28	27
F/M Plane Angle	22	21
Craniomandibular Angle	50	48
Maxillary Plane	1	0
Convexity	3	1
U/Incisor to Vertical	13	26
L/Incisor to Vertical	29	35
L/Incisor to A/Po	1	2
L/Lip to Aesthetic Plane	3	−2
6 to Pterygoid vertical	10	12

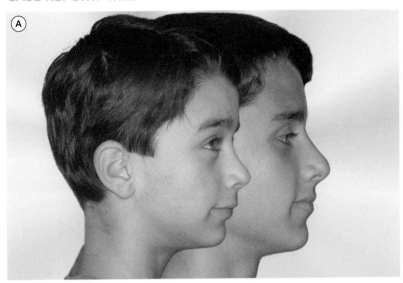

Fig. 10.6 Treatment:
A Profiles at ages 14 years 1 month (before treatment) and 16 years 2 months (after treatment).
B–D Occlusion before treatment.
E, F (68,69) Archforms before treatment.
G, H Appearance before treatment.

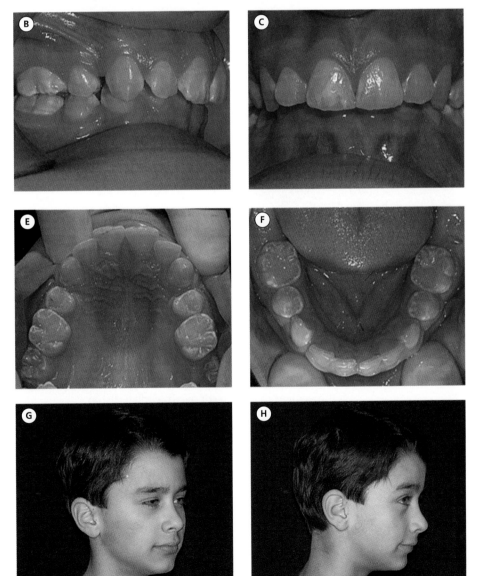

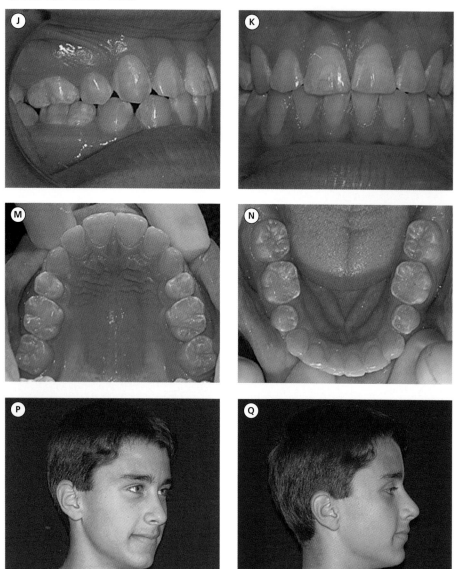

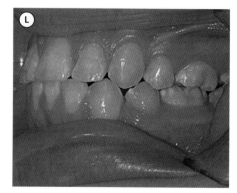

Fig. 10.6 Treatment (cont.):
J–L Occlusion after treatment.
M, N Archforms after treatment.
P, Q Appearance after treatment.

CASE REPORT: M.Z. AGED 14 YEARS 1 MONTH

by Gary Baker DMD

This case illustrates the protocol for combination therapy following extraction of premolars. Mandibular retrusion is evident in the facial appearance of this patient who previously had four first premolars extracted as part of a serial extraction programme to relieve severe crowding in both arches.

Favourable improvement in the profile is accounted for by a good mandibular growth response with positive vertical changes in the lower face, in addition to mandibular advancement by Twin Blocks (Fig. 10.6). Note the improvement in the incisor overbite relationship.

Total active treatment: 24 months
Fixed appliances: upper arch, 21 months; lower arch, 14 months
Twin Blocks: 6 months
Final detailing/Hawley retainers: 3 months.

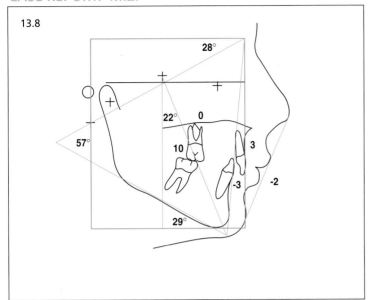

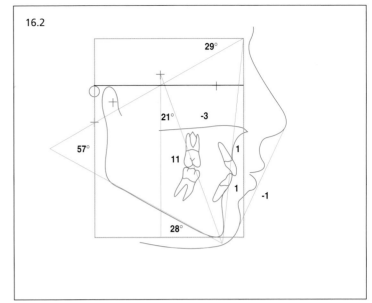

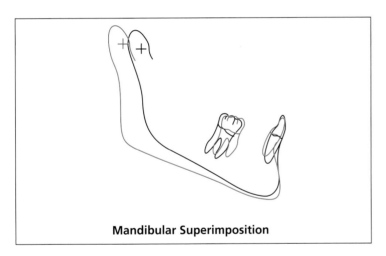

Mandibular Superimposition

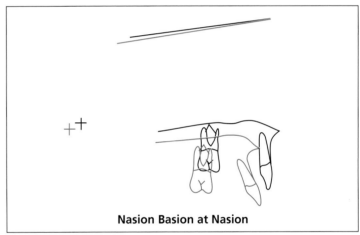

Nasion Basion at Nasion

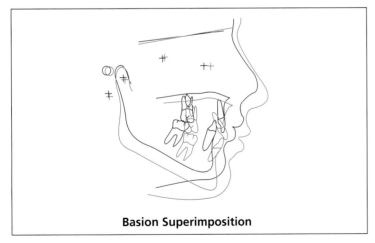

Basion Superimposition

MZ Age	14.1	16.2
Cranial Base Angle	28	29
Facial Axis Angle	22	21
F/M Plane Angle	29	28
Craniomandibular Angle	57	57
Maxillary Plane	0	−3
Convexity	3	1
U/Incisor to Vertical	6	27
L/Incisor to Vertical	20	31
L/Incisor to A/Po	−3	1
L/Lip to Aesthetic Plane	−2	−1
6 to Pterygoid vertical	10	11

CHAPTER 11

The Twin Block Traction Technique

ORTHOPAEDIC TRACTION

In most cases, full functional correction of occlusal relationships can be achieved with Twin Blocks without the addition of any orthopaedic or traction forces. Where the response to functional correction is poor, the addition of orthopaedic traction force may be considered.

In the early stages of development of the Twin Block technique a method was devised to combine functional therapy with orthopaedic traction. This approach should be limited to the treatment of severe malocclusion, where growth is unfavourable for conventional fixed or functional therapy. Functional therapy combined with traction achieves rapid correction of malocclusion.

The indications are confined to a minority of cases with growth patterns where maxillary retraction is the treatment of choice. For example:

- In the treatment of severe maxillary protrusion.
- To control a vertical growth pattern by the addition of vertical traction to intrude the upper posterior teeth.
- In adult treatment where mandibular growth cannot assist the correction of a severe malocclusion.

The Concorde facebow

Before Twin Blocks were developed, the author used extraoral traction with removable appliances as a means of anchorage to retract upper buccal segments to correct Class II malocclusion (Cousins & Clark, 1965). In the early years using Twin Blocks, tubes were added to clasps for extraoral traction on the upper appliance to be worn at night so as to reinforce the functional component for correction of a Class II buccal segment relationship.

A method was developed to combine extraoral and intermaxillary traction by adding a labial hook to a conventional facebow and extending an elastic back to attach to the lower appliance in the incisor region (Clark, 1982). This development was based on previous experience of

functional appliances that were worn part time and were slow and unpredictable in correcting arch relationships.

The Concorde facebow is a new means of applying intermaxillary and extraoral traction to restrict maxillary growth and, at the same time, to encourage mandibular growth in combination with functional mandibular protrusion. A conventional facebow is adapted by soldering a recurved labial hook to extend forwards to rest outside the

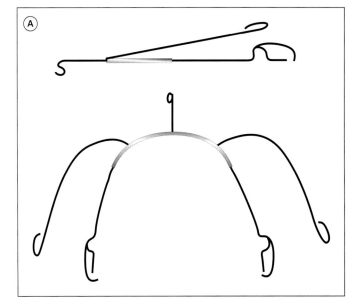

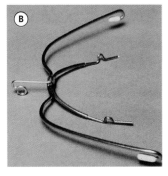
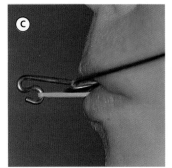

Fig. 11.1 A–C Concorde facebow.

lips as an anchor point to combine intermaxillary and extraoral traction. Patient comfort and acceptance is similar to a conventional facebow. Intermaxillary traction was added to the appliance system to ensure that if the patient postured out of the appliance during the night, the intermaxillary traction force would increase. This ensured that the appliance was effective 24 hours per day (Fig. 11.1).

The labial hook is positioned extraorally, 1 cm clear of the lips in the midline. This enables an elastic back to pass intraorally to attach anteriorly to the lower appliance to apply intermaxillary traction as a horizontal force vector. This has the advantage of eliminating the unfavourable upward component of force in conventional intermaxillary elastic traction, which can extrude lower molars and cause tipping of the occlusal plane.

When distal extraoral traction is applied to a removable appliance, the outer bow of the facebow should be adjusted to lie slightly above the inner bow in order to apply a slight upward component of force to help retain the upper appliance. Fixation of the appliance must be excellent before any orthopaedic force is applied to a removable appliance, and poor fixation contraindicates the addition of traction, except to a fixed attachment.

The traction components are worn at night only to reinforce the action of the occlusal inclined plane. If the patient fails to posture the mandible to the corrected occlusal position during the night, the intermaxillary traction force is automatically increased to compensate and to ensure that favourable intermaxillary forces are applied continuously. The aim is to make the appliances active 24 hours per day to maximise the orthopaedic response.

Careful case selection is essential before using a combination of Twin Blocks with orthopaedic traction. This is a very powerful mechanism for maxillary retraction and, as the majority of Class II malocclusions are due to mandibular retrusion, it is contraindicated in most cases. The headgear effect tends to tip the occlusal plane and palatal plane down anteriorly and to retrocline the upper incisors, which may cause unfavourable autorotation of the mandible. Extraoral traction should be used selectively, bearing in mind that most patients respond to treatment without the addition of traction components.

Later experience in using Twin Blocks confirmed that the addition of a traction component was not necessary to achieve correction of the buccal segment relationship, and extraoral traction is no longer used to reinforce the action of the inclined planes. Study of early cases showed that the headgear effect caused unneccessary maxillary retraction.

Occasionally (Orton, 1990), high pull traction may be indicated to intrude the upper posterior teeth in cases with a severe vertical growth pattern, in an effort to achieve a forward mandibular rotation by intruding upper molars. The same objective can be achieved more simply by using vertical intraoral elastics to intrude the posterior teeth.

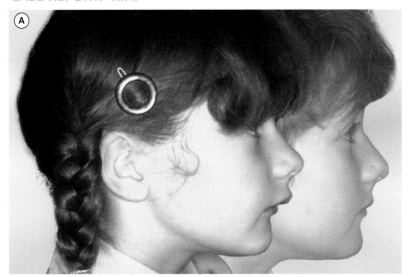

Fig. 11.2 Treatment:
A Profiles at ages 9 years 6 months (before treatment) and 10 years 7 months (after 8 months of treatment).
B, C Occlusion before treatment at age 9 years 6 months (note the anterior open bite).
D Occlusion after 8 months of treatment.

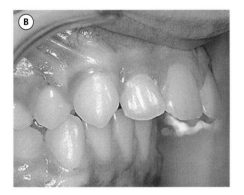
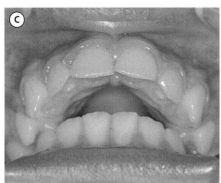
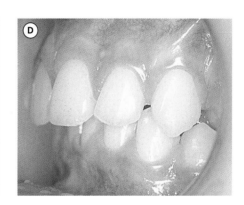

TWIN BLOCKS COMBINED WITH ORTHOPAEDIC TRACTION

Treatment of maxillary protrusion

CASE REPORT: K.A. AGED 9 YEARS 6 MONTHS

A severe Class II skeletal base relationship is due to maxillary protrusion. A previous thumb sucking habit has resulted in an anterior open bite which is perpetuated by a tongue thrust and the lower lip is trapped in a 14 mm overjet. The addition of the Concorde facebow with extraoral and intermaxillary traction applied a retraction force to the maxilla, while the action of the occlusal inclined planes advanced the mandible. This combination of mechanics resulted in a rapid response to treatment, in spite of spasmodic appliance wear (Fig. 11.2).

Twin Blocks and Concorde facebow: 8 months
Support and retention: 6 months.

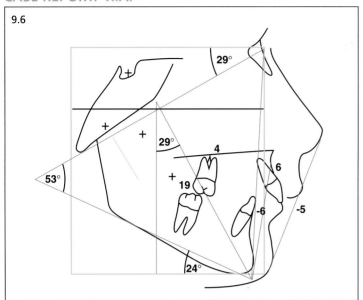

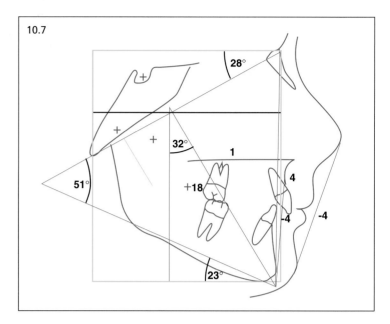

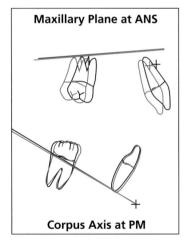

Maxillary Plane at ANS

Corpus Axis at PM

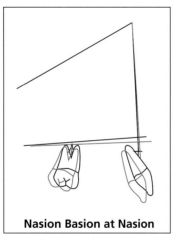

Nasion Basion at Nasion

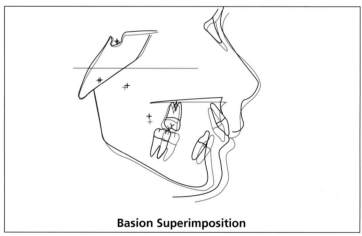

Basion Superimposition

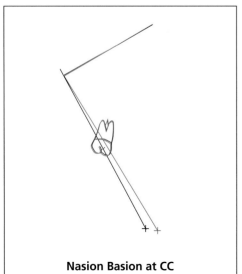

Nasion Basion at CC

K.A.	Age	9.6	10.7
Cranial Base Angle		29	28
Facial Axis Angle		29	32
F/M Plane Angle		24	23
Craniomandibular Angle		53	51
Maxillary Plane		4	1
Convexity		6	4
U/Incisor to Vertical		27	24
L/Incisor to Vertical		29	28
Interincisal Angle		124	128
6 to Pterygoid Vertical		19	18
L/Incisor to A/Po		−6	−4
L/Lip to Aesthetic Plane		−5	−4

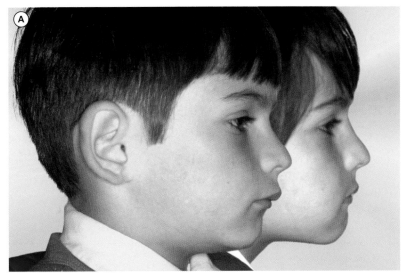

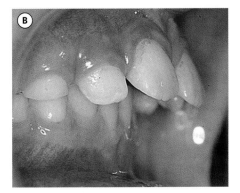
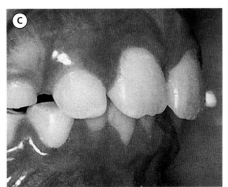

Fig. 11.3 Treatment:
A Profiles at ages 9 years 5 months (before treatment) and 9 years 11 months (after treatment).
B, C Occlusion after 5 months of treatment at age 9 years 11 months.

CASE REPORT: W.F. AGED 9 YEARS 5 MONTHS

This patient presents a 12 mm overjet and deep overbite with a full unit distal occlusion in the mixed dentition. At this stage of development there may be a resting phase in growth, when the patient does not gain significantly in height. The mandible follows the growth pattern of a long bone, therefore mandibular growth is also limited. In appropriate cases maxillary retraction may be required to contribute to the correction of a distal occlusion. The Concorde facebow with intermaxillary and extraoral traction is effective in accelerating correction to compensate for a lack of mandibular growth (Fig. 11.3).

Twin Blocks and Concorde facebow: 9 months
Support and retention: 9 months.

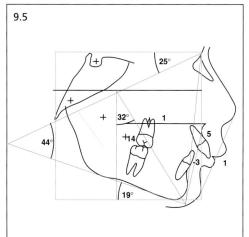

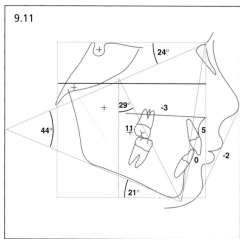

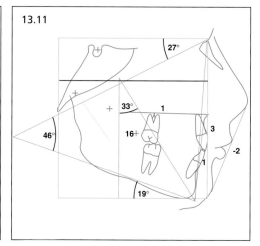

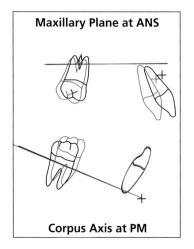

Maxillary Plane at ANS

Corpus Axis at PM

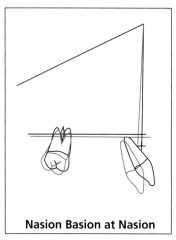

Nasion Basion at Nasion

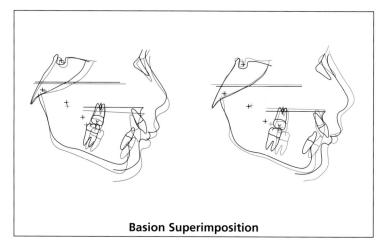

Basion Superimposition

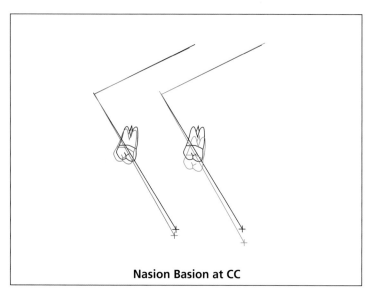

Nasion Basion at CC

W.F.	Age	9.5	9.11	13.11
Cranial Base Angle		25	24	27
Facial Axis Angle		32	29	33
F/M Plane Angle		19	21	19
Craniomandibular Angle		44	44	46
Maxillary Plane		1	−3	−1
Convexity		5	5	3
U/Incisor to Vertical		32	18	16
L/Incisor to Vertical		30	34	39
Interincisal Angle		118	128	125
6 to Pterygoid Vertical		14	11	16
L/Incisor to A/Po		−3	0	1
L/Lip to Aesthetic Plane		1	−2	−2

CASE REPORT: K.S.

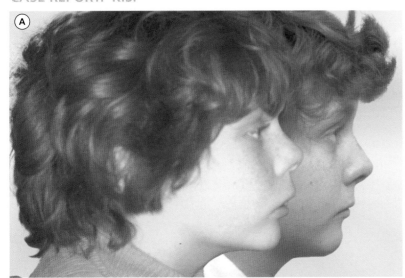

Fig. 11.4 Treatment:
A Profiles at ages 11 years 6 months (before treatment) and 14 years 2 months (after treatment).
B, C Occlusion before treatment.
D Occlusion 2 years out of retention.
E Facial appearance before treatment.
F Concorde facebow used during treatment.
G Facial appearance after treatment: aged 14 years 2 months.

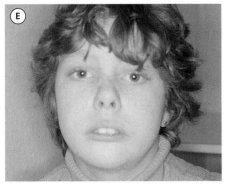
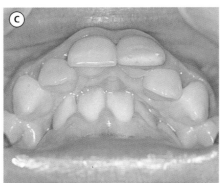
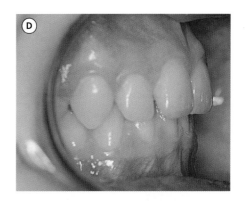
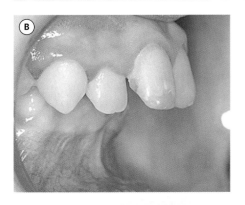
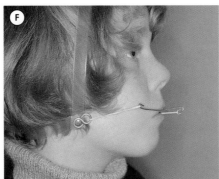
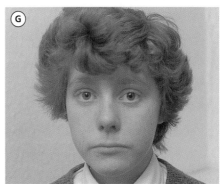

CASE REPORT: K.S. AGED 11 YEARS 6 MONTHS

The growth response slows significantly in girls after the onset of menstruation. This tends to reduce the mandibular response to functional treatment. The addition of orthopaedic traction may be required to achieve correction of a severe distal occlusion.

This is an early example of Twin Block treatment for a girl with a severe Class II division 1 malocclusion with excessive overbite. The case was complicated by previous loss of $\overline{6|}$, and was treated by extraction of $4|4$ and $\overline{4|}$ to achieve better symmetry (Fig. 11.4). Treatment was effective in reducing an overjet of 12 mm and an excessive overbite of 9 mm to produce an acceptable occlusion. A Concorde facebow resulted in flattening of the profile by maxillary retraction, combined with a favourable mandibular advancement. The skeletal correction reduced the convexity from 8 mm before treatment to 3 mm out of retention at age 18.

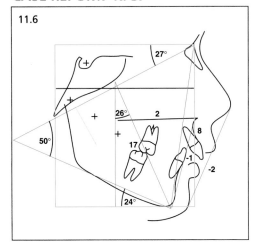

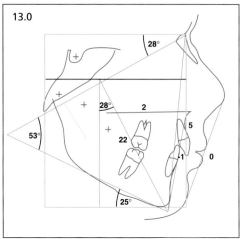

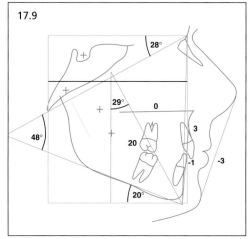

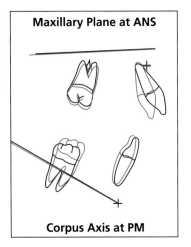

Maxillary Plane at ANS

Corpus Axis at PM

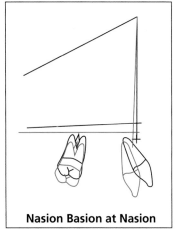

Nasion Basion at Nasion

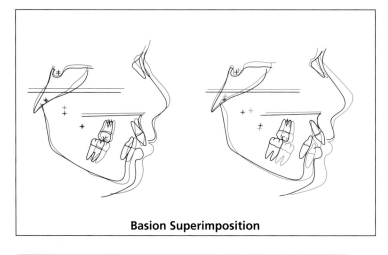

Basion Superimposition

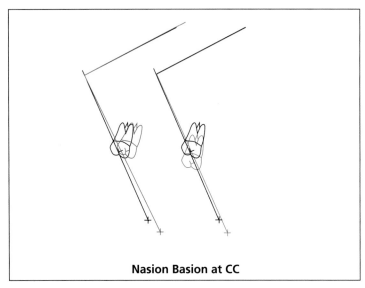

Nasion Basion at CC

K.S.	Age	11.6	13.0	17.9
Cranial Base Angle		27	28	28
Facial Axis Angle		26	28	29
F/M Plane Angle		24	25	20
Craniomandibular Angle		50	53	48
Maxillary Plane		2	2	0
Convexity		8	5	3
U/Incisor to Vertical		32	14	17
L/Incisor to Vertical		26	20	17
Interincisal Angle		122	146	146
6 to Pterygoid Vertical		17	22	20
L/Incisor to A/Po		−1	−1	−1
L/Lip to Aesthetic Plane		−2	0	−3

DIRECTIONAL CONTROL OF ORTHOPAEDIC FORCE

Additional orthopaedic forces may help to control vertical growth by applying an intrusive orthopaedic force to the upper posterior teeth. A high pull headgear is used to apply an intrusive force to the upper molars to resist the vertical component of growth and to reduce the anterior open bite. The Concorde facebow is a unique method of delivering an intrusive force to upper molars and, at the same time, a protrusive force to the mandible and the lower dentition.

The direction of extraoral force is especially important in the treatment of patients with a vertical growth pattern. A vertical orthopaedic force to the upper appliance applies an intrusive force to the upper posterior teeth and palate, and limits downward maxillary growth.

Intrusion of the upper posterior teeth allows the bite to close by a favourable forward rotation of the mandible, and facilitates correction of mandibular retrusion in vertical growth discrepancies.

The addition of traction is optional in reduced overbite cases, and many cases respond well to treatment without traction. Traction is indicated in severe discrepancies with vertical growth which are unfavourable for functional correction. A vertical component of traction force is particularly effective in controlling this type of malocclusion.

The Concorde facebow is adjusted so that it lies just below the level of the upper lip at rest, with the ends of the outer bow sloping slightly upwards above the level of the inner bow. The resulting extraoral traction applies an upward component of force that helps to retain the upper appliance.

This girl presented a severe mandibular retrusion with 10 mm convexity and mild maxillary protrusion. An overjet of 10 mm was perpetuated by a tongue thrust and a tooth apart swallow, resulting in an incomplete overbite. The lower incisors normally erupt into contact with the upper incisors or the soft tissue of the palate, unless they are prevented from doing so by intervening soft tissues or by a thumb or finger sucking habit. Reduced overbite may present as a small separation of the lower incisors from the palate. This is due to an atypical swallowing pattern as the tongue thrusts between the teeth to contact the lower lip to form an anterior oral seal in a 'tooth apart' swallow. The soft-tissue pattern improves when the mandible postures forwards and an anterior seal is formed by closing the lips together over the teeth. The soft tissues adapt quickly to full-time appliance wear as the patient eats with the appliance in the mouth. This produces an effective anterior oral seal, whereby it is more economical for the circumoral muscles to form the seal by lip closure than by lip to tongue contact.

The overjet reduced from 10 mm to 2 mm in 3 months. During this period a slight posterior open bite developed. To maintain an intrusive occlusal force on the posterior teeth, Twin Blocks continued to be worn full time without reducing the occlusal blocks. This helps to resolve an anterior open bite. The Concorde facebow was worn at night for the first 6 months of treatment. During the support phase an anterior inclined plane was designed for retention with the lower incisors occluding on the cingulae of the upper incisors as the buccal teeth settle into occlusion.

The rapid correction occurred in this case mainly by mandibular advancement, and was accompanied by an increase in the upper pharyngeal space from 3 mm to 10 mm after 4 months of treatment.

Twin Blocks and Concorde facebow: 4 months
Support phase: 6 months
Retention: 4 months
Treatment time: 14 months
Final records: 6 years 9 months out of retention
(Figs 11.5, 11.6).

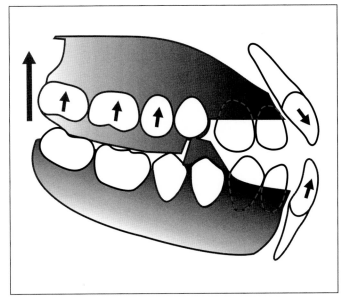

Fig. 11.5 Vertical extraoral traction force to intrude upper posterior teeth.

CASE REPORT: L.G.

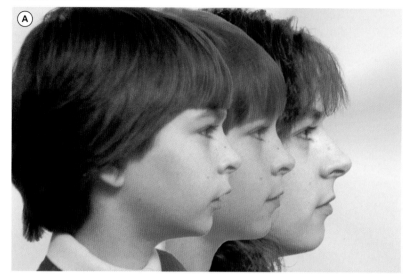

Fig. 11.6 Treatment:
A Profiles at ages 10 years 8 months (before treatment), 10 years 11 months (after 3 months treatment) and 18 years 4 months.
B Occlusion before treatment.
C Twin Blocks.
D Occlusion before treatment.
E–G Occlusion after 3 months of treatment.

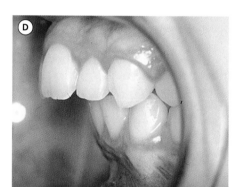

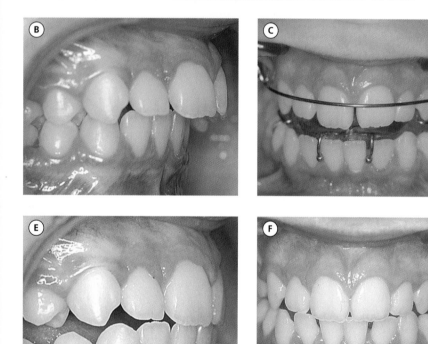

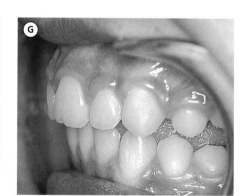

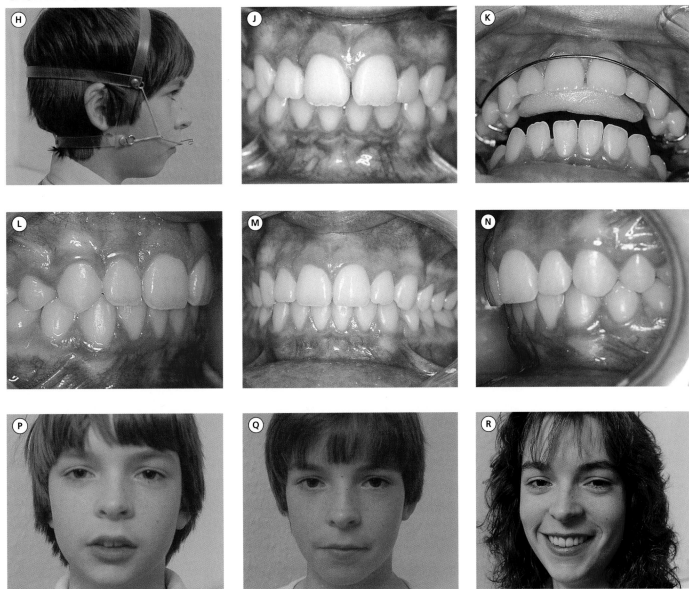

Fig. 11.6 Treatment (cont.):
H Concorde facebow and combination headgear with high pull.
J Occlusion after 9 months of treatment.
K Addition of an anterior inclined plane.
L–N Occlusion at age 11 years 6 months.
P Facial appearance before treatment at age 10 years 8 months.
Q Facial appearance after 3 months of treatment.
R Facial appearance at age 18 years 4 months.

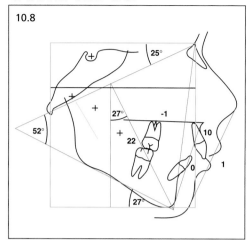

10.8

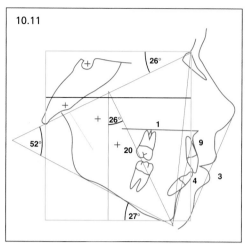

10.11

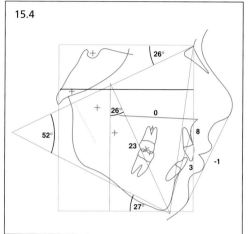

15.4

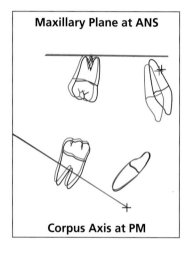

Maxillary Plane at ANS

Corpus Axis at PM

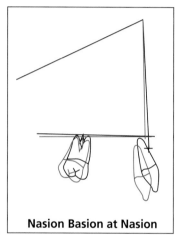

Nasion Basion at Nasion

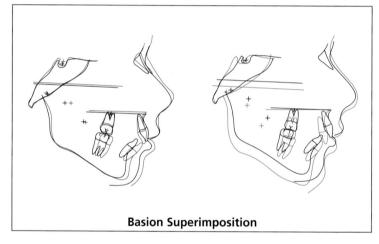

Basion Superimposition

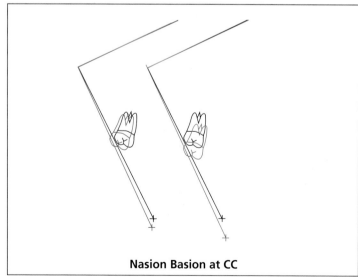

Nasion Basion at CC

L.G.	Age	10.8	10.11	15.4
Cranial Base Angle		25	26	26
Facial Axis Angle		27	26	26
F/M Plane Angle		27	27	27
Craniomandibular Angle		52	52	52
Maxillary Plane		−1	1	0
Convexity		10	9	8
U/Incisor to Vertical		19	18	17
L/Incisor to Vertical		46	47	41
Interincisal Angle		115	115	122
6 to Pterygoid Vertical		22	20	23
L/Incisor to A/Po		0	4	3
L/Lip to Aesthetic Plane		1	3	−1

REFERENCES

Clark, W.J. (1982). The twin-block traction technique. *Eur. J. Orthod.*, **4:** 129–38.

Clark, W.J. (1988). The twin-block technique. *Am. J. Orthod. Dentofac. Orthop.*, **93:** 1–18.

Cousins, A.J.P. & Clark, W.J. (1965). Extra-oral traction. Theoretical considerations and the development of the removable appliance system. *Trans. BSSO*, 29–38.

Orton, H.S. (1990). *Functional Appliances in Orthodontic Treatment*. London, Quintessence.

Treatment of Anterior Open Bite and Vertical Growth Patterns

The anterior open bite is frequently due to a combination of skeletal and soft-tissue factors. A full clinical and cephalometric diagnosis is necessary to establish the aetiology of the problem. This includes evaluation of the airway, which is a factor in achieving lip competence after treatment.

Airway obstruction may be due to enlargement of tonsils or adenoids and should be referred for evaluation or treatment when required. The upper pharyngeal airway is measured from the posterior pharyngeal wall to the outline of the upper half of the soft palate. An upper airway of 12 mm is typical in the mixed dentition. This increases with age to a mean of 17.4 mm in the adult (McNamara & Brudon, 1993). Narrowing of the pharyngeal airway appears to be improved by mandibular advancement during the first few months of Twin Block treatment. Long-term observation after treatment confirms that the increase in upper pharyngeal width is maintained and lip competence is also achieved consistently during Twin Block treatment.

The prognosis for correction of anterior open bite depends on the degree of skeletal and soft-tissue imbalance. In addition, assessment of the direction of facial growth to identify a horizontal or vertical growth tendency helps to establish the prognosis for treatment.

Early treatment is frequently effective in controlling the functional imbalance associated with adverse soft-tissue behaviour patterns. Tongue thrust is often a necessary functional adaptation required to form an effective anterior oral seal by means of tongue contact with a trapped lower lip. This type of tongue thrust is usually adaptive after expanding the maxilla and correcting arch relationships. Learning to eat with Twin Blocks in the mouth encourages the formation of a good lip seal. When the overjet is reduced, a lip seal can be formed more efficiently without the support of the tongue. The oral musculature then adapts accordingly.

A more persistent anterior open bite is related occasionally to a tongue thrust which does not adapt to corrective treatment and can be one of the most difficult orthodontic problems to resolve. This condition is related frequently to a lisp and a habitual forward tongue position, causing a bimaxillary protrusion. Some patients have a pernicious habit of licking the lips, which may be dry and cracked as a result. This is often associated with a tongue thrust and may be difficult to resolve.

Reduced overbite or anterior open bite is often related to unfavourable vertical growth and requires careful management. Throughout treatment, all posterior teeth must remain in occlusal contact with the opposing bite blocks to prevent overeruption. It is important to avoid overeruption of posterior teeth, as this would accentuate the vertical growth tendency and tend to open the bite even more. Intrusion of posterior teeth helps to reduce anterior open bite and encourages a favourable mandibular rotation to close the mandibular plane angle (Fig. 12.1A).

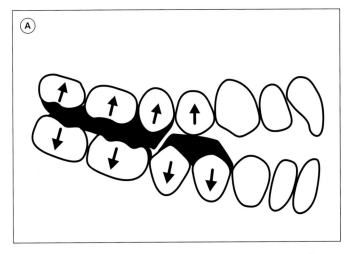

Fig. 12.1 A Maintain occlusal contact to intrude posterior teeth.

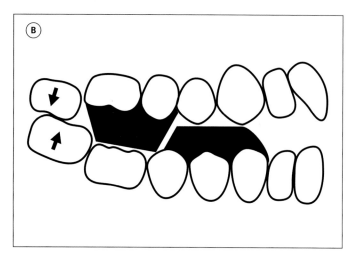

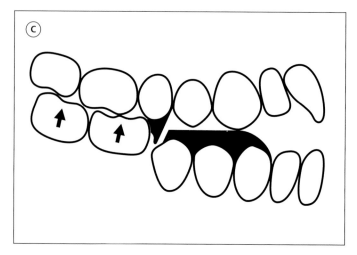

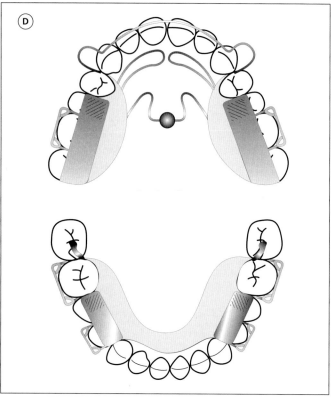

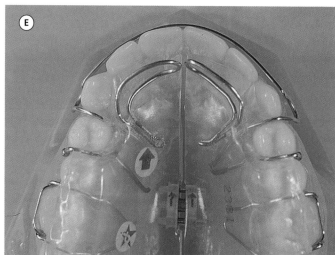

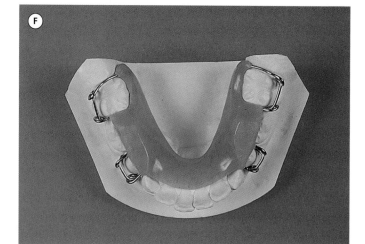

Fig. 12.1 (cont.):
B PITFALL – Do not allow second molars to overerupt. Extend occlusal cover or occlusal rests distally to second molars.
C PITFALL – Do not trim upper block in reduced overbite cases. This increases the anterior open bite.
D Appliance design with spinner.
E Upper appliance with tongue guard (recurved wires).
F Lower appliance with clasps extended to lower molars.

PITFALLS IN TREATMENT OF ANTERIOR OPEN BITE

The worst complications of Twin Block treatment of anterior open bite arise from careless management of the occlusal blocks, by allowing eruption of posterior teeth. This results in an increase in the anterior open bite. Two common mistakes are therefore to be avoided.

First, it is necessary to be attentive to avoid overeruption of second molars behind the appliance (Fig. 12.1B). It is all too easy to make this mistake by failing to check for eruption of second molars at every visit. If the patient attends once every 6 weeks, a lapse of concentration at one visit can allow the second molars to erupt unimpeded for 3 months. Prevention is better than cure for this problem. Attention to appliance design is effective, and if second molars are likely to erupt during treatment it is appropriate to include occlusal rests, even before these teeth erupt, in order to control their eruption.

The second complication is equally damaging. If the upper block is trimmed occlusally in the treatment of anterior open bite this will allow the lower molars to erupt, again propping the bite open and increasing the anterior open bite (Fig. 12.1C). Fortunately, anterior open bite cases are in the minority, but as a result it is easy to become accustomed to trimming the upper block as a matter of routine. To avoid the problem it is strongly suggested that a clear note or colour code is placed on the patient's record card to draw attention to the anterior open bite and as a reminder not to trim the blocks at any stage during treatment.

Patients with anterior open bite and a vertical growth pattern tend to have weak musculature and may have difficulty in consistently maintaining a forward posture to engage the occlusal inclined planes of the bite blocks. They are prone to posture out of the appliance, which reduces the effectiveness in correcting both sagittal and vertical discrepancies. These patients may benefit from phased progressive activation to allow the muscles to adapt more gradually to mandibular advancement. Vertical elastics or attracting magnets can help overcome this problem (see case reports below).

BITE REGISTRATION

It is important to relate the degree of activation to the freedom of movement of the mandible by measuring the protrusive path. The overjet is measured with the mandible retruded and in the position of maximum protrusion. The activation must not exceed 70% of the total protrusive path. It is especially important in vertical growth patterns to ensure that the patient can maintain comfortably the protrusive position and, if necessary, to settle for a lesser amount of initial activation.

The yellow Projet or Exactobite is designed to register a 4 mm interincisal clearance, resulting in approximately 5 mm clearance between the cusps of the first premolars or deciduous molars. It is necessary to accommodate blocks of sufficient thickness between the posterior teeth to open the bite beyond the free-way space so as to intrude the posterior teeth. The objective is to make it difficult for the patient to disengage the blocks. The process of bite registration is similar in other respects to the method described for treatment of deep overbite.

Appliance design: Twin Blocks to close the bite

Appliance design is modified to achieve vertical control and close the anterior open bite. The lower appliance extends distally to the lower molar region with clasps on the lower first molars and occlusal rests on the second molars to prevent their eruption. The acrylic may be trimmed slightly to relieve contact with the lingual surfaces of the upper and lower anterior teeth so that they are free to erupt to reduce the anterior open bite (Fig. 12.1 D–F).

A palatal spinner may be added to the upper appliance to help control an anterior tongue thrust. The spinner is an acrylic bead that is free to rotate round a transpalatal wire positioned in the palate. The objective is to encourage the tongue to curl upwards and backwards instead of thrusting forwards. This is especially effective in younger patients and the spinner should be used as early as possible to control tongue thrust.

A spinner may be incorporated in an upper appliance with a midline screw without interfering with the action of the midline screw to expand the arch. The spinner may be mounted on a piece of steel tubing supported by wires extending from either side of the midline. Alternatively, the spinner may be attached by a wire that extends towards the midline from one side, and is then recurved on itself to retain the spinner in position (Fig. 12.2 A,B).

Young children respond to the suggestion that the spinner is a toy for the tongue to play with. They learn first to spin it with the finger, then with the tongue. Anything that moves in the mouth is irresistible to the tongue. This is a very positive mechanism for controlling tongue thrust by retraining the tongue to move up into the palate rather than thrusting forwards between the teeth.

A tongue guard is a more passive obstruction to discourage the tongue from thrusting forwards against the lingual surfaces of the upper incisors. It is in the form of a recurved wire extending from the premolar region towards the midline and is recurved to its point of attachment. This wire lies in the vertical plane and is clear of the lingual surface of the upper incisors to allow them to settle lingually.

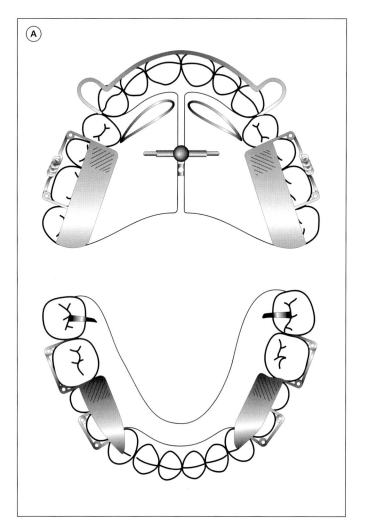

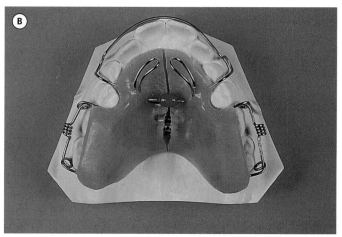

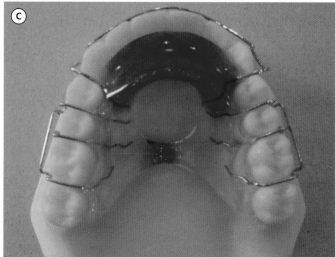

Fig. 12.2 A, B Spinner on tubing. **C** Modified anterior inclined plane with palate-free area to control tongue thrust.

An effective method of controlling tongue thrust is to provide a target area to train the tongue to adopt the correct position in swallowing. The upper appliance may incorporate a hole in the area of the palatal rugae and the tongue is naturally attracted to this area. This may be combined with a shelf to restrict forward movement of the tongue, and with instruction this helps the patient to improve the swallowing pattern. It is necessary to devote a few minutes every day practising with a glass of water to in order to train the tongue to adopt the correct position in the palate during swallowing. The same target area should be continued in the support appliance.

In treatment of anterior open bite a labial bow is usually added to retract the upper incisors if they have been significantly proclined by tongue and lip action. In the treatment of reduced overbite it is essential that no trimming is done on the blocks, and that occlusal contact of the posterior teeth is maintained on the blocks throughout treatment.

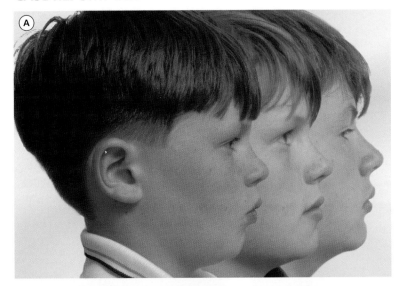

Fig. 12.3 Treatment:
A Profiles at ages 10 years 10 months (before treatment), 11 years 10 months (12 months after treatment) and 13 years 11 months.
B–D Occlusion before treatment.

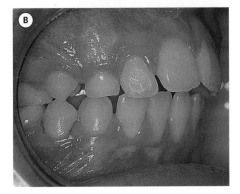

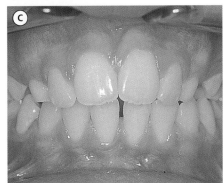

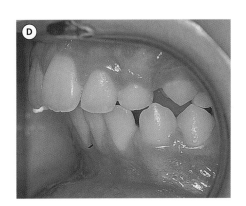

CASE REPORT: D.P. AGED 10 YEARS 10 MONTHS

This boy had a history of thumb sucking and presented an anterior open bite associated with a tongue thrust (Fig. 12.3 A–M). The underlying skeletal pattern was brachyfacial with a convexity of 5 mm and mild mandibular retrusion. The overjet was 10 mm with a full unit distal occlusion.

The overjet reduced from 10 mm to 4 mm after 3 months of treatment, at which stage the appliance was reactivated by the addition of cold cure acrylic to the mesial aspect of the upper block. During the course of treatment the blocks were not trimmed, but were maintained in occlusal contact with all the posterior teeth. This had the effect of intruding the posterior teeth to produce a slight posterior open bite, and allowed a positive overbite to develop anteriorly. The upper pharyngeal space increased from 6 mm to 10 mm.

Twin Blocks: 10 months
Support and retention: 1 year.

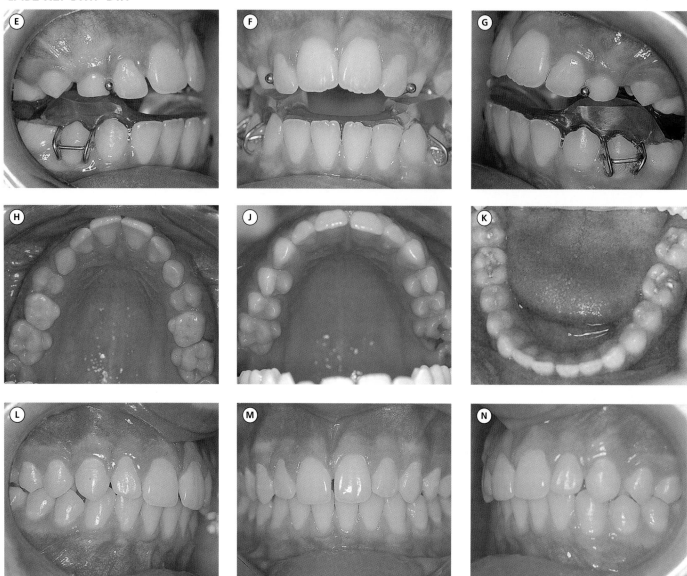

Fig. 12.3 Treatment (cont.):
E–G Twin Blocks.
H Contracted upper arch due to thumbsucking.
J, K Upper and lower archforms after treatment.
L, M Occlusion at age 13 years 11 months.
N Occlusion at age 13 years 11 months.

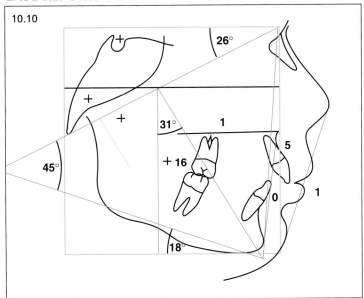

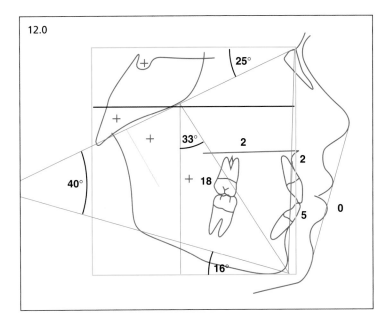

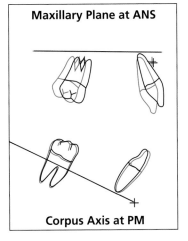

Maxillary Plane at ANS

Corpus Axis at PM

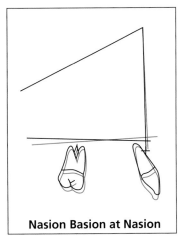

Nasion Basion at Nasion

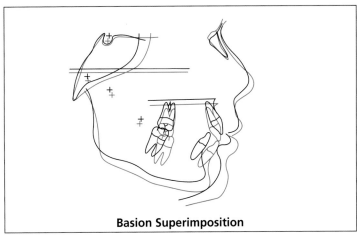

Basion Superimposition

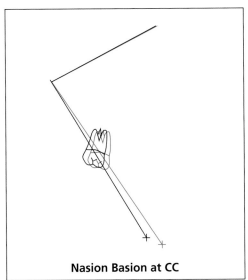

Nasion Basion at CC

D.P.	Age	10.10	12.0
Cranial Base Angle		26	25
Facial Axis Angle		31	33
F/M Plane Angle		18	16
Craniomandibular Angle		45	40
Maxillary Plane		1	2
Convexity		5	2
U/Incisor to Vertical		27	23
L/Incisor to Vertical		37	40
Interincisal Angle		116	117
6 to Pterygoid Vertical		16	18
L/Incisor to A/Po		0	5
L/Lip to Aesthetic Plane		1	0

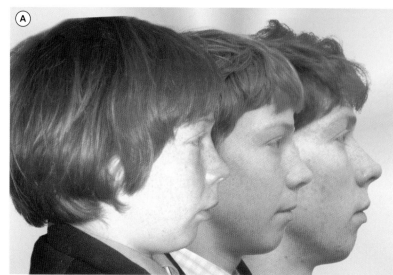

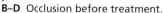

Fig. 12.4 Treatment:
A Profiles at ages 14 years 1 month (before treatment), 14 years 9 months (after 8 months of treatment) and 18 years.
B–D Occlusion before treatment.

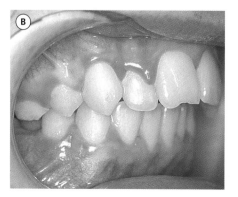

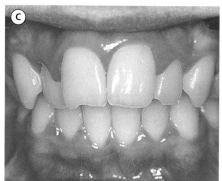

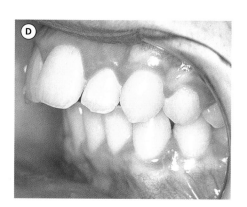

CASE REPORT: S.S. AGED 14 YEARS 1 MONTH

This patient presented a Class II division 1 malocclusion in the permanent dentition with a severe dolichofacial growth pattern, resulting in a severe mandibular retrusion. A convexity of 11 mm and a high mandibular plane angle were associated with an anterior open bite and increased lower facial height. Vertical control was achieved by the Twin Block, followed by retention with a bionator to close the open bite (Fig. 12.4). The upper pharyngeal space increased from 9 mm to 14 mm during treatment.

The Twin Block achieves a more rapid response in the active phase to correct the anteroposterior arch relationships. During this period the patient enjoys the freedom of wearing a less restricting two-piece appliance, with better speech and less interference with normal function.

This is followed by a short period of day- and night-time

wear of the bionator, to encourage closure of the anterior open bite by preventing the tongue from resting between the teeth. The bionator continues as a retainer with a favourable functional component. This approach observes the principle of using a functional retainer that supports the objectives of treatment.

Twin Blocks: 5 months
Bionator: 4 months full time, 12 months night time.

This patient has a severe vertical growth pattern which is still present after treatment. This limits the improvement that can be achieved in the facial profile. The dental relationship is corrected to class I, however, and a further improvement could be achieved by a genioplasty, which is a simpler approach than major surgical correction involving both the maxilla and the mandible.

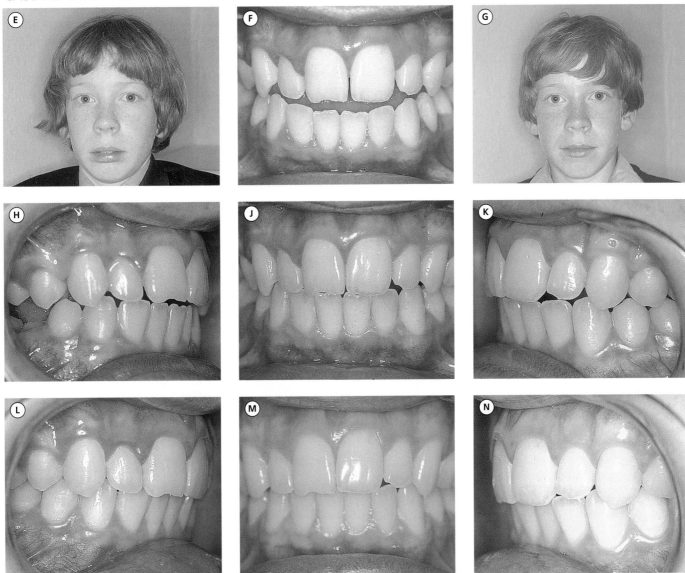

Fig. 12.4 Treatment (cont.):
E Facial appearance before treatment at age 14 years 1 month.
F, G Facial appearance and occlusion after 4 months of treatment at age 14 years 5 months.
H–K Occlusion after 8 months of treatment at age 14 years 9 months.
L–N Occlusion out of retention at age 18 years.

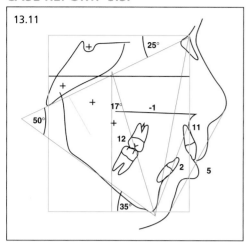

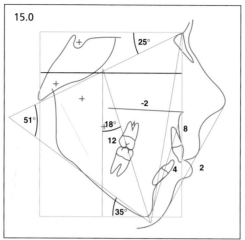

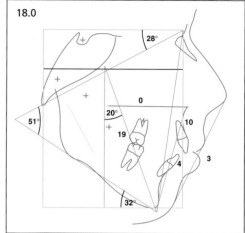

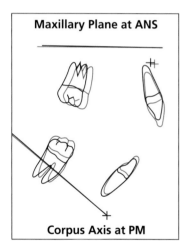

Maxillary Plane at ANS

Corpus Axis at PM

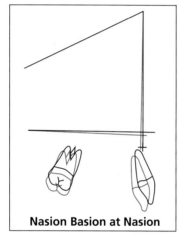

Nasion Basion at Nasion

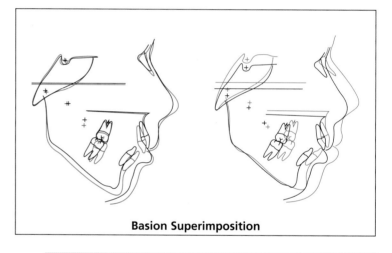

Basion Superimposition

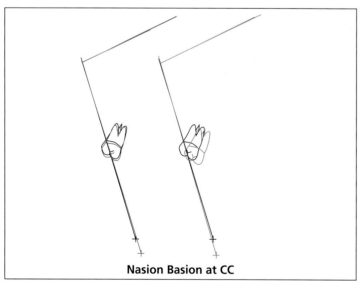

Nasion Basion at CC

S.S.	Age	13.11	15.0	18.0
Cranial Base Angle		25	25	28
Facial Axis Angle		17	18	20
F/M Plane Angle		35	35	32
Craniomandibular Angle		50	51	51
Maxillary Plane		−1	−2	0
Convexity		11	8	10
U/Incisor to Vertical		16	13	16
L/Incisor to Vertical		43	42	45
Interincisal Angle		121	125	119
6 to Pterygoid Vertical		12	12	19
L/Incisor to A/Po		2	4	4
L/Lip to Aesthetic Plane		5	2	3

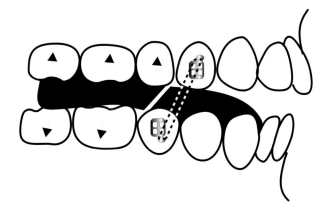

Fig. 12.5 Intraoral traction to close anterior open bite.

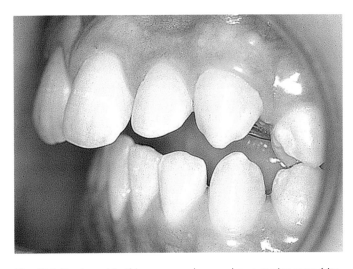

Fig. 12.6 Treatment in this case was slow, and an anterior open bite persisted because the patient did not close consistently into the blocks.

INTRAORAL TRACTION TO CLOSE ANTERIOR OPEN BITE

Intraoral elastics may be used to accelerate bite closure as an efficient alternative to high-pull extraoral traction. This simple mechanism is very effective in closing anterior open bites. The method was brought to the author's attention by Dr Christine Mills who first used the system in orthodontic practice in Vancouver. Vertical elastics were first applied to help patients maintain occlusal contact on the appliances overnight. The author observed at a study group in Vancouver that the elastics had the additional benefit of closing the bite (Fig. 12.5).

The intrusive effect of the bite blocks is reinforced by running a vertical elastic between upper and lower teeth on both sides. Elastics may be attached directly to the upper and lower appliances or to brackets or bands with gingival hooks. An effective vector is produced by passing an elastic from between the brackets on the upper first deciduous molar and lower second deciduous molar (or the upper first and lower second premolars). The elastics are worn at night to maintain occlusal contact of the posterior teeth on the bite blocks to intrude posterior teeth. All posterior teeth must contact the occlusal blocks to prevent eruption and to deliver intrusive forces.

To maximise the effects of elastic traction, the elastics may be worn full time. It is important that the construction bite should open the bite beyond the rest position to ensure that the patient cannot comfortably posture out of the blocks.

Intraoral vertical elastics have the additional advantage of increasing occlusal contact on the inclined planes. This is an important factor in patients who have weak musculature and do not occlude positively on the occlusal inclined planes. These are generally patients with a vertical growth pattern who do not respond well to functional therapy, because their

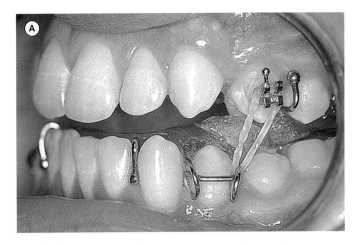

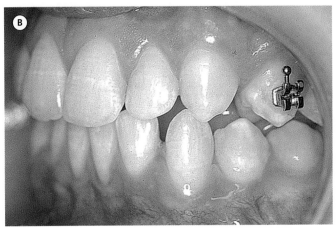

Fig. 12.7 A Intraoral vertical elastics to intrude posterior teeth. When vertical elastics were added an immediate improvement in response was noted.
B The anterior open bite reduced and the overjet and distal occlusion corrected.

potential for horizontal growth is poor. The addition of a mechanical component of elastic traction is effective in improving the response to treatment by assisting muscle action in maintaining contact on the occlusal inclined planes. The elastics worn in this manner were light and passive as long as the jaws were closed properly into the appliance. However, as soon as the patient's mandible dropped open, the elastics were stretched, which in turn caused the appliance to become dislodged from either the upper or the lower dentition. The patient was thus reminded of the importance of keeping the mandible closed in the proper forward position while sleeping. This helps by intruding the posterior teeth and also accelerates the correction of distal occlusion (Figs 12.6, 12.7 A,B). This is particularly important in patients with restricted airways due to enlarged tonsils and adenoids as well as in those patients with chronic nasal congestion due to allergies or sinus problems. Such patients tend to sleep with the mouth open and this in turn

favours vertical growth of the jaws as well as excessive eruption of the dentition.

VERTICAL ELASTICS TO CORRECT ANTERIOR OPEN BITE

This patient failed to respond to Twin Block treatment and the position after 9 months showed an anterior open bite with contact only on the first permanent molars. No adjustment was made to the appliance, except that the patient was instructed to wear vertical intra-oral elastics, which passed from clasps on the lower premolars to the loop of the labial bow on the upper appliance.

This had the immediate effect of improving progress, and treatment was completed successfully within a further 6 months. The occlusion proved to be stable out of retention for a patient who did not initially respond to treatment.

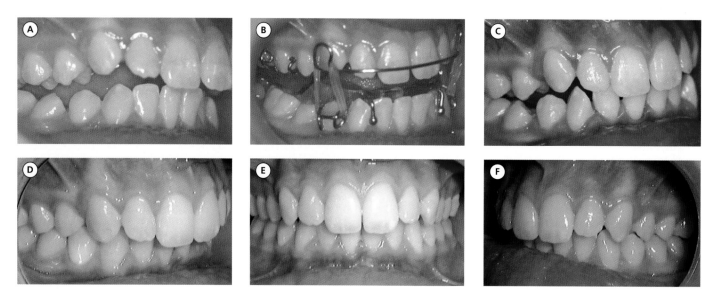

Fig. 12.8:
A Occlusion with anterior open bite is not responding after 9 months treatment.
B Vertical elastics added to accelerate correction.
C Progress improved after 4 months with vertical elastics.
D–F The occlusion is stable out of retention.

CASE REPORT: B.G.

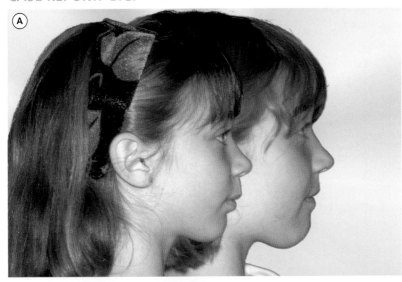

Fig. 12.9 Case records show the progress during treatment of this severe malocclusion:
A Profiles at ages 8 years 1 month (before treatment) and 8 years 9 months (after treatment).
B–D Occlusion before treatment.
E–G Occlusion after treatment.

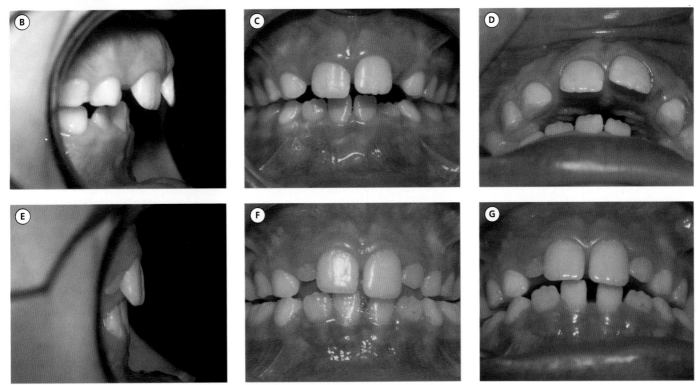

The following patients were treated by Dr Christine Mills in her orthodontic practice in Vancouver. The addition of vertical intra-oral elastics is a significant factor in the favourable changes observed in these patients. The elastics were worn only at night.

CASE REPORT: B.G. AGED 8 YEARS 1 MONTH

This girl has a retrognathic profile (SNA = 76°) and a facial axis angle of 15°, indicating an extreme vertical growth pattern. An anterior open bite relates to the skeletal pattern and vertical growth. After 8 months of treatment with Twin Blocks the facial axis angle has improved to 18° as a result of forward mandibular translation, and the ANB angle is reduced from 8° to 5°. Mandibular superimposition clearly shows that the angulation of condylar growth is in a distal direction, thus contributing to the forward mandibular rotation. This is a very favourable response in a patient with a difficult growth pattern. The improvement is reflected in the facial profile (Fig. 12.9).

8.1

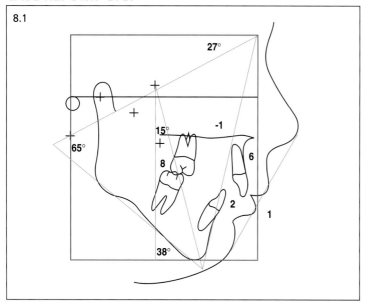

8.9

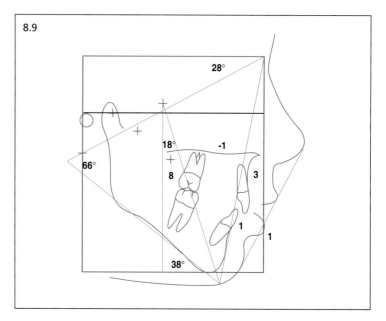

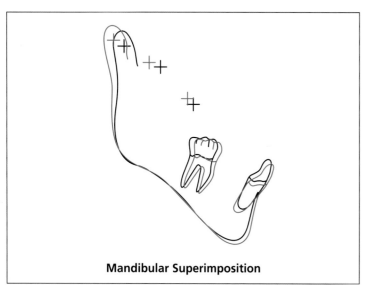

Mandibular Superimposition

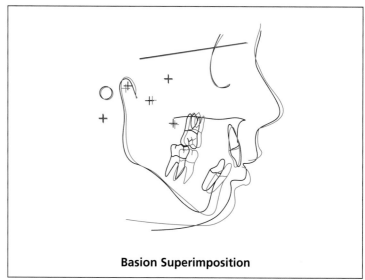

Basion Superimposition

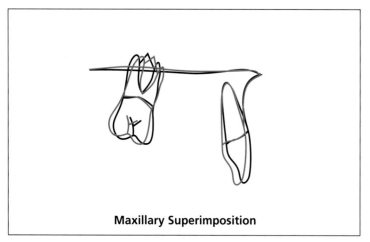

Maxillary Superimposition

B.G.	Age	8.1	8.9
Cranial Base Angle		27	28
Facial Axis Angle		15	18
F/M Plane Angle		38	38
Craniomandibular Angle		65	66
Maxillary Plane		−1	−1
Convexity		6	3
U/Incisor to Vertical		10	5
L/Incisor to Vertical		33	37
L/Incisor to A/Po		2	1
L/Lip to Aesthetic Plane		1	1
6 to Pterygoid vertical		8	8

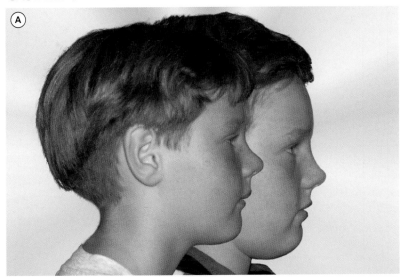

Fig. 12.10 Treatment:
A Profiles at ages 9 years 8 months (before treatment) and 10 years 9 months (after treatment).
B–D Occlusion before treatment.
E–G Occlusion after treatment.

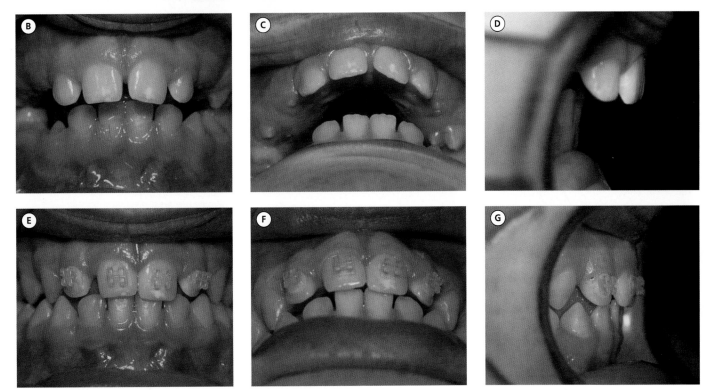

CASE REPORT: C.R. AGED 9 YEARS 8 MONTHS

by Christine Mills

This patient presents a substantial open bite and excessive overjet in mixed dentition, which can prove difficult to manage. Treatment is successful in correcting the open bite, reducing the overjet and correcting the distal occlusion. The ANB angle reduces from 5° to 1° and the anterior open bite is closed after 1 year of treatment (Fig. 12.10).

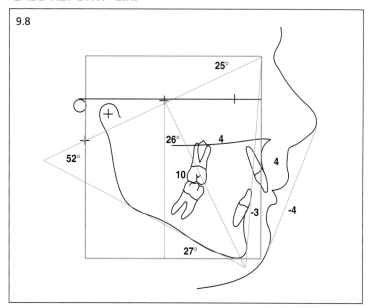

9.8

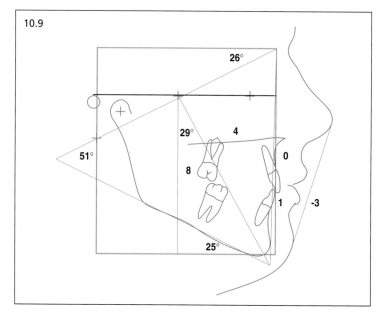

10.9

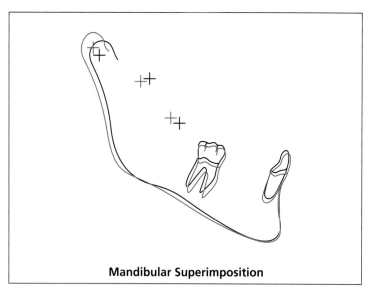

Mandibular Superimposition

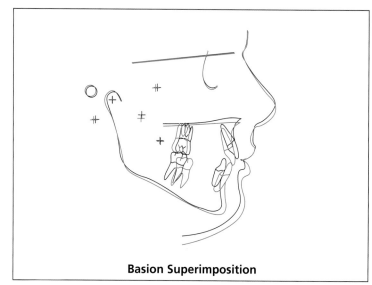

Basion Superimposition

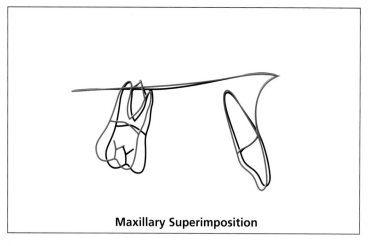

Maxillary Superimposition

C.R. Age	9.8	10.9
Cranial Base Angle	25	26
Facial Axis Angle	28	29
F/M Plane Angle	27	25
Craniomandibular Angle	52	51
Maxillary Plane	4	4
Convexity	3	0
U/Incisor to Vertical	26	20
L/Incisor to Vertical	23	26
L/Incisor to A/Po	–3	1
L/Lip to Aesthetic Plane	–4	–3
6 to Pterygoid vertical	10	8

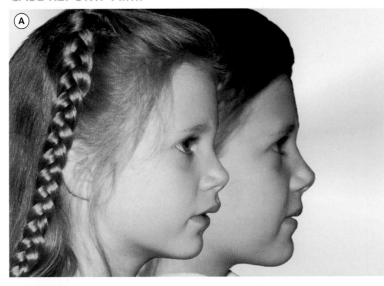

(A)

Fig. 12.11 Case records show the progress during treatment of this severe malocclusion:
A Profiles at ages 8 years 8 months (before treatment) and 9 years 4 months (after treatment).
B–E Occlusion before treatment.
F, G Occlusion after treatment.

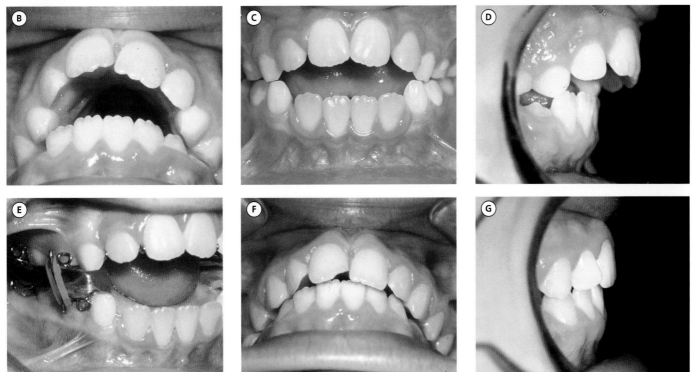

CASE REPORT: A.M. AGED 8 YEARS 8 MONTHS

by Christine Mills

A severe vertical growth pattern is related in this case to an anterior open bite with an extreme facial axis angle of 16° and a mandibular plane angle of 38°. This pattern would normally present a very poor prognosis for functional correction, but responded favourably to Twin Block treatment. The overjet of 10 mm was reduced to 2 mm after 8 months' treatment and within the same time frame the open bite was completely resolved. Favourable skeletal changes are confirmed by an increase in the facial axis angle from 16° to 20°, while the mandibular plane angle reduced from 38° to 35°. The primary factor in successful treatment can be attributed to intrusion of the upper molars, which in turn allowed the mandible to rotate forward, accounting for a reduction in the ANB angle by 4.7°.

These are exceptional skeletal changes in a short period of time, allowing this difficult malocclusion to be corrected by simple treatment. In aesthetic terms there is a significant improvement in facial appearance (Fig. 12.11).

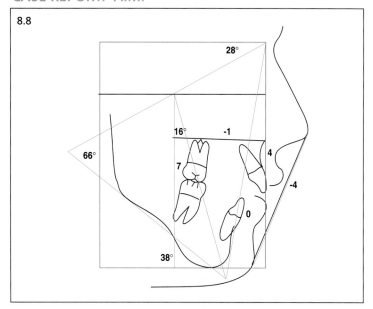

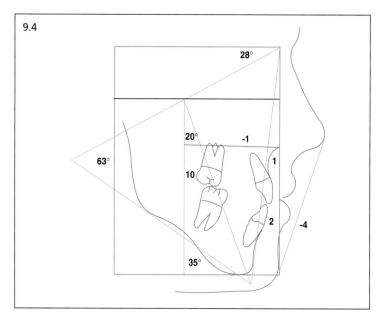

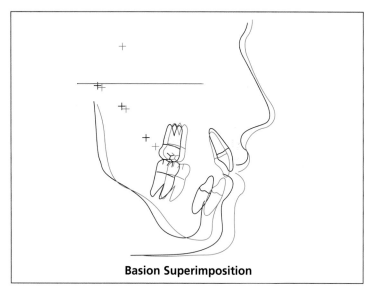

Basion Superimposition

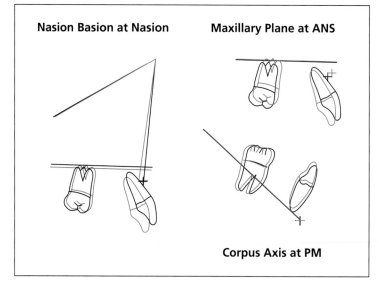

Nasion Basion at Nasion

Maxillary Plane at ANS

Corpus Axis at PM

A.M.	Age	8.8	9.4
Cranial Base Angle		28	28
Facial Axis Angle		16	20
F/M Plane Angle		38	35
Craniomandibular Angle		66	63
Maxillary Plane		−1	−1
Convexity		4	1
U/Incisor to Vertical		27	20
L/Incisor to Vertical		28	25
L/Incisor to A/Po		0	2
L/Lip to Aesthetic Plane		−4	−5
6 to Pterygoid vertical		7	10

CASE REPORT: M.S.

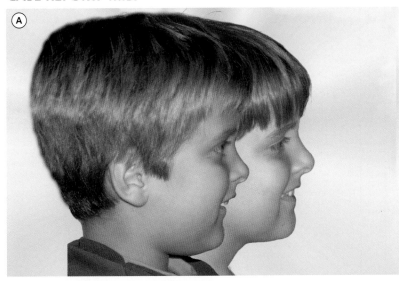

Fig. 12.12 Treatment:
A Profiles at ages 10 years 0 months (before treatment) and 11 years 1 month (after treatment).
B Occlusion before treatment.
C Occlusion after treatment.
D Occlusion before treatment.
E Appearance after treatment.

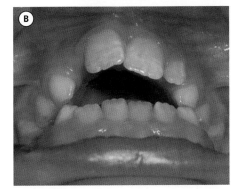

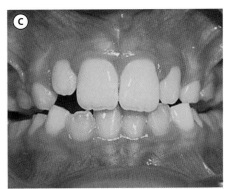

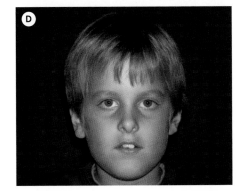

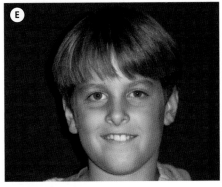

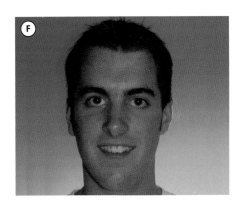

CASE REPORT: M.S. AGED 10 YEARS

by Christine Mills

Vertical growth is again associated with an anterior open bite due to a facial axis angle of 22°. After 1 year of treatment the ANB angle is reduced from 6° to 2°, the open bite is closed with positive improvements in archform, occlusion and facial appearance (Fig. 12.12). Functional retention is important in mixed dentition treatment, for example using an occluso-guide. This can be followed by a short period with fixed appliances to complete.

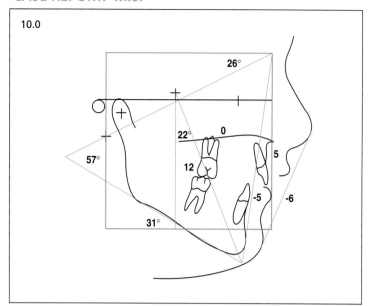

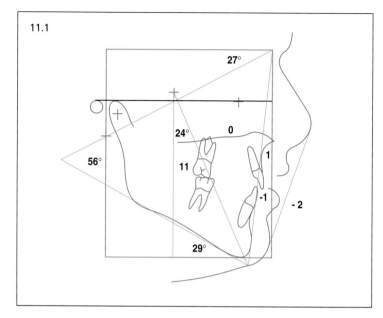

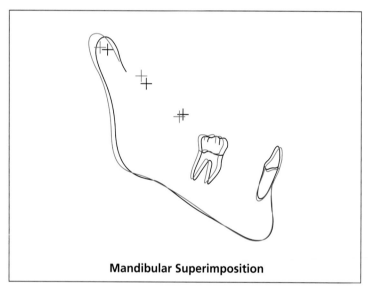

Mandibular Superimposition

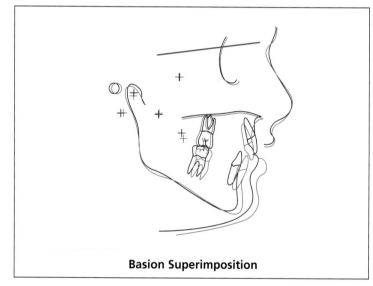

Basion Superimposition

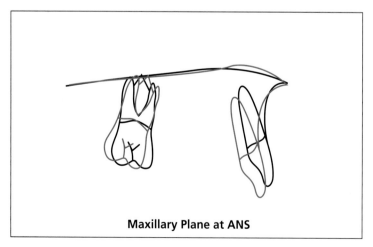

Maxillary Plane at ANS

M.S. Age	10.0	11.1
Cranial Base Angle	26	27
Facial Axis Angle	22	24
F/M Plane Angle	31	29
Craniomandibular Angle	57	56
Maxillary Plane	0	0
Convexity	5	1
U/Incisor to Vertical	14	17
L/Incisor to Vertical	19	24
L/Incisor to A/Po	−5	−1
L/Lip to Aesthetic Plane	−6	−2
6 to Pterygoid vertical	12	11

TREATMENT OF VERTICAL GROWTH

CASE REPORT: H.D. AGED 12 YEARS 2 MONTHS

This patient presented a severe dolichofacial growth pattern and was past the adolescent or pubertal growth spurt at the start of treatment. Convexity was 9 mm due to severe mandibular retrusion with an increased mandibular plane

CASE REPORT: H.D.

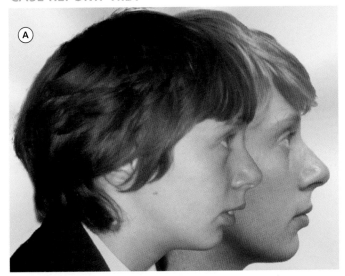

angle of 28°. As a result the response to treatment was slower than normal due to a limited growth response combined with the vertical direction of growth (facial axis angle = 24°). The overjet was 14 mm with excessive overbite and the lower incisors were 4 mm lingual to the A–Po line. The Concorde facebow was used to accelerate the response to treatment (Fig. 12.13 A–F).

Clinical management

The Twin Blocks were made with occlusal contact on all posterior teeth to apply an intrusive force to minimise vertical growth. No trimming was done on the blocks. The Concorde facebow was worn intermittently at night for the first 5 months to maintain a forward component of force on the mandible via the horizontal labial elastic.

Twin Blocks: 12 months
Support and retention: 12 months.

An alternative approach to consider when a deep overbite is associated with a vertical growth pattern would be to level and align the lower arch with a fixed appliance, so as to reduce the overbite before the Twin Block stage. The mandible may then be advanced with a smaller vertical component of activation in order to reduce the vertical component of growth during treatment.

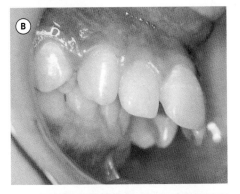

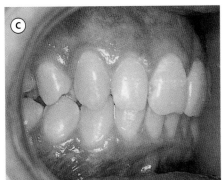

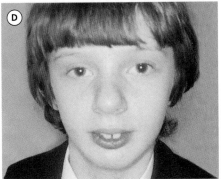

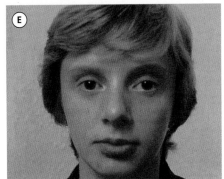

Fig. 12.13 Treatment:
A Profiles at ages 12 years 2 months (before treatment) and 15 years 7 months (after treatment).
B, C Occlusal change at age 12 years 2 months and 15 years 1 month.
D Facial appearance before treatment at age 12 years 2 months.
E Facial appearance at age 15 years 7 months.

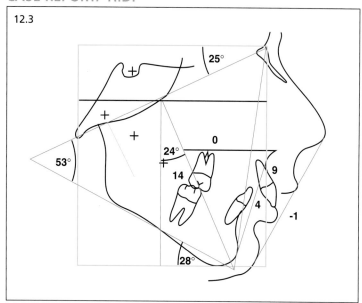

12.3

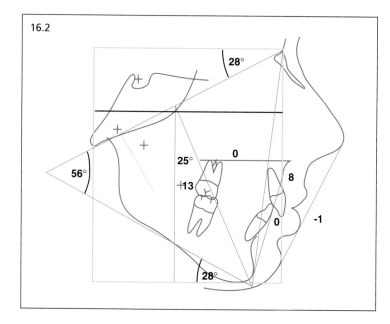

16.2

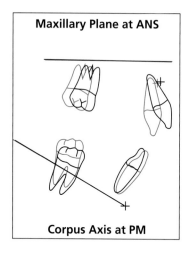

Maxillary Plane at ANS

Corpus Axis at PM

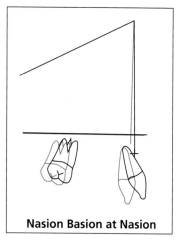

Nasion Basion at Nasion

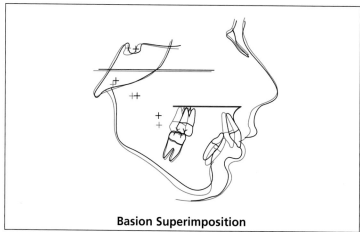

Basion Superimposition

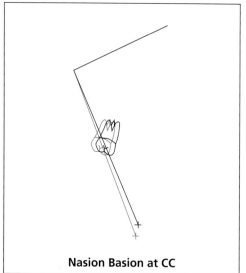

Nasion Basion at CC

H.D.	Age	12.3	16.2
Cranial Base Angle		25	28
Facial Axis Angle		24	25
F/M Plane Angle		28	28
Craniomandibular Angle		53	56
Maxillary Plane		0	0
Convexity		9	8
U/Incisor to Vertical		22	8
L/Incisor to Vertical		24	36
Interincisal Angle		134	134
6 to Pterygoid Vertical		14	13
L/Incisor to A/Po		4	0
L/Lip to Aesthetic Plane		−1	−1

CASE REPORT: L.J. AGED 9 YEARS 10 MONTHS

An example of the response to treatment in a girl with a dolichofacial growth pattern. An overjet of 11 mm, associated with convexity of 8 mm, is mainly due to maxillary protrusion, with moderate mandibular retrusion. The Concorde facebow was therefore used to assist correction. The Frankfort mandibular plane angle is 29° and the maxillary plane has an upward cant of 5° resulting in increased lower facial height and a maxillo-mandibular plane angle of 34° (Fig. 12.14).

Clinical management

The Twin Blocks were made with occlusal contact on all posterior teeth to apply an intrusive force to minimise vertical growth. The response to treatment was slow in this case, because the patient did not appear to posture her mandible consistently forward on the inclined planes. This was probably related to weak musculature associated with vertical growth. The overjet and distal occlusion were corrected within a year and support and retention with an anterior inclined plane produced a satisfactory result which was stable 5 years out of retention.

Twin Blocks: 12 months
Support: 3 months
Retention: 1 year.

CASE REPORT: L.J.

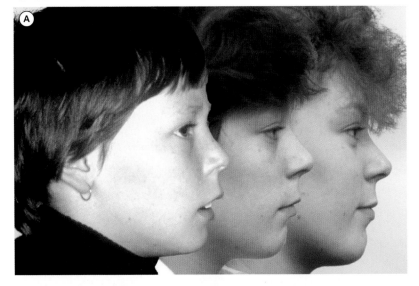
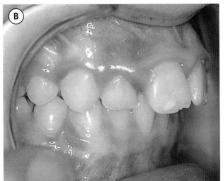
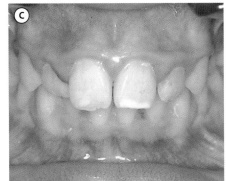
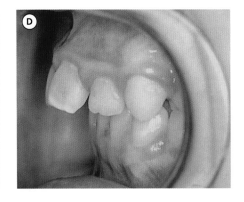

Fig. 12.14 Treatment:
A Profiles at ages 9 years 11 months (before treatment), 14 years (1 year 10 months out of retention) and 16 years 10 months).
B–D Occlusion before treatment.

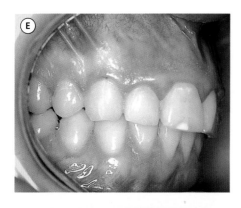

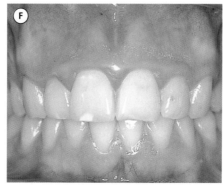

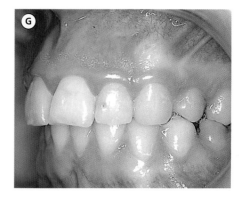

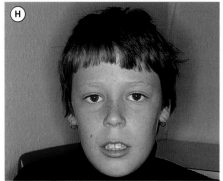

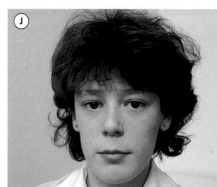

Fig. 12.14 Treatment (cont.):
E–G Occlusion 5 years out of retention.
H, J Facial appearance before and after treatment.

Magnetic force

Magnetic force is an alternative method of increasing forces for intrusion of opposing posterior teeth by incorporating magnets in the inclined planes on the posterior bite blocks. Either attracting or repelling magnets may be used and both are effective. Repelling magnets increase the opposing forces in the occlusal bite blocks to intrude opposing teeth. This principle has been investigated by Dellinger (1986).

Attracting magnets increase the frequency of occlusal contacts on the inclined planes. Occlusal forces are the activating mechanism of Twin Blocks and increasing the forces of occlusion is effective in accelerating both anteroposterior and vertical correction. The application of magnets in Twin Block treatment is discussed further in Chapter 19.

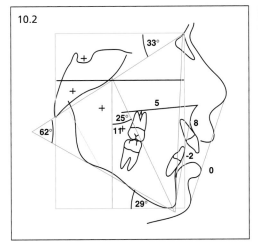

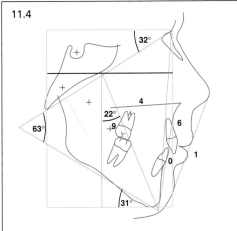

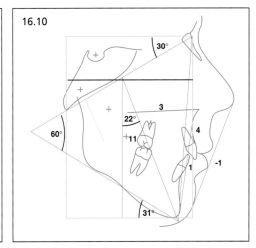

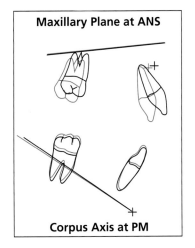

Maxillary Plane at ANS

Corpus Axis at PM

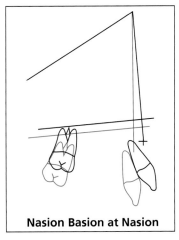

Nasion Basion at Nasion

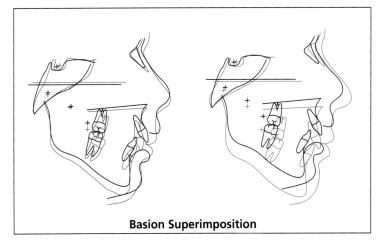

Basion Superimposition

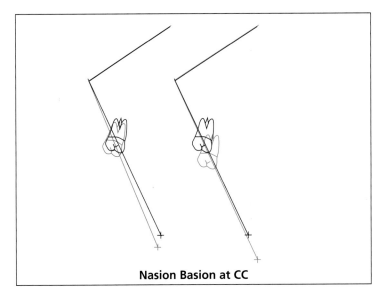

Nasion Basion at CC

L.J.	Age	10.2	11.4	16.10
Cranial Base Angle		33	32	30
Facial Axis Angle		25	22	22
F/M Plane Angle		29	31	31
Craniomandibular Angle		62	63	60
Maxillary Plane		5	4	3
Convexity		8	6	4
U/Incisor to Vertical		28	11	23
L/Incisor to Vertical		31	30	32
Interincisal Angle		121	139	123
6 to Pterygoid Vertical		11	9	11
L/Incisor to A/Po		−2	0	1
L/Lip to Aesthetic Plane		0	1	−1

RESPONSE TO TREATMENT OF ANTERIOR OPEN BITE

by Christine Mills with reference to a thesis by Colleen Adams

Introduction

Invariably, when outstanding clinical results are demonstrated with functional appliances, sceptics in the profession suggest that these results are more likely the result of a 'good growth pattern' than the therapeutic effect of the appliance itself. Detractors argue that the Class II skeletal correction was more a matter of luck than of actual treatment effect.

The real litmus test of functional appliance therapy comes with the severe skeletal Class II patient who has a vertical growth pattern and an anterior open bite. These are cases that orthodontists tend to view as their greatest challenge. Luck with the growth pattern rarely enters into the equation when correcting these patients.

When such an unfavourable skeletal pattern is encountered in an adult patient, it is expedient to enlist the services of a good oral surgeon. However, in the case of an 8-year-old child with a Class II open bite, the decision is not so straightforward. Should one wait 8–10 years to correct the patient surgically with methods that are somewhat invasive but nevertheless predictable and effective? Or is it reasonable to attempt growth modification at a much earlier age to achieve the correction of the malocclusion? If you choose to treat early, are vertical growers less likely to respond well to treatment than those with horizontal growth patterns?

Some light has been shed on this subject by the findings of Dr Colleen Adams in her Master's thesis research at the University of Alberta in Edmonton, Canada (Adams 2000). Dr Adams investigated the role played by the Twin Block appliance in controlling the vertical dimension during Class II treatment, and she has attempted to clarify the relationship between changes in the vertical dimension and the anteroposterior correction achieved during Twin Block therapy.

Methods and materials

In order to test the efficacy of the Twin Block appliance, eight of the most vertical growers with anterior open bite malocclusions were selected from a group of 59 consecutively treated severe Class II Twin Block patients from the private practice of the author. The combination of a severe Class II skeletal pattern and an unfavourable vertical growth pattern in these patients created a challenge for orthodontic treatment. All of the patients were in the mixed dentition stage of development.

A matched control group was obtained from the Bolton–Brush growth study to achieve the best possible match based on age, sex, severity of the Class II relation and vertical skeletal indicators.

It was found that there was a high degree of matching of the vertical indicators with no significant differences between the treatment and control groups. When the Class II indicators were compared, there were no significant differences in the ANB angles, although there was a trend for higher ANB angles in the treatment groups as compared to the control groups.

Measurements

A constructed grid as described by Mamandras & Allen (1990) was incorporated into the customised computer analysis to assess various linear and angular measurements. A horizontal reference plane was constructed through sella at an angle of 8° below sella–nasion to be used as an X-axis for measuring vertical changes in various skeletal landmarks. A perpendicular plane through sella served as the Y-axis for measuring anteroposterior changes of the various anatomic structures.

Summary and conclusions

The fact that the treatment group in this study had more significant Class II discrepancies than even the most severe cases available from the Bolton–Brush growth study is an important consideration. It may be that the treatment group and the control groups would have grown differently because of this pre-treatment disparity. Nevertheless, the Twin Block appliance was effective in achieving correction of these difficult Class II open bite malocclusions. The Twin Block's ability to control the vertical dimension by inhibiting molar eruption was helpful in preventing any increase in the mandibular plane angle as the mandible grew forward.

While there was no apparent withholding effect on the maxilla, there was a substantial forward growth effect on the mandible. When the SNA angles were compared, there were no significant differences in the changes experienced between T1 and T2 for the two groups. Both showed decreases in angle SNA (0.6° for the Twin Block group and 0.4° for the controls). With angle SNB, there was a statistically significant difference ($P = 0.004$) with this angle increasing 2.2° in the treatment group as compared to an increase of only 0.1° in the controls. The above changes in turn resulted in a decrease in angle ANB in the treatment group by 2.8° as compared to a decrease of 0.5° in the controls ($P = 0.005$).

The 6.7 mm overjet correction in the Twin Block group can be attributed to a combination of three factors:

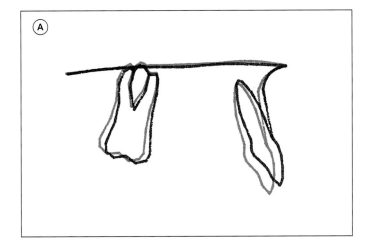

Fig. 12.15 Superimposition of composite tracing, for vertical growth pattern, open bite patients treated with Twin Blocks.
A Maxilla.
B Mandible.
C Superimposition on anterior cranial base. T_1-T_2 = 12.6 months.

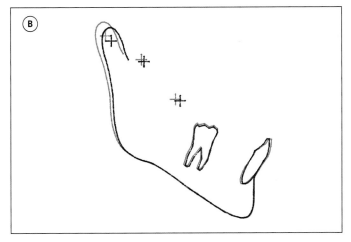

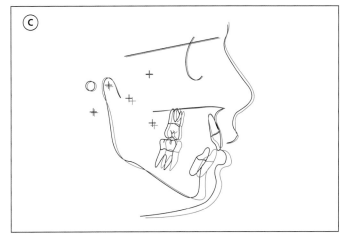

1. Forward mandibular growth (4.1 mm).
2. Forward tipping of the lower incisors (0.8 mm).
3. Lingual tipping of the upper incisors (1.8 mm).

Although the sample size is small and the results must therefore be interpreted with caution, nevertheless the trends displayed in this study indicate a very favourable treatment response with the Twin Block appliance in these Class II open bite patients with vertical growth patterns (Fig. 12.15).

The author (Dr Mills) does however recommend long-term retention of these types of patients by using the Twin Block for night wear so that the original unfavourable vertical growth pattern is not re-expressed following the Phase I correction. In addition, airway problems, mouth breathing habits and abnormal tongue function should be addressed early in treatment in order to minimise the risk of post-treatment instability. In those patients where the primary aetiological factor in the malocclusion is an unfavourable hereditary growth pattern, the Twin Block can correct the symptom but not eliminate the cause. Until a method of genetically reprogramming the growth pattern becomes available, functional appliance treatment and orthognathic surgery will continue to be our most viable treatment options.

REFERENCES

Adams, C. (2000). The Twin Block Appliance: a cephalometric analysis of vertical control. Master thesis, University of Alberta, Edmonton, Canada.

Dellinger, E.L. (1986). A clinical assessment of the active vertical corrector, a non-surgical alternative for skeletal open bite treatment. *Am. J. Orthod.*, **89**: 428–36.

McNamara, Jr, J.A. & Brudon, W.L. (1993). *Orthodontic and Orthopedic Treatment in the Mixed Dentition*. Ann Arbor, Needham Press.

Mamandras, A.H. & Allen, L.P. (1990). Mandibular response to the bionator appliance. *Am. J. Orthod. Dentofac. Orthop.*, **97**:113–120.

CHAPTER 13

Treatment of Class II Division 2 Malocclusion

Retroclined upper incisors are responsible for holding the mandible in a distal position in Angle's Class II division 2 malocclusion. Twin Blocks have the effect of unlocking the malocclusion by releasing the mandible from an entrapped position of distal occlusion and thereby encouraging a rapid transition to Class I arch relationship.

Correction of Class II division 2 malocclusion is achieved by releasing the mandible downwards and forwards and encouraging the lower molars to erupt. At the same time, the upper incisors are advanced to achieve a normal upper to lower incisor relationship that is cleared far enough forwards to accommodate the progressively advancing mandibular arc of closure (Fig. 13.1).

The upper lateral incisors are frequently proclined and rotated in this malocclusion and functional correction of the distal occlusion is followed by a finishing stage with fixed appliances to correct incisor rotations and detail the occlusion. Brackets may be fitted on the upper anterior teeth during the Twin Block stage and this is effective in shortening the period of treatment, resulting in an easy transition into fixed appliances.

BITE REGISTRATION

The construction bite in Class II division 2 malocclusion is registered with the incisors in edge-to-edge occlusion. When the overbite is excessive, the clearance between the posterior teeth is correspondingly increased. These patients require more vertical development, so that the occlusal bite blocks tend to be thicker in the premolar region to allow clearance of the upper and lower incisors.

Harvold demonstrated that control of vertical development allows the correction of a Class II molar relationship to Class I by manipulation of the functional occlusal plane. An occlusal table is used to inhibit the eruption of upper molars while the mandibular buccal

segments are allowed to erupt vertically in harmony with vertical growth of the lower face.

Vertical development is the primary factor in correction of the Class II division 2 malocclusion, with minimum advancement of the mandible. The overjet is frequently normal, or may be reduced, and the construction bite is registered with the incisors in edge-to-edge occlusion.

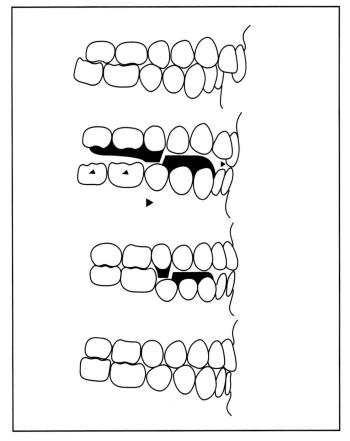

Fig. 13.1 Management of Class II division 2.

The amount of mandibular advancement is limited in Class II division 2 malocclusion as this malocclusion is normally associated with a mild Class II skeletal relationship with a horizontal growth pattern and a well-developed chin. It is important in treating this malocclusion not to overcorrect the mandibular position which would result in a 'dished in' or Class III profile.

APPLIANCE DESIGN: TWIN BLOCK SAGITTAL APPLIANCE

Sagittal development

In the treatment of Class II division 2 malocclusion, sagittal arch development is necessary to increase arch length and to advance retroclined incisors.

Sagittal appliances were formerly used in anteroposterior development of archform (Witzig & Spahl, 1987) as an initial stage of treatment to improve archform before functional correction of arch-to-arch relationships. The distalisation of the posterior quadrants is about 20–25% of the total arch development; the other 75–80% of the movement is exhibited by the anteriors as they tip forwards. This 20–80% ratio of posterior movement to anterior movement is a product of the anchorage of the second molars (Spahl, 1993).

Functional correction may now proceed simultaneously with sagittal arch development by adding sagittal screws to upper and lower Twin Blocks to combine the features of Twin Block and sagittal appliances.

The design of the upper Twin Block is modified by the addition of two sagittal screws set in the palate for antero-posterior arch development. The screws expand the arch by advancing the upper incisors and, at the same time, drive the upper buccal segments distally and buccally along the line of the arch (Fig. 13.2 A,B).

In appliance construction it is important that the screws are positioned in the horizontal plane and angled along the line of the buccal segments to achieve the desired expansion. If the screws are angled downwards anteriorly, the appliance tends to ride down off the upper incisors as the screws are opened.

The sagittal design is suitable for both upper and lower arches to increase arch length. In the lower arch there is a choice of positioning the screws forwards in the canine region when small curved screws may be used, or in the premolar region when straight screws may be used to open premolar spaces.

Combined transverse and sagittal development

Many patients with malocclusion present archforms that are restricted in both transverse and anteroposterior dimensions.

The Class II division 2 malocclusion and variations often require a combination of transverse and anteroposterior arch development in order to free the mandible from a distal occlusion.

Examination of the occlusion and study models in such cases shows retroclined upper and lower incisors. Deficient arch width is associated with distal occlusion, and crowding is present in the upper incisor or canine region. Sometimes all four upper incisors are retroclined and the upper canines are crowded buccally. The upper anterior teeth cause interference when the lower model is advanced and it is not possible to engage the molars in Class I occlusion because of occlusal interference. Appliances must be designed to improve archform in order to free the mandible from distal occlusion (see Figs. 13.3 & 13.4). It was formerly necessary to complete separate stages of treatment to improve archform before proceeding to functional correction.

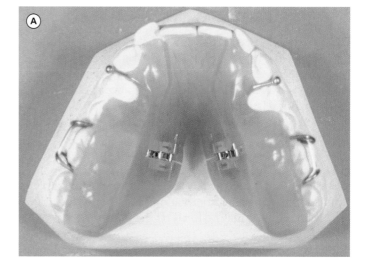

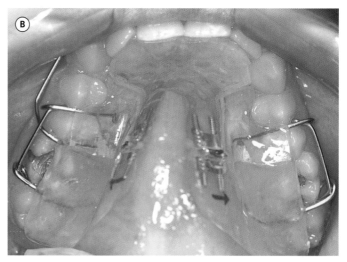

Fig. 13.2 A, B Sagittal Twin Blocks for correction of Class II division 2.

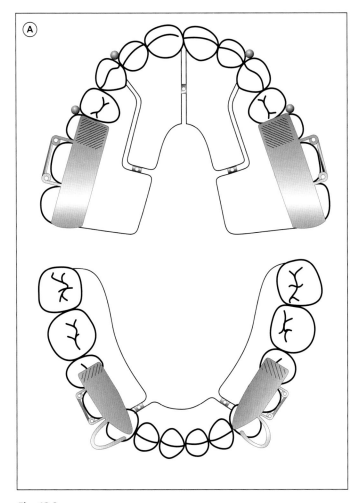

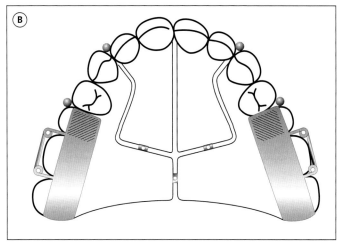

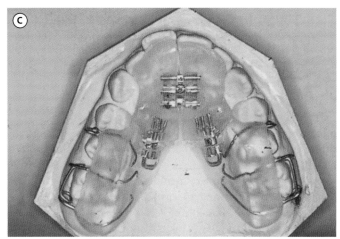

Fig. 13.3
A, B Triple screw sagittal appliances.
C A triple screw sagittal Twin Block appliance.

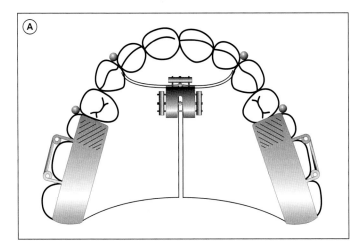

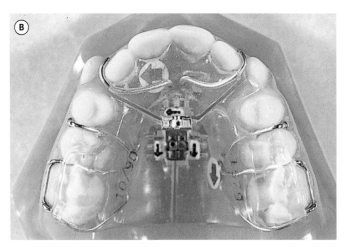

Fig. 13.4 Three-way screw for combined transverse and anteroposterior arch development.

The triple-screw sagittal Twin Block appliance is designed to improve archform in anteroposterior and transverse dimensions and simultaneously correct arch relationships for patients presenting complex problems of arch development. This appliance is a very powerful mechanism for interceptive treatment and arch development (Fig. 13.3 A,B).

Alternatively, the three-way screw combines transverse and sagittal arch development. This incorporates two screws housed in a single unit and operated independently to expand in the transverse and sagittal dimensions. The three-way screw must be positioned in the midline behind the anterior teeth. It has the disadvantage of being bulky to accommodate in this area, but is effective if the patient will tolerate the bulk in the anterior part of the palate (Fig. 13.4).

THE TWIN BLOCK SAGITTAL APPLIANCE

CASE REPORT: H.McL. AGED 14 YEARS 5 MONTHS

In this typical Class II division 2 malocclusion in the permanent dentition, the major correction of arch relationships was achieved in 6 months with Twin Blocks. Brackets were fitted to improve alignment of the upper anterior teeth during this stage, before progressing to a simple fixed appliance to complete treatment.

The advantage of using a Twin Block sagittal appliance in the management of Class II division 2 malocclusion is that the major correction of arch relationships is achieved quickly and consistently. There is the additional advantage of controlling the vertical dimension to increase lower facial height. Subsequent fixed appliance treatment to complete orthodontic correction is simplified by this approach.

Clinical management

Both palatal screws are opened two quarter-turns per week, once midweek and once at the weekend. This maintains contact of the appliance on the lingual of the upper incisors, and is effective in advancing these teeth to release the mandible from its retrusive position, locked in distal occlusion. The palatal acrylic adjacent to the attached gingiva and rugae of the premaxillary area may need slight reduction to allow the plate to abut against the lingual surfaces of the crowns of the upper anteriors.

The same sequence of trimming the occlusal blocks applies in the management of deep overbite in treatment of Class II division 2 as in Class II division 1 malocclusion (Fig. 13.5). The upper bite block is progressively trimmed posteriorly to clear the occlusion for molar eruption in the

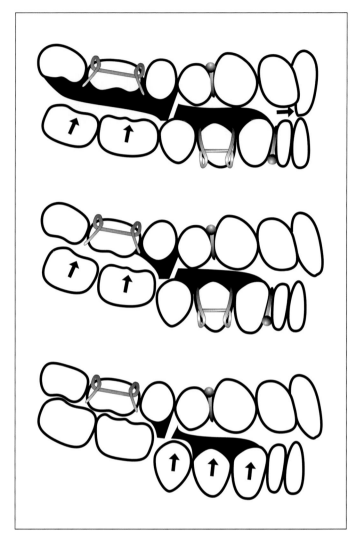

Fig. 13.5 Sequence of trimming blocks for Class II division 2.

early stages (Fig. 13.7E). When the molars are in occlusion, the lower appliance is gradually trimmed occlusally to allow lower premolar eruption to reduce the lateral open bite.

After 5 months of treatment, brackets were placed on the upper anterior teeth to initiate alignment at the end of the Twin Block phase. At the next visit, the lower appliance was left out and a Wilson lingual arch was fitted to hold the position in the lower arch. An anterior inclined plane with an occlusal stop for the lower incisors was worn for 6 months to maintain the vertical correction and allow the buccal teeth to settle fully into occlusion. The removable appliance was then discarded and treatment was completed in 6 months with a simple upper fixed appliance, followed by retention (Fig. 13.6).

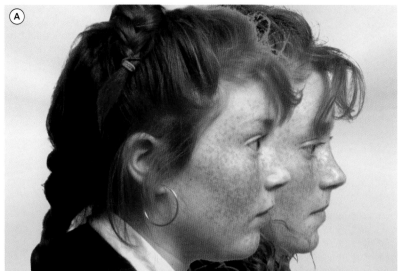

Fig. 13.6 Treatment:
A Profiles at ages 14 years 5 months (before treatment) and 15 years 2 months (9 months after treatment).
B–D Occlusion before treatment.
E, F Twin Block appliances with screws to advance the upper incisors. Brackets were added to the upper incisors at the end of the Twin Block phase.
G Support phase after 4 months of treatment.
H, J, K Upper archform and occlusion after 9 months of treatment.

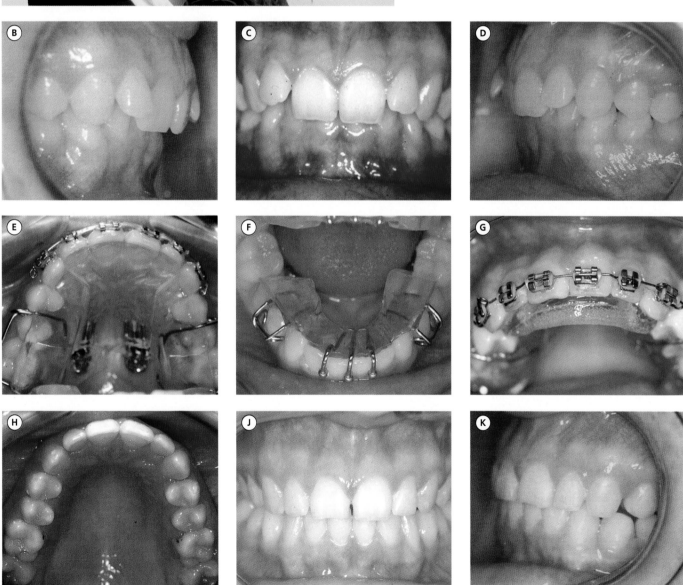

CASE REPORT: H.K.

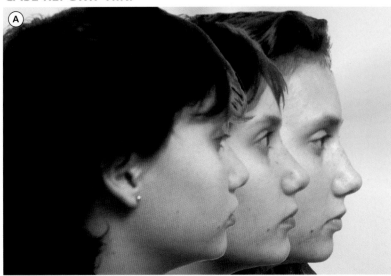

Fig. 13.7 Treatment:
A Profiles at ages 14 years 8 months (before treatment), 14 years 11 months (after 3 months of treatment) and 16 years 6 months.
B–D Occlusion before treatment.
E Occlusion cleared for molar eruption.

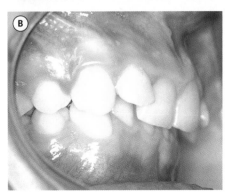

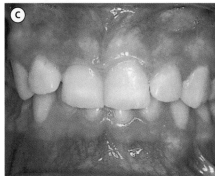

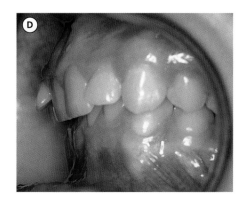

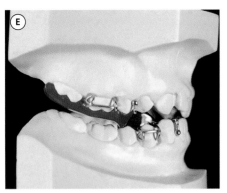

CASE REPORT: H.K. AGED 14 YEARS 6 MONTHS

Another typical Class II division 2 malocclusion with a Class I skeletal pattern and a full unit Class II dental occlusion as the mandible is trapped in distal occlusion by retroclined upper incisors. The lower incisors are also retroclined and are positioned 4 mm lingual to the A–Po line. After initial proclination of the upper incisors, an upper sectional fixed appliance was added during the Twin Block stage to align the upper anterior teeth concurrently with correction of the distal occlusion and vertical development to correct the deep overbite. A simple upper fixed appliance was used with a Wilson lower lingual arch to complete the treatment (Fig. 13.7).

Twin Blocks: 5 months
Support appliance/lingual arch: 6 months
Upper fixed appliance: 6 months
Final records: 1 year out of retention.

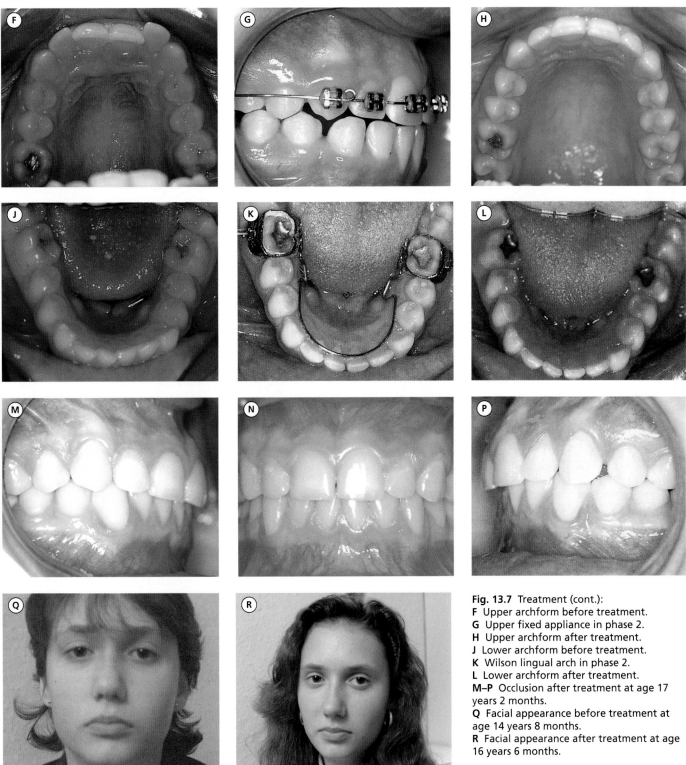

Fig. 13.7 Treatment (cont.):
F Upper archform before treatment.
G Upper fixed appliance in phase 2.
H Upper archform after treatment.
J Lower archform before treatment.
K Wilson lingual arch in phase 2.
L Lower archform after treatment.
M–P Occlusion after treatment at age 17 years 2 months.
Q Facial appearance before treatment at age 14 years 8 months.
R Facial appearance after treatment at age 16 years 6 months.

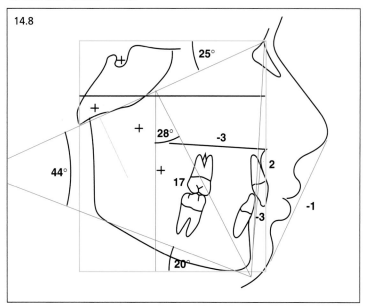

14.8

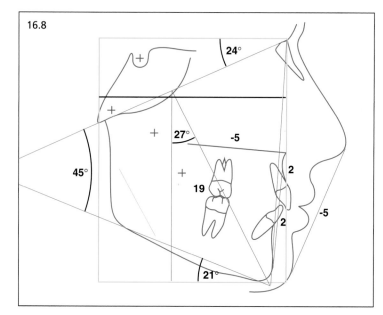

16.8

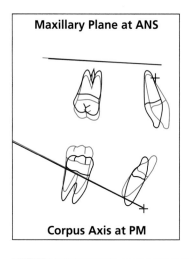
Maxillary Plane at ANS

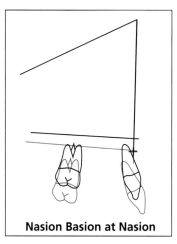
Corpus Axis at PM

Nasion Basion at Nasion

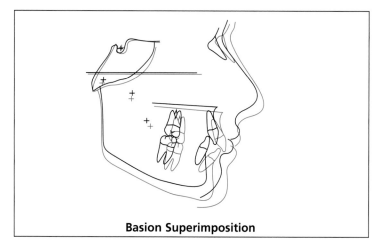
Basion Superimposition

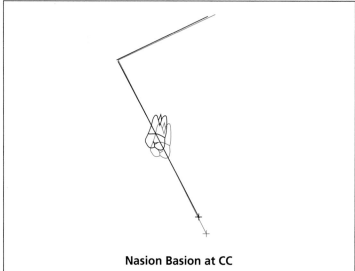
Nasion Basion at CC

H.K.	Age	14.8	16.8
Cranial Base Angle		25	24
Facial Axis Angle		28	27
F/M Plane Angle		20	21
Craniomandibular Angle		44	45
Maxillary Plane		−3	−5
Convexity		2	2
U/Incisor to Vertical		12	22
L/Incisor to Vertical		21	43
Interincisal Angle		157	135
6 to Pterygoid Vertical		17	19
L/Incisor to A/Po		−3	2
L/Lip to Aesthetic Plane		−1	−5

CASE REPORT: S.W.

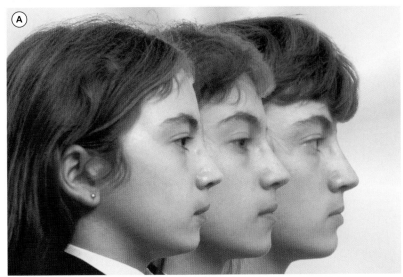

Fig. 13.8 Treatment:
A Profiles at ages 12 years 9 months (before treatment), 13 years 3 months (after 6 months with Twin Blocks) and 14 years 9 months.
B–D Occlusion before treatment.
E–G Orthodontic phase after 6 months of treatment.

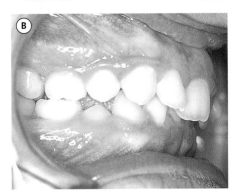

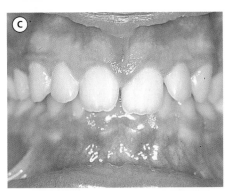

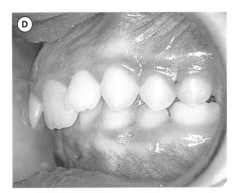

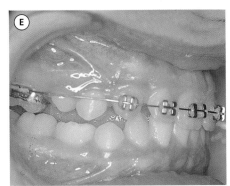

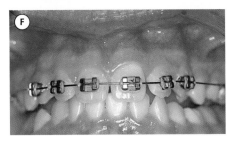

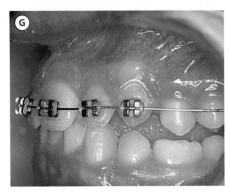

CASE REPORT: S.W. AGED 12 YEARS 9 MONTHS

This girl is an example of treatment of a Class II division 2 malocclusion in the late mixed dentition with a combination of Twin Blocks and fixed appliances. There is a brachyfacial tendency and a mild mandibular retrusion, with a normal maxilla.

Bite registration

The intention of treatment in this Class II division 2 malocclusion is to limit forward translation of the mandible because the Class II skeletal discrepancy is mild. Therefore the bite is registered in an edge-to-edge incisor relationship and the upper incisors are advanced during the Twin Block stage to develop a positive overjet. Correction of the distal

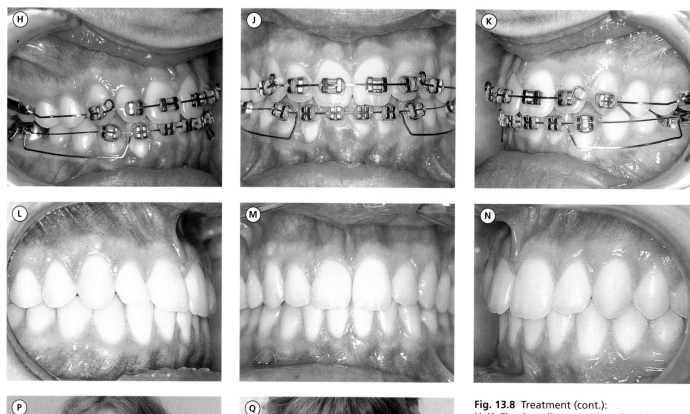

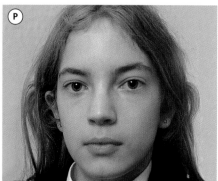

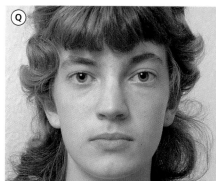

Fig. 13.8 Treatment (cont.):
H–K Fixed appliances to complete the treatment.
L–N Occlusion at age 17 years 3 months.
P Facial appearance before treatment at age 12 years 9 months.
Q Facial appearance after treatment at age 14 years 9 months.

occlusion is achieved by encouraging vertical development of the lower molars that erupt forwards into a Class I occlusion with the upper molars.

Anterior brackets are fitted during the Twin Block phase. This allows an easy transition to a fixed appliance in the finishing stage. Sectional fixed appliances are used with utility arches in a bioprogressive approach to complete treatment (Fig. 13.8).

Twin Blocks: 5 months
Fixed appliances: 15 months.

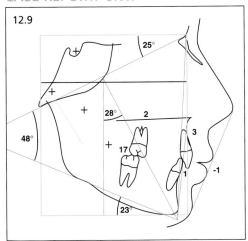

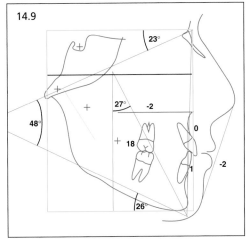

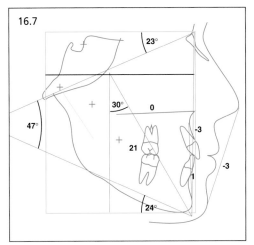

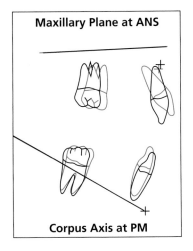

Maxillary Plane at ANS

Corpus Axis at PM

Nasion Basion at Nasion

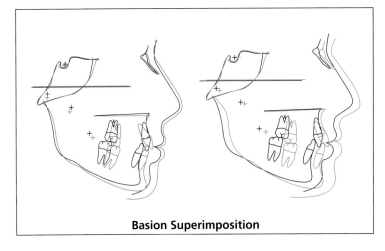

Basion Superimposition

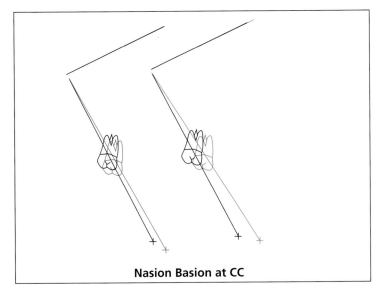

Nasion Basion at CC

S.W.	Age	12.9	14.9	16.7
Cranial Base Angle		25	23	23
Facial Axis Angle		28	27	30
F/M Plane Angle		23	26	24
Craniomandibular Angle		48	48	47
Maxillary Plane		2	−2	0
Convexity		3	0	−
U/Incisor to Vertical		8	27	29
L/Incisor to Vertical		23	23	20
Interincisal Angle		149	130	131
6 to Pterygoid Vertical		17	18	21
L/Incisor to A/Po		−2	1	1
L/Lip to Aesthetic Plane		1	−2	−3

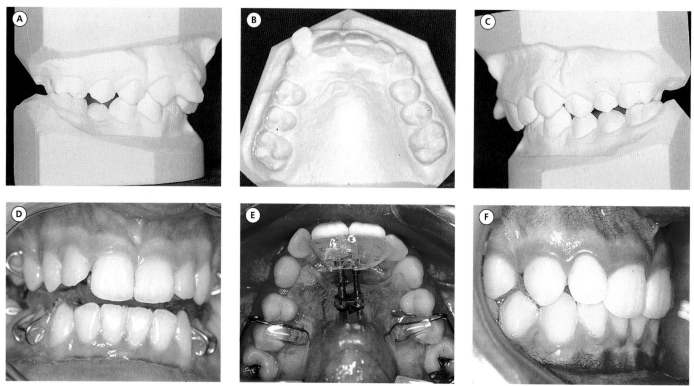

Fig. 13.9 Treatment:
A, B Occlusion before treatment at age 12 years 6 months.
C, D Screw to advance the upper incisors.
E Twin Block appliances.
F Occlusion after 1 year.

THE CENTRAL SAGITTAL TWIN BLOCK

Combination therapy by Twin Blocks and fixed appliances

CASE REPORT: S.Wn. AGED 12 YEARS 6 MONTHS

This boy presented a Class II division 2 malocclusion in the permanent dentition with severely retroclined upper incisors and an excessive overbite. A central sagittal Twin Block was used to advance the upper incisors, to reduce the overbite and to correct the distal occlusion. This appliance incorporates only a single screw lingual to the upper incisors to advance the retroclined incisors.

Failure to include lateral expansion during the first phase of sagittal correction can result in the development of a lateral crossbite in the buccal segments, and it is normally better to combine transverse and sagittal expansion during the Twin Block phase.

In this case, lateral expansion in the upper arch was carried out during the support phase, using a three-way expansion screw to combine anteroposterior and lateral arch development, with a Wilson lower lingual arch to improve the lower archform. The major correction is completed during the Twin Block phase, and the overbite is controlled in the support phase. This was followed by fixed appliances to complete the treatment. It is worth noting that consecutive use of removable and fixed appliances extends the period of treatment, whereas concurrent use of fixed appliances with Twin Blocks reduces the treatment time (Fig. 13.9).

Twin Blocks: 12 months
Arch development: 12 months
Fixed appliances: 12 months.

CASE REPORT: S.Wn.

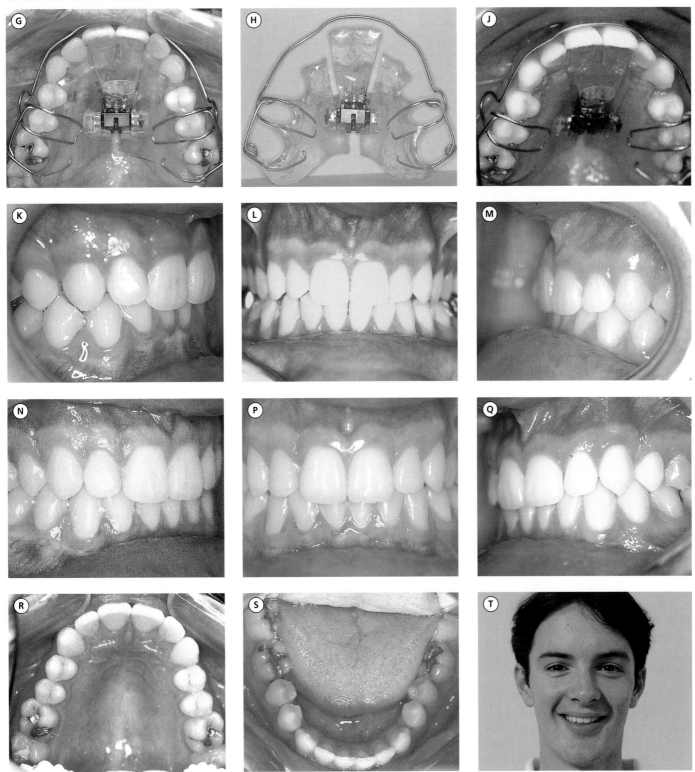

Fig. 13.9 Treatment (cont.):
G–J Phase 2 appliance with a three-way expansion screw.
K–M Occlusion before fitting the fixed appliances at age 14 years 8 months.

N–Q Occlusion at age 17 years 11 months.
R–T Occlusal views and facial appearance at age 17 years 11 months.

CASE REPORTS

by Forbes Leishman

The following three patients were treated by Dr Forbes Leishman in orthodontic practice in Auckland, New Zealand. They demonstrate the management of Class II division 2 malocclusion by a combination of Twin Blocks and fixed appliances.

CASE REPORT: J.C.

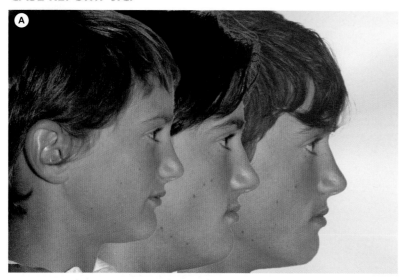

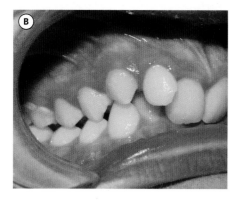 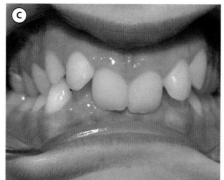 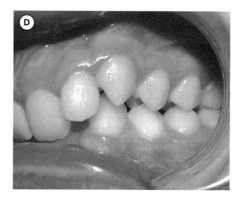

Fig. 13.10 Treatment:
A Profiles at ages 12 years 6 months (before treatment) and 17 years (after treatment).
B–D Occlusion before treatment.

CASE REPORT: J.C. AGED 12 YEARS 6 MONTHS

A strong brachyfacial pattern is the underlying skeletal configuration for a severe Class II division 2 malocclusion with reduced lower facial height. Treatment was initiated with an upper removable appliance to procline the upper central incisors in combination with a lower fixed appliance to procline the lower incisors. This was followed by Twin Blocks to correct the distal occlusion and initiate correction of the overbite and the excessive curve of Spee. During the support phase a bite plate was used with fixed appliances and elastics extending from upper laterals to lower molars and then to upper molars to combine vertical closure with a Class II

intermaxillary component. Levelling of the arches was then completed with fixed appliances. This approach encouraged a good vertical growth response, which together with the mandibular advancement produced favourable changes in the profile. Final records show the position out of retention at age 20 years 1 month (Fig. 13.10).

Upper removable and lower fixed appliances: 5 months
Twin Blocks: 6 months
Bite plane: 6 months
Fixed appliances: 18 months
Total treatment time: 3 years followed by retention.

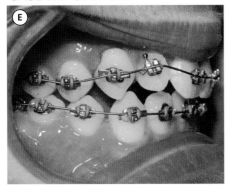

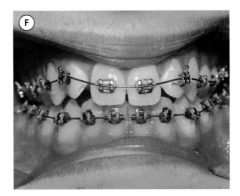

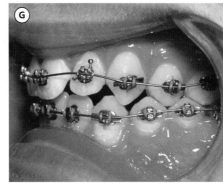

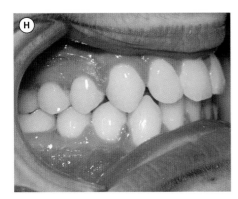

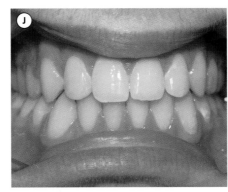

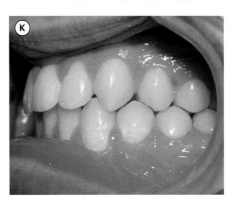

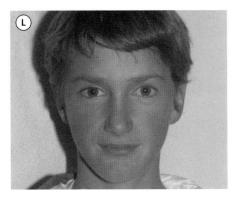

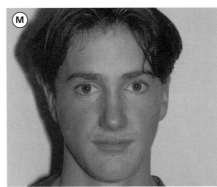

Fig. 13.10 Treatment (cont.):
E–G Fixed appliance in orthodontic phase.
H–K Occlusion after treatment.
L Facial appearance before treatment.
M Facial appearance after treatment.

CASE REPORT: J.C.

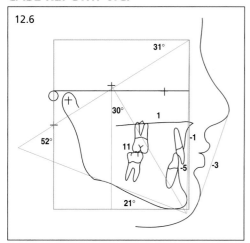

12.6

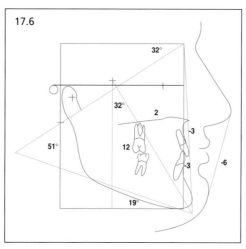

17.6

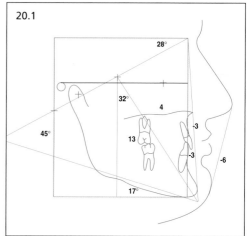

20.1

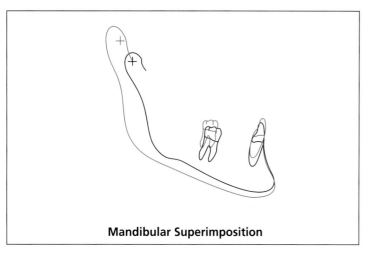

Mandibular Superimposition

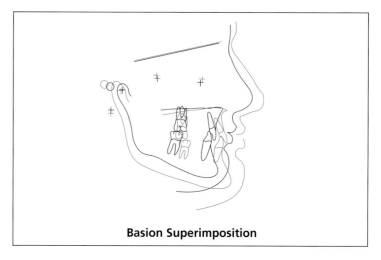

Basion Superimposition

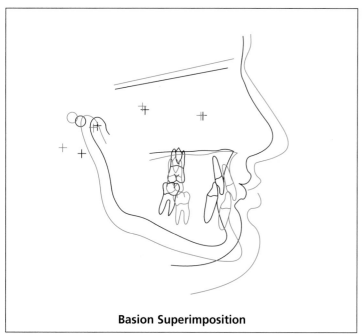

Basion Superimposition

J.C. Age	12.6	17.6	20.1
Cranial Base Angle	31	32	28
Facial Axis Angle	30	32	32
F/M Plane Angle	21	19	17
Craniomandibular Angle	52	51	45
Maxillary Plane	1	2	4
Convexity	–1	–3	–3
U/Incisor to Vertical	12	22	21
L/Incisor to Vertical	11	16	12
L/Incisor to A/Po	–5	–3	–3
L/Lip to Aesthetic Plane	–3	–6	–6
6 to Pterygoid vertical	11	12	13

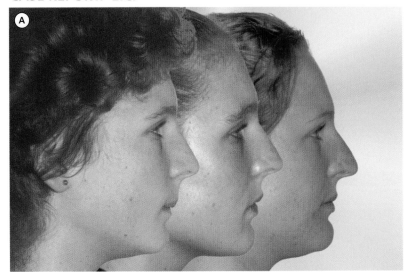

Fig. 13.11 Treatment:
A Profiles at ages 11 years 11 months (before treatment), 13 years 8 months (after treatment) and 21 years 5 months (out of retention).
B–D Occlusion before treatment.

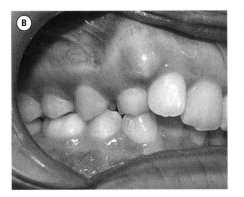

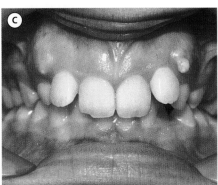

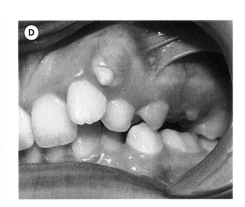

The following case records show the treatment of two sisters, both of whom have severe Class II division 2 malocclusions. This type of malocclusion can be effectively treated in late mixed dentition or early permanent dentition by a combination of Twin Blocks and fixed appliances, either concurrently or in consecutive phases.

CASE REPORT: E.C. AGED 11 YEARS 11 MONTHS

by Forbes Leishman

The first sister is treated in late mixed dentition and presents a severe Class II division 2 malocclusion with a typical brachyfacial pattern and 5 mm convexity due to mandibular retrusion. The mandible is trapped in a distal position by severely retroclined upper central incisors before treatment, accentuating the retrusive profile. Typically maxillary width is also contracted, as an additional factor contributing to deficient mandibular development. An obtuse naso-labial

angle compromises facial aesthetics by accentuating nasal growth, while the dentition and the mandible are not free to develop normally. Treatment was initiated with an upper removable appliance to procline the upper incisors, followed by the Twin Block phase, and finally fixed appliances. Comparison of the profile before and after treatment demonstrates the improvement in facial aesthetics when the angulation of the upper incisors is corrected and the mandible is released to develop forward. The naso-labial angle improves and mandibular development brings the chin forward to improve facial balance (Fig. 13.11).

Upper removable appliance: 5 months
Twin Blocks: 6 months
Fixed appliances: 10 months
Total treatment time: 1 year 9 months followed by retention
Final records: show the position out of retention at age 21 years 5 months.

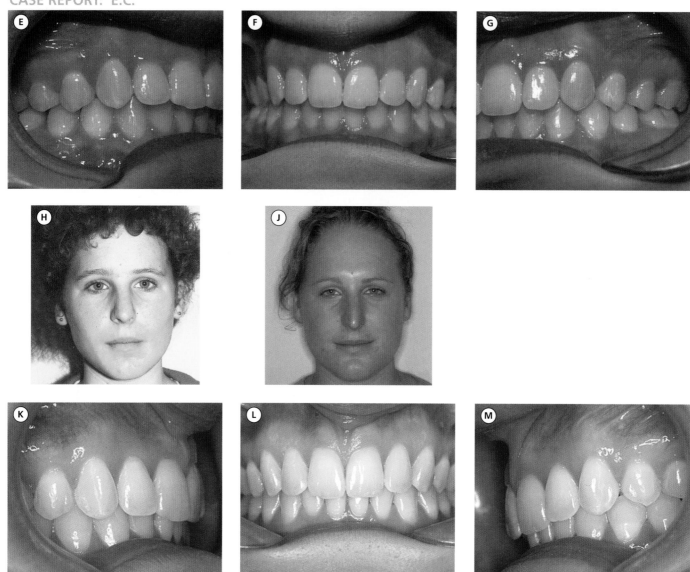

Fig. 13.11 Treatment (cont.):
E–G Orthodontic phase after 21 months of treatment.
H Facial appearance before treatment.
J Facial appearance after treatment.
K–M Occlusion out of retention.

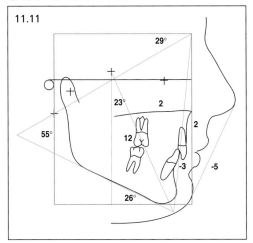

11.11

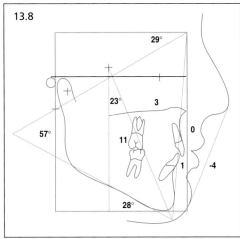

13.8

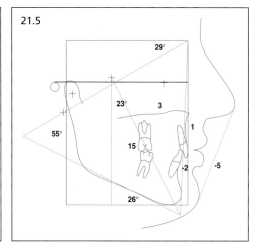

21.5

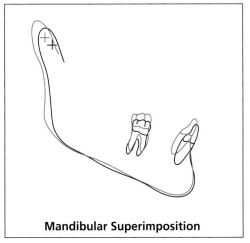

Mandibular Superimposition

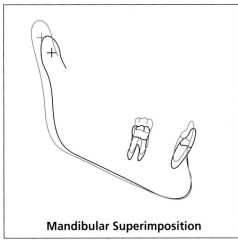

Mandibular Superimposition

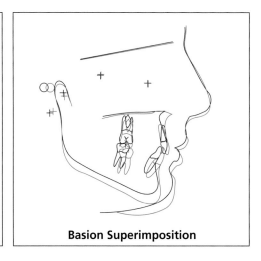

Basion Superimposition

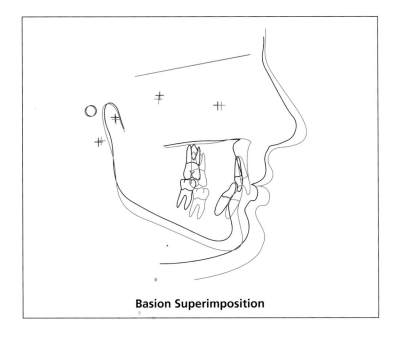

Basion Superimposition

E.C. Age	11.11	13.8	21.5
Cranial Base Angle	29	29	29
Facial Axis Angle	23	23	23
F/M Plane Angle	26	28	26
Craniomandibular Angle	55	57	55
Maxillary Plane	2	3	3
Convexity	2	0	1
U/Incisor to Vertical	2	16	13
L/Incisor to Vertical	28	39	22
L/Incisor to A/Po	–3	1	–2
L/Lip to Aesthetic Plane	–5	–4	–5
6 to Pterygoid vertical	12	11	15

CASE REPORT: K.C.

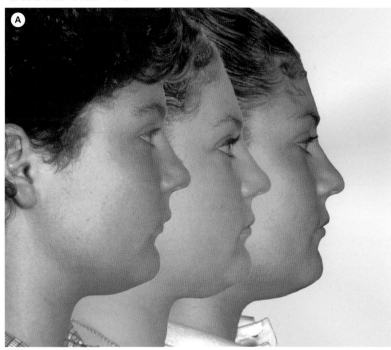

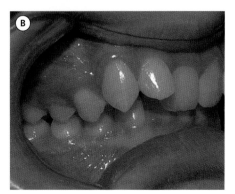

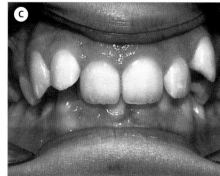

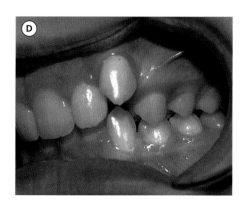

Fig. 13.12 Treatment:
A Profiles at ages 12 years 8 months (before treatment), 14 years 11 months (after treatment) and 18 years 11 months (out of retention).
B–D Occlusion before treatment.

CASE REPORT: K.C. AGED 12 YEARS 9 MONTHS

The previous patient's sister was treated slightly later after the permanent canines had erupted. Once again the profile before treatment shows evidence of mandibular retrusion. A partial bonded upper fixed appliance was used in the early stages to correct the alignment and torque values of the upper labial segment, followed by Twin Blocks, and a final stage with fixed appliances. Vertical development, combined with mandibular advancement, again make a significant contribution to the improvement in facial balance (Fig. 13.12).

Upper limited fixed appliance: 7 months
Twin Blocks: 7 months
Fixed appliances: 14 months
Total treatment time: 2 years 4 months followed by retention
Final records: show the position out of retention at age 18 years 11 months

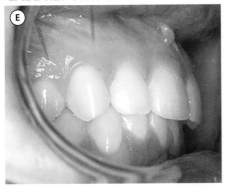

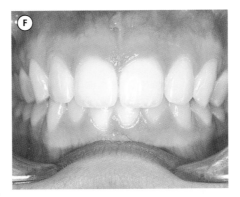

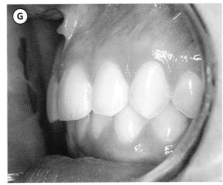

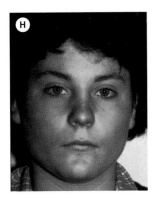

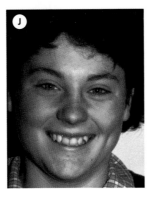

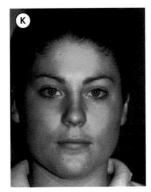

Fig. 13.12 Treatment (cont.):
E–G Occlusion out of retention.
H, K Facial appearance before treatment.
J Facial appearance after treatment.

CASE REPORT: K.C.

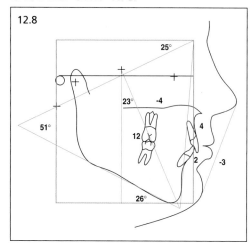

12.8

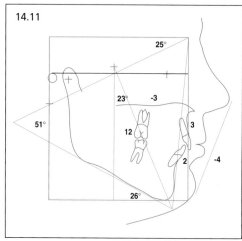

14.11

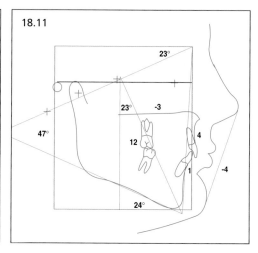

18.11

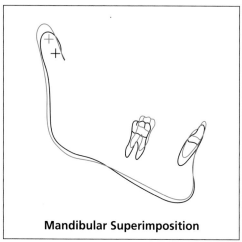

Mandibular Superimposition

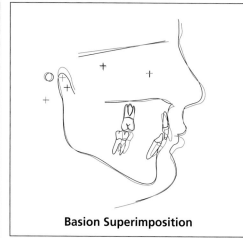

Basion Superimposition

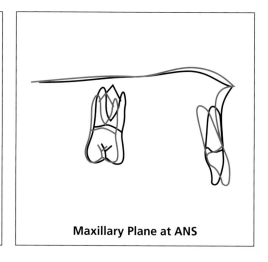

Maxillary Plane at ANS

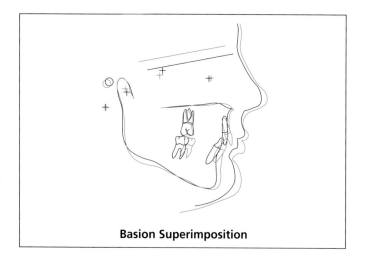

Basion Superimposition

K C Age	12.8	14.11	18.11
Cranial Base Angle	25	25	23
Facial Axis Angle	23	23	23
F/M Plane Angle	26	26	24
Craniomandibular Angle	51	51	47
Maxillary Plane	−4	−3	−3
Convexity	4	3	4
U/Incisor to Vertical	17	17	16
L/Incisor to Vertical	40	40	32
L/Incisor to A/Po	2	2	1
L/Lip to Aesthetic Plane	−3	−4	−4
6 to Pterygoid vertical	12	12	12

REFERENCES

Spahl, T.J. (1993). The Spahl split vertical eruption acceleration appliance system. *Functional Orthod.*, **10**(1): 10–24.

Witzig, J.W. & Spahl, T.J. (1987). The great second molar debate. In *The Clinical Management of Basic Maxillofacial Orthopedic Appliances*, Vol. 1 – *Mechanics*. Massachusetts, PSG, pp. 155–216.

CHAPTER 14

Treatment of Class III Malocclusion

REVERSE TWIN BLOCKS

Functional correction of Class III malocclusion is achieved in Twin Block technique by reversing the angulation of the inclined planes, harnessing occlusal forces as the functional mechanism to correct arch relationships by maxillary advancement, while using the lower arch as the means of anchorage. The position of the bite blocks is reversed compared to Twin Blocks for Class II treatment. The occlusal blocks are placed over the upper deciduous molars and the lower first molars.

Reverse Twin Blocks are designed to encourage maxillary development by the action of reverse occlusal inclined planes cut at a 70° angle to drive the upper teeth forwards by the forces of occlusion and, at the same time, to restrict forward mandibular development (Fig. 14.1). The maxillary appliance should include provision for three-way expansion to increase the size of the maxilla in both sagittal and transverse dimensions.

Prior to initiation of Class III Twin Block treatment it is important to ensure that the patient's condyles are not displaced superiorly and/or posteriorly in the glenoid fossae at full occlusion. In treatment with the reverse Twin Block, the occlusal force exerted on the mandible is directed downwards and backwards by the reverse inclined planes. No damaging force is exerted on the condyles because the bite is hinged open with the condyles down and forward in the

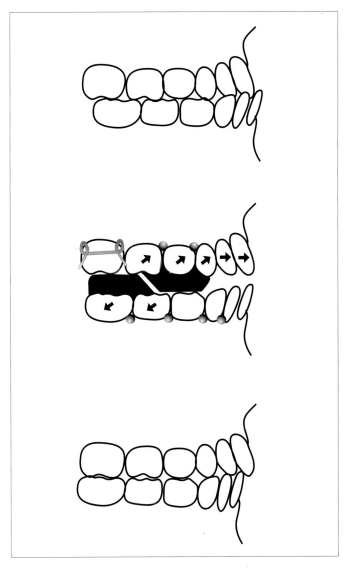

Fig. 14.2 Management of Class III malocclusion.

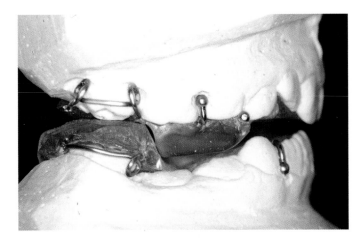

Fig. 14.1 Reverse Twin Blocks.

fossae and the inclined planes are directed downwards and backwards on the mandibular teeth. The force vector in the mandible passes from the lower molar towards the gonial angle. This is the area of the mandible best able to absorb occlusal forces (Fig. 14.2).

CASE SELECTION

The skeletal Class III malocclusion is one of the most difficult to treat by an orthodontic or orthopaedic approach, and case selection is especially important before undertaking treatment. Early treatment is often indicated in this type of malocclusion to counter the unfavourable developmental pattern. In severe cases treatment may be initiated in the deciduous dentition or early mixed dentition. Orthopaedic correction is more likely to succeed by maxillary advancement rather than mandibular retraction, as it is difficult to reduce the potential for mandibular growth, except by surgery.

The simplest clinical guideline is whether or not the patient can occlude squarely edge-to-edge on the upper and lower incisors. The ease with which the patient can achieve this position is an indication of the prognosis for correction. The most favourable cases for correction present a postural Class III where the incisors can meet comfortably edge-to-edge, but the patient is forced to move the mandible forward in order to occlude on the posterior teeth.

If an edge-to-edge occlusion is achieved only with difficulty the prognosis for orthodontic correction is poor, while orthopaedic correction would depend on a good response to maxillary protraction, perhaps using a reverse pull headgear. If the patient cannot close edge-to-edge on the incisors it is likely that surgical correction will be required. If in doubt a combined orthodontic and surgical opinion should be sought.

The degree of skeletal discrepancy is an important diagnostic factor in case selection. When convexity moves into the negative range the patient should be informed of the possibility that surgery may be required to achieve a stable correction. The prognosis reduces in direct proportion to the increase in negative convexity. In some cases the Class III occlusion may respond to treatment in the mixed dentition, but relapse may occur during the pubertal growth spurt, when the position needs to be reviewed.

Combination therapy with Twin Blocks reinforced by reverse pull traction to advance the maxilla may be successful in the younger patient. An initial stage of rapid maxillary expansion is often indicated to free up the maxillary sutures prior to applying forward traction to the maxilla (McNamara

1993). The rapid maxillary expander may be modified to incorporate reverse blocks designed to occlude with the lower reverse Twin Block.

BITE REGISTRATION

It is not possible to build in the same degree of anteroposterior activation in the construction bite for functional correction of a Class III malocclusion compared to a Class II correction, because there is less scope for distal displacement of the mandible.

The blue exactobite is normally used to register a construction bite with the teeth closed to the position of maximum retrusion, leaving sufficient clearance between the posterior teeth for the occlusal bite blocks. This is achieved by recording a construction bite with 2 mm interincisal clearance in the fully retruded position. In treatment of the brachyfacial Class III additional vertical activation may be applied by opening the bite further in the construction bite if required by using the yellow Exactobite to register 4 mm interincisal clearance. This may result in an increase in the lower facial height.

TREATMENT OF CLASS III MALOCCLUSION WITH REVERSE TWIN BLOCKS

CASE REPORT: S.L. AGED 11 YEARS

This case is an example of the response to treatment with reverse Twin Blocks in permanent dentition for a mild Class III skeletal discrepancy with a postural element. A three-screw sagittal appliance was used in this case. The construction bite is registered in the maximum retruded position, which is edge-to-edge with 4 mm interincisal clearance. Activation to correct the lingual occlusion is achieved by opening the bite on the articulator and constructing the appliances so that contact is made only on the reverse inclined planes, with no contact on the occlusal surface of the blocks. This has the effect of increasing the advancing forces on the maxilla as the forces of occlusion drive the upper appliance forward and the blocks settle into occlusion with the opposing teeth. Treatment was completed in 10 months, followed by 5 months of retention. The final records show the position 1 year out of retention (Fig. 14.3).

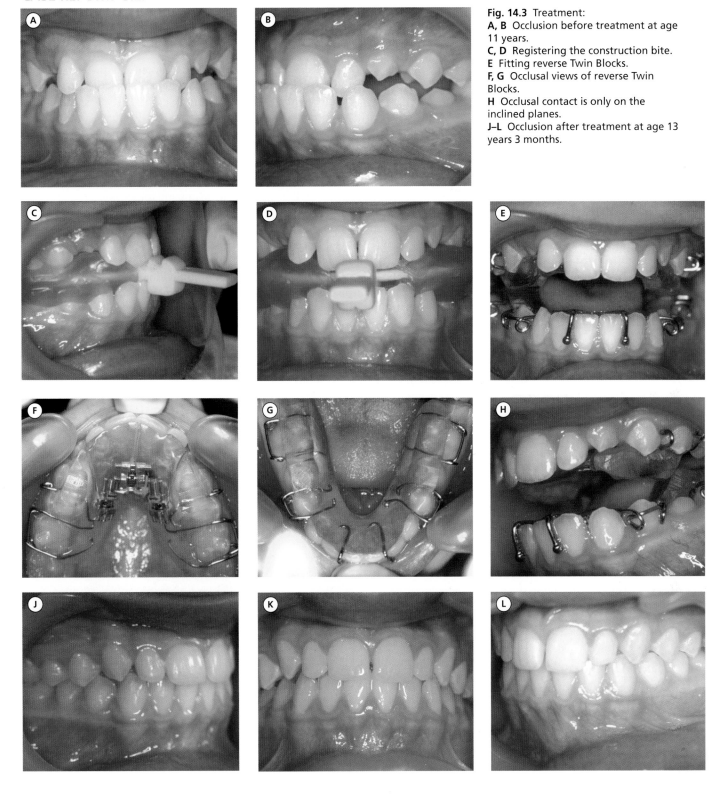

Fig. 14.3 Treatment:
A, B Occlusion before treatment at age 11 years.
C, D Registering the construction bite.
E Fitting reverse Twin Blocks.
F, G Occlusal views of reverse Twin Blocks.
H Occlusal contact is only on the inclined planes.
J–L Occlusion after treatment at age 13 years 3 months.

REVERSE TWIN BLOCKS: APPLIANCE DESIGN

The sagittal design is used to advance the upper incisors to correct the lingual occlusion in treatment of Class III malocclusion (Fig. 14.4).

In many cases, the maxilla is contracted laterally in addition to occluding in a distal relationship to the mandible. This is an indication for combined sagittal and transverse expansion using a three-screw sagittal appliance which includes a midline screw to complement the action of the sagittal screws.

An alternative design uses a three-way expansion screw to combine transverse and sagittal expansion. This is also effective in expanding a contracted maxilla and in correcting lingual occlusion if used in combination with reverse inclined planes (Fig. 14.5). Alternatively, a triple screw sagittal may be used for three-way maxillary development, as described for treatment of Class II division 2 malocclusion (see Fig. 13.4 A,B).

REVERSE TWIN BLOCKS: MANAGEMENT

With the sagittal appliance design, because of the curvature of the palate it is easier for the patient to operate the screws from the fitting surface of the appliance. The screws should be positioned so that both are opened by turning in the same direction. This is less confusing for a young patient. The lower appliance is retained with clasps on the lower molars and additional interdental clasps as required.

Opening the screws has the reciprocal effect of driving the upper molars distally and advancing the incisors. Distal movement of the upper molars is resisted by occlusion of the lower bite blocks on the reverse inclined planes. Therefore the net effect of opening the screws is a forward driving force on the upper dental arch. The position of the cut for the screws will influence their action on individual teeth. The cuts may be positioned distal to the lateral incisors to advance only the four upper incisors. Positioning the cuts mesial to the upper molars would increase the distalising component of force on the molars, but distal movement is resisted by occlusion with the lower bite blocks, and the reciprocal force acts to advance the entire upper arch mesial to the molars, using the lower arch as anchorage.

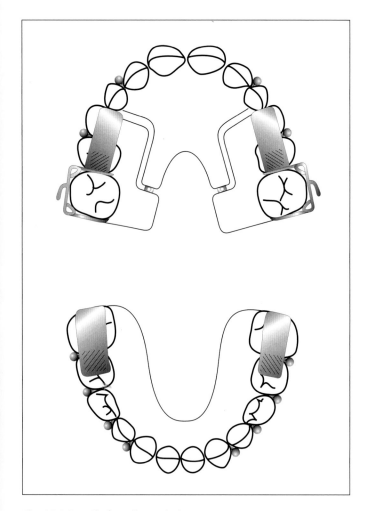

Fig. 14.4 Detail of appliance design.

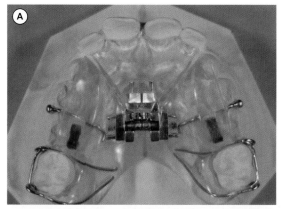

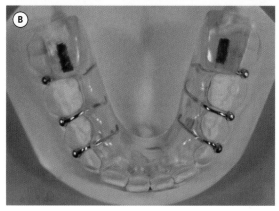

Fig. 14.5 A, B Three-way screw appliance design.

LIP PADS

To enhance the forward movement of the upper labial segment, lip pads may be added to support the upper lip clear of the incisors with an action similar to that of the Frankel III. The lip pads need not be joined in the midline provided they are carried on heavy gauge wires that are self-supporting to hold the pads clear of the gingivae in order to avoid gingival irritation. It is important to attach the lip pads to the anterior segment of the appliance so that they advance as the screws are opened, otherwise the pads become compressed against the gingivae in the labial segment. In addition, they may be adjusted forwards clear of the gingivae as the incisors are advanced (Fig. 14.6).

CASE REPORT: T.C. AGED 8 YEARS 2 MONTHS

A mild Class III skeletal pattern with negative maxillary convexity of –1 mm resulted in lingual occlusion of all four upper incisors and the upper lateral incisors were displaced lingual to the central incisors. Retroclined upper incisors were associated with an obtuse naso-labial angle, and proclination of the incisors improved the profile during treatment. A positive growth response to mixed dentition treatment resulted in an improvement in convexity to +5 mm. A lip pad was added to the upper reverse Twin Block with twin sagittal screws to improve the maxillary response. The favourable improvement in facial balance was partly due to a clockwise rotation of the mandible, with a significant rotation of the facial axis. The facial axis angle changed from 26° before treatment to 19° after treatment, and 22° out of retention. Similar changes were observed in the mandibular plane angle. The downward rotation of the mandible improved the profile. The lingual occlusion was corrected after 5 months and reverse Twin Block treatment was completed after 12 months, followed by retention for a further 12 months. Final records show the position 1 year out of retention after the transition into the permanent dentition (Fig. 14.7).

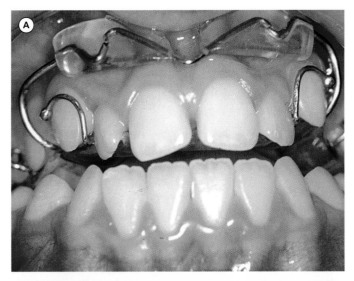

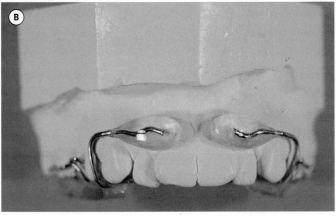

Fig. 14.6 A, B Lip pads must be supported clear of the gingivae. The action is similar to the upper lip pads on the Frankel III.

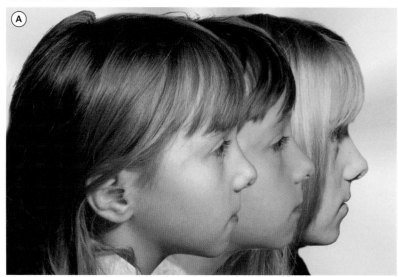

Fig. 14.7 Treatment:
A Profiles at ages 8 years 2 months (before treatment), 10 years 1 month (after treatment) and 11 years 4 months (out of retention).
B–D Occlusion before treatment.
E, G Upper archforms at age before treatment and after treatment.
F Occlusion after treatment.
H, J Occlusion out of retention.

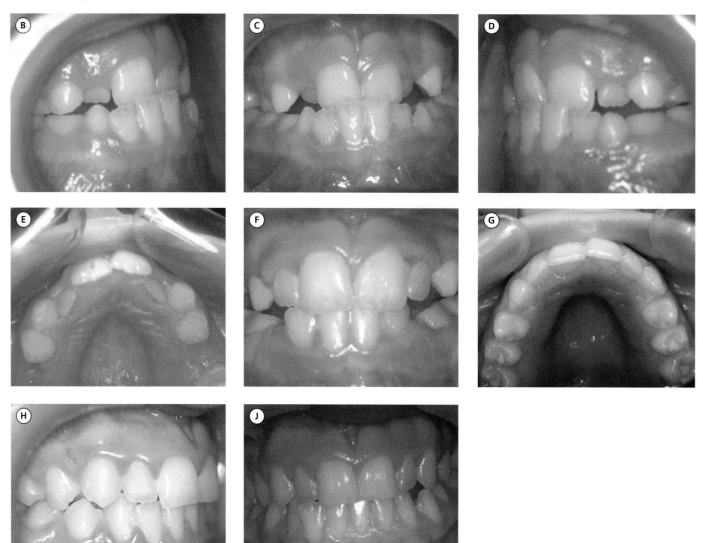

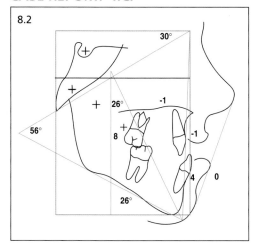

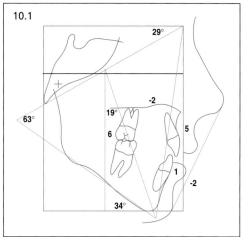

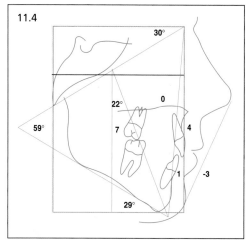

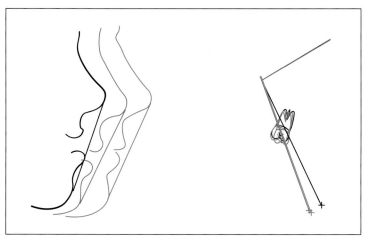

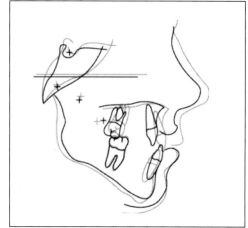

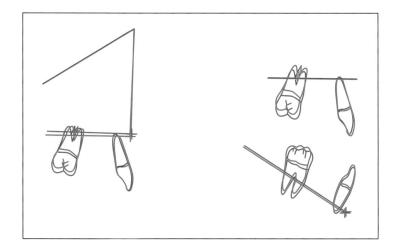

T.C. Age	8.2	10.1	11.4
Cranial Base Angle	30	29	30
Facial Axis Angle	26	19	22
F/M Plane Angle	26	34	29
Craniomandibular Angle	56	63	59
Maxillary Plane	−1	−2	0
Convexity	−1	5	4
U/Incisor to Vertical	5	13	14
L/Incisor to Vertical	24	27	27
L/Incisor to A/Po	4	1	1
L/Lip to Aesthetic Plane	0	−2	−3
6 to Pterygoid vertical	8	6	7

CASE REPORT: A.J.

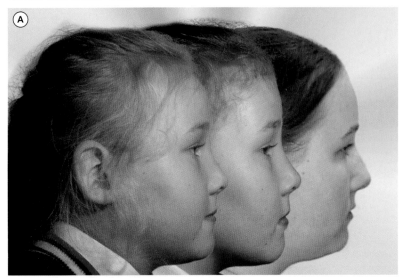

Fig. 14.8 Treatment:
A Profiles at ages 6 years 11 months (before treatment), 8 years 7 months (after treatment) and 13 years 7 months (out of retention).
B–D Occlusion before treatment.
E–G Occlusion after treatment at age 8 years 7 months.

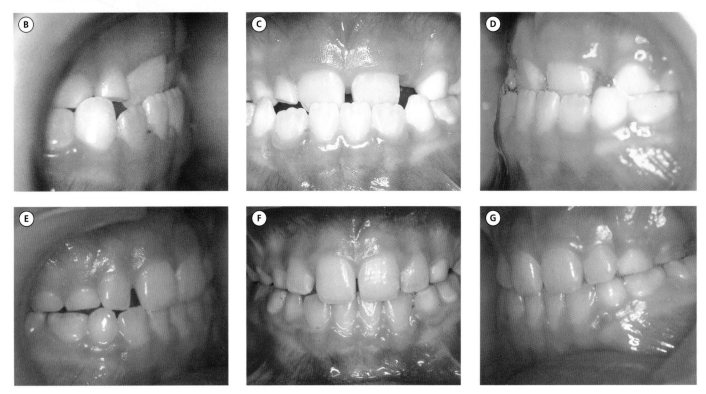

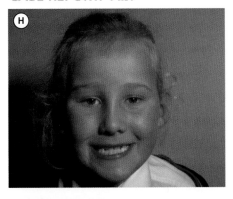

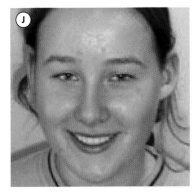

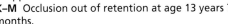

Fig. 14.8 Treatment (cont.):
H Appearance before treatment at age 6 years 11 months.
J Appearance out of retention.
K–M Occlusion out of retention at age 13 years 7 months.

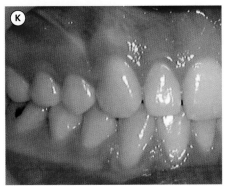

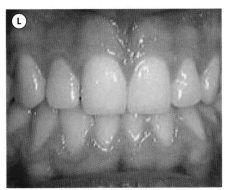

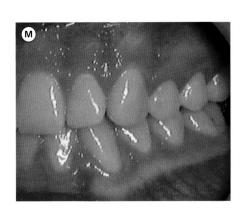

CASE REPORT: A.J. AGED 6 YEARS 11 MONTHS

Treatment was indicated in early mixed dentition for this young girl, who presented a contracted maxilla with lingual occlusion of the upper incisors and a mild Class III skeletal pattern with a reduced overbite. Treatment with reverse Twin Blocks included three-way expansion of the maxilla and was completed after 12 months.

Retention continued for 1 year to stabilise the position in view of the reduced overbite. Final records show the position at age 15 when a settled occlusion has developed without further treatment in the permanent dentition (Fig. 14.8).

CASE REPORT: M.L. AGED 7 YEARS 5 MONTHS

This young girl presented a severe dental Class III malocclusion soon after eruption of the permanent incisors. The 2|2 were displaced lingual to 1|1 , and there was a lingual occlusion of the upper labial segment with a reverse overjet of 3 mm and no forward posture on closure. The skeletal relationship showed a convexity of –1 with a normal mandible and moderate maxillary retrusion (Fig. 14.9 A–Q).

A short period of treatment was successful in reversing the Class III growth tendency, and establishing a Class I occlusion that was maintained 6 years out of retention without further treatment.

Twin Blocks: 5 months
Retention: 3 months
Treatment time: 8 months.

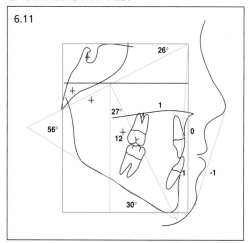

6.11

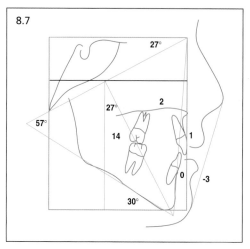

8.7

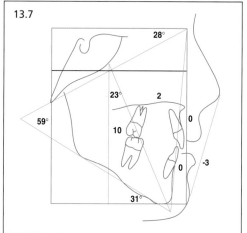

13.7

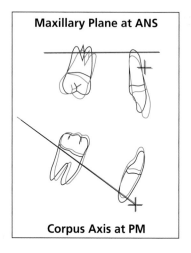

Maxillary Plane at ANS

Corpus Axis at PM

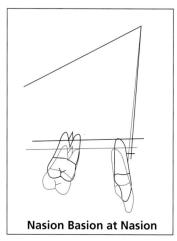

Nasion Basion at Nasion

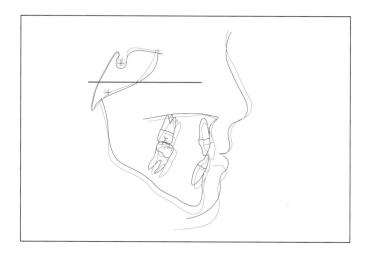

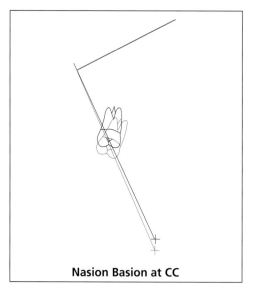

Nasion Basion at CC

AJ Age	6.11	8.7	13.7
Cranial Base Angle	26	27	28
Facial Axis Angle	27	27	23
F/M Plane Angle	30	30	31
Craniomandibular Angle	56	57	59
Maxillary Plane	1	2	2
Convexity	0	1	0
U/Incisor to Vertical	5	15	18
L/Incisor to Vertical	26	21	22
L/Incisor to A/Po	1	0	0
L/Lip to Aesthetic Plane	−1	−3	−3
6 to Pterygoid vertical	12	14	10

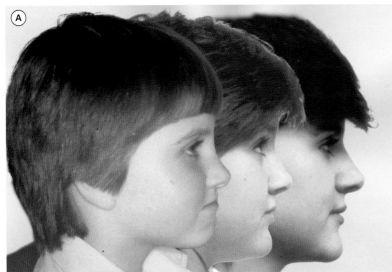

Fig. 14.9 Treatment:
A Profiles at ages 7 years 5 months (before treatment), 8 years 1 month (8 months after treatment) and 14 years 3 months.
B–D Occlusion before treatment.
E Facial appearance before treatment at age 7 years 5 months.
F Occlusion after 8 months.
G Facial appearance at age 14 years 3 months.
H–K Occlusion 6 years out of retention at age 14 years 3 months.

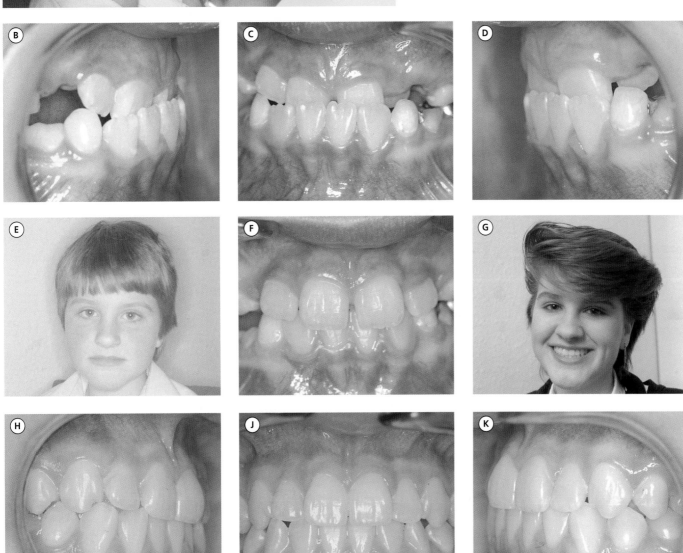

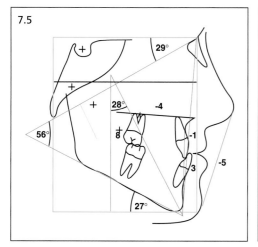

7.5

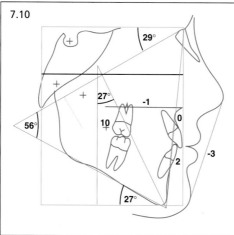

7.10

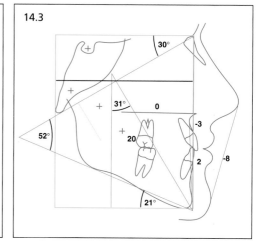

14.3

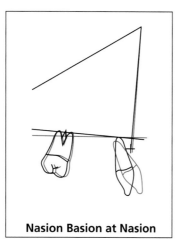

Maxillary Plane at ANS

Corpus Axis at PM

Nasion Basion at Nasion

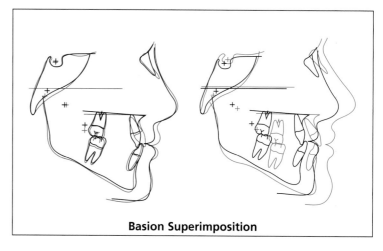

Basion Superimposition

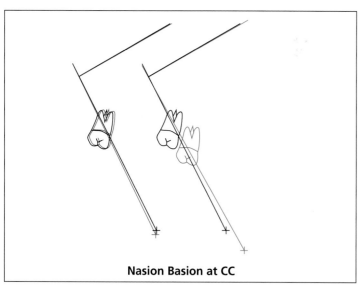

Nasion Basion at CC

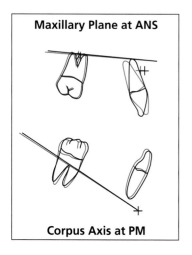

M.L.	Age 7.5	7.10	14.3
Cranial Base Angle	29	29	30
Facial Axis Angle	28	27	31
F/M Plane Angle	27	27	21
Craniomandibular Angle	56	56	52
Maxillary Plane	−4	−1	0
Convexity	−1	0	−3
U/Incisor to Vertical	11	29	30
L/Incisor to Vertical	26	26	18
Interincisal Angle	143	125	132
6 to Pterygoid Vertical	8	10	20
L/Incisor to A/Po	3	2	2
L/Lip to Aesthetic Plane	−5	−3	−8

EARLY TREATMENT OF SEVERE CLASS III MALOCCLUSION WITH REVERSE TWIN BLOCKS

A study to establish the efficiency of reverse Twin Blocks for the early treatment of Class III malocclusion was carried out at University College, London (Kidner, Di Biase *et al.*, 1998). The appliance design did not include any additional provision for advancement of the upper incisors. Fourteen subjects with severe Class III malocclusion were selected according to criteria established by Loh & Kerr (1985). The treatment effects were as follows:

- Retroclination of lower incisors.
- Proclination of upper incisors.
- Increase in SNA (mean values 79.4° before treatment, 79.8° after treatment).
- Decrease in SNB (from 81.2° to 79.6°).
- Increase in ANB (from –1.9° to +0.2°).
- Increase in MM angle (from 25° to 26.5°).
- Decrease in overbite.

The study concluded that the appliance was well tolerated, and treatment time was 75% less than with the FR III (Loh & Kerr, 1985). Compensation was achieved with minimal skeletal changes. Results compared favourably with the FR III appliance.

The superimposed tracings before and after treatment indicate that correction is achieved by proclining upper incisors, retroclining lower incisors, while the mandible rotates slightly downwards and backwards to improve the skeletal relationship.

REVERSE PULL FACIAL MASK

The reverse pull facial mask applies an additional component of orthopaedic force to advance the maxilla by elastic traction (Delaire, 1971, 1976; Delaire *et al.*, 1972; Petit, 1982, 1983, 1984, 1991; McNamara, 1987, 1993). This mechanism can be attached to the upper Twin Block to maximise the forward component of force on the maxilla, converting the technique to a functional orthopaedic system. The addition of three-way expansion in the appliance design enhances treatment of maxillary deficiency. Sagittal screws cut anterior to the upper molars have the effect of increasing the activation of the inclined planes to advance the premaxillary segment by driving the blocks distally against the resistance of the lower inclined planes (Fig. 14.10 A, B).

The elastic force applied should be increased gradually from the time the facial mask is fitted and as the patient adapts to the pressure. A starting pressure using bilateral 3/8 in, 8 oz elastics is recommended for the first 2 weeks. The force may then be increased by using 1/2 in, 14 oz elastics, and later to a maximum by 5/16 in, 14 oz elastics. If the patient experiences pain or soft-tissue irritation, the elastic force should be reduced to a more comfortable level.

The face mask is most effective if worn for a short period of 4–6 months using heavy forces. The additional functional forces make it unnecessary to wear the facial mask during the day and it can be applied as a night-time auxilliary force.

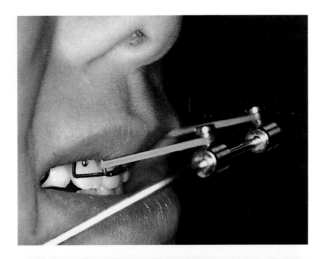

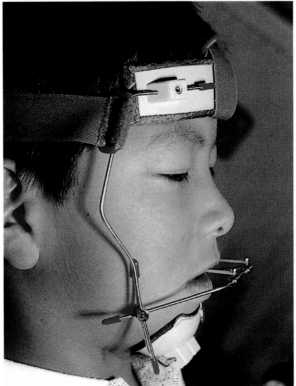

Fig. 14.10 A, B An example of facial mask for maxillary advancement.

REFERENCES

Delaire, J. (1971). Confection du masque orthopedique. *Rev. Stomat. Paris*, **72:** 579–84.

Delaire, J. (1976). L'articulation fronto-maxillaire. Bases theoretiques et principles generaux d'application de forces extra-orales postero-anterieures sur masque orthopedique. *Rev. Stomat. Paris*, **77:** 921–30.

Delaire, J., Verson, P., Lumineau, J.P., Gegha-Negrea, A., Talmont, J. & Boisson, M. (1972). Quelques resultats des tractions extra-orales à apput fronto-mentonnier dans le traitement orthopedique des malformations maxillo mandibulaires de Class III et des sequelles osseuses des fentes labio-maxillaires. *Rev. Stomat. Paris*, **73:** 633–42.

Kidner, G., Di Biase, A., Bali, J. & Di Biase, D. (1998). Reverse Twin Blocks for early treatment of Class III malocclusion. Poster exhibit, EOS Congress.

Loh, M.K. & Kerr, W.J.S. (1985). The Function Regulator III: Effects and indications for use. *Br. Dent. J.*, **12:** 153–157.

McNamara, J.A. (1987). An orthopedic approach to the treatment of class III malocclusion in young patients. *J. Clin. Orthod.*, **21:** 598–608.

McNamara, J.A. (1993). Orthopedic facial mask therapy. In *Orthodontic and Orthopedic Treatment in the Mixed Dentition*. Ann Arbor, Needham Press, pp. 283–95.

Petit, H.P. (1982). Syndromes prognathiques: schemas de traitement 'global' autour de masques facieux. *Rev. Orthop. Dent. Faciale*, **16:** 381–411.

Petit, H.P. (1983). Adaptation following accelerated facial mask therapy. In *Clinical Alteration of the Growing Face*, eds J.A. McNamara, Jr, J.A. Ribbens & R.P. Howe. Monograph No. 14, Craniofacial Growth Series. Ann Arbor, University of Michigan.

Petit, H.P. (1984). Orthopédie et/ou Orthodontie. *Orthod. Fr.*, **55:** 527–33.

Petit, H.P. (1991). Normalisation morphogenetique, apport de l'orthopédie. *Orthod. Fr.*, **62:** 549–57.

CHAPTER 15

Orthodontics, Orthopaedics or Surgery?

Treatment of severe Class II malocclusion may involve a choice between orthodontics, orthopaedics or surgery. Some patients may require a combination of these disciplines. A severe skeletal discrepancy cannot normally be treated by orthodontics alone, except to a compromise result, where the skeletal component is not corrected. Correction of severe maxillary protrusion may be achieved by the application of orthopaedic forces through a facebow and headgear, aiming to restrict forward maxillary growth. This approach is often more successful in the younger child, but has the disadvantage of being time consuming, as treatment can be slow and extend over a lengthy period of time.

Orthodontic force levels are not sufficient to encourage a significant increase in mandibular growth. Treatment of mandibular retrusion ideally requires a combination of orthodontics with either orthopaedic force to stimulate mandibular growth, or surgery to correct the mandibular deficiency. A choice between these alternatives is usually made according to the belief and experience of the practitioner. Opinions remain divided on philosophical grounds regarding the efficacy of functional mandibular protrusion as a mechanism for improving the mandibular growth response.

In the early 1960s the author shared the same experience as most orthodontists engaged in a postgraduate orthodontic training programme. The perceived knowledge from research on growth seemed to indicate that it was not possible to enhance mandibular growth, and the existing pattern of craniofacial growth was thought to be genetically predetermined. According to the genetic paradigm, the only feasible approach to the treatment of a retrusive mandible was to retract the maxilla to match the position of the retrusive mandible, or alternatively to correct the skeletal discrepancy surgically, with the attendant risk factors and the excessive cost of combined surgical and orthodontic treatment. The latter approach

became more popular in North America, while functional appliances remained popular in Europe, partly due to social and financial factors.

During the twentieth century the debate regarding the potential of functional appliances to stimulate mandibular growth remained unresolved. Early experience with night-time functional appliances did not produce encouraging results. The design of functional appliances continued to evolve as modifications were made to reduce the bulk of acrylic in order to increase the number of hours of day-time wear. Only in the latter part of the century did research begin to examine the effects of full-time functional appliances, with more positive results.

A fundamental aim of a dentofacial orthopaedic approach is to enhance mandibular growth by functional mandibular protrusion. The crucial question remains: 'Does full-time appliance wear bring us closer to achieving this objective?' Improved functional technique offers a more pragmatic solution for the patient who prefers not to undergo major surgery. This approach has the additional advantage that the cost to the patient and the provider of the service is significantly reduced compared to the more expensive surgical alternative.

The purpose of this chapter is to examine the potential for an orthopaedic/orthodontic correction for patients who might otherwise be considered suitable for surgical/orthodontic correction. The following patients were treated by Dr Forbes Leishman in his orthodontic practice in Auckland, New Zealand. They are examples of the treatment of severe malocclusions by a combination of Twin Blocks followed by fixed appliances, demonstrating the potential of the orthopaedic/orthodontic interface as an alternative to the surgical approach. These cases show a level of expertise in dentofacial orthopaedics that offers a valid alternative to the surgical approach.

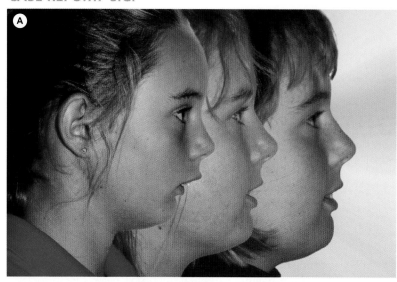

Fig. 15.1 Progress during treatment of this severe malocclusion:
A Profiles at ages 11 years 8 months (before treatment), 12 years 4 months (after treatment) and 23 years 8 months (out of retention).
B Overjet of 20 mm before treatment with anterior open bite.
C, D Occlusion before treatment.
E, F Corrected occlusion at age 14 years 6 months.

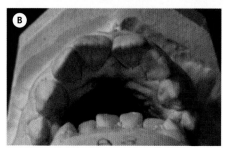

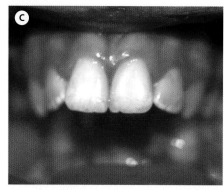

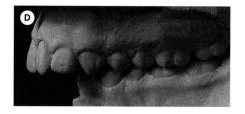

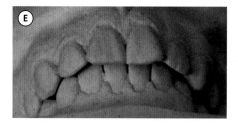

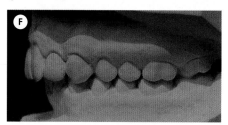

CASE REPORT: S.G. AGED 11 YEARS 8 MONTHS

by Forbes Leishman

The first patient undoubtedly falls within guidelines normally considered for surgical correction. Before treatment she presented an overjet of 20 mm and an anterior open bite associated with thumb sucking. The lower incisors were retroclined and positioned 7 mm lingual to the A–Po line. The skeletal pattern is moderate brachyfacial with a combination of maxillary protrusion and mandibular retrusion. A convexity of 8 mm is combined with a Class II molar relationship discrepancy of 11 mm, equivalent to a full molar width. In most orthodontic offices surgery would be considered the best option in a malocclusion of this severity. This patient was not keen to embark on major surgery, and preferred the functional approach.

After 8 months of treatment with Twin Blocks the overjet reduced to 8 mm, with the lower incisors positioned 3.5 mm lingual to A–Po. A subsequent orthodontic phase of treatment produced an excellent Class I occlusion. A favourable response during treatment resulted in a reduction in convexity from 8 mm to 4 mm. The patient was followed through post treatment to age 23 years 8 months, a total of 12 years from the commencement of treatment. In the post-treatment period the overjet increased from 4 mm to 6 mm, while the convexity remained 4 mm. At age 23 there is mild crowding in the lower arch with excellent stability of the Class I occlusion. A functional orthopaedic approach followed by orthodontics achieved facial balance and a good profile. These changes were maintained out of retention and treatment of this severe malocclusion was completed without the need for surgery (Fig. 15.1).

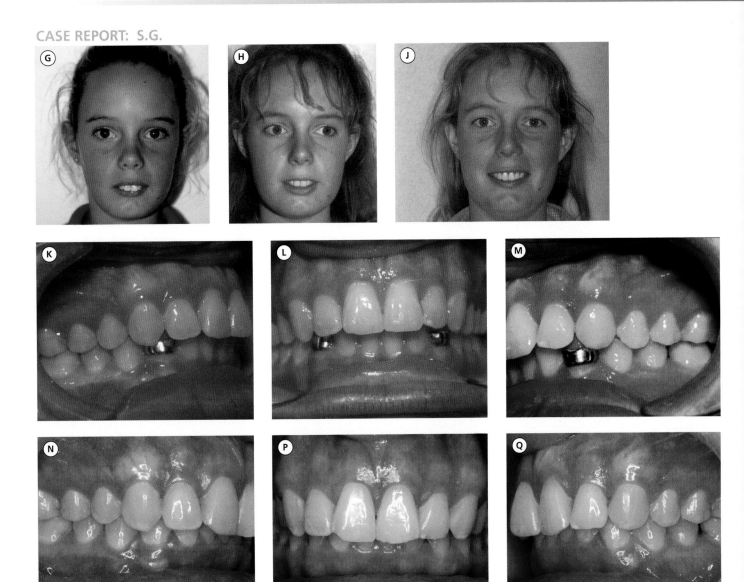

Fig. 15.1 (cont.)
G Facial appearance before treatment.
H Facial appearance after treatment at age 12 years 4 months.
J Age 23 years, 8 months.
K, L, M Occlusion after treatment at age 14 years 6 months.
N, P, Q Occlusion out of retention at age 23 years 8 months.

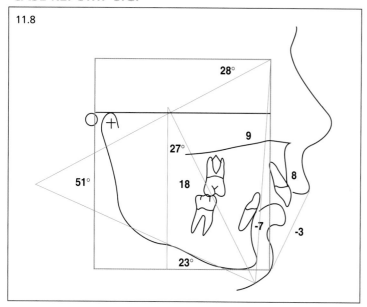

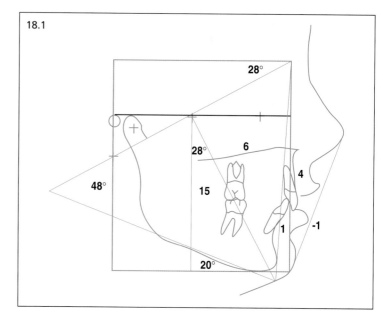

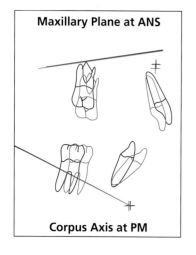

Maxillary Plane at ANS

Corpus Axis at PM

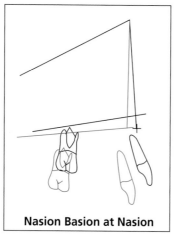

Nasion Basion at Nasion

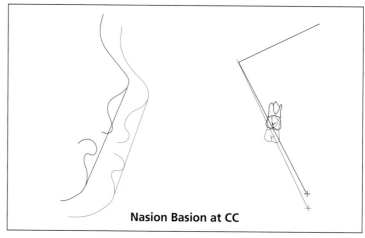

Nasion Basion at CC

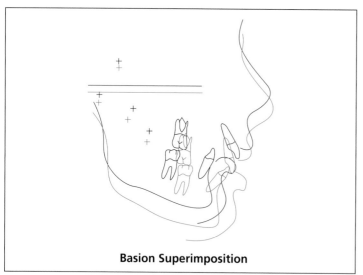

Basion Superimposition

S.G. Age	11.8	18.1
Cranial Base Angle	28	28
Facial Axis Angle	27	28
F/M Plane Angle	23	20
Craniomandibular Angle	51	48
Maxillary Plane	9	6
Convexity	8	4
U/Incisor to Vertical	24	15
L/Incisor to Vertical	27	42
L/Incisor to A/Po	−7	1
L/Lip to Aesthetic Plane	−3	−1
6 to Pterygoid vertical	18	15

CASE REPORT: T.K.

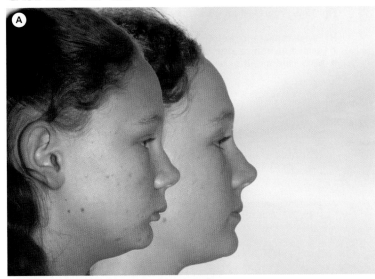

Fig. 15.2 Progress during treatment of this severe malocclusion:
A Profiles at ages 14 years 9 months (before treatment) and 20 years 2 months (out of retention).
B–D Occlusion before treatment.
E–G Occlusion after treatment at age 17 years 3 months.

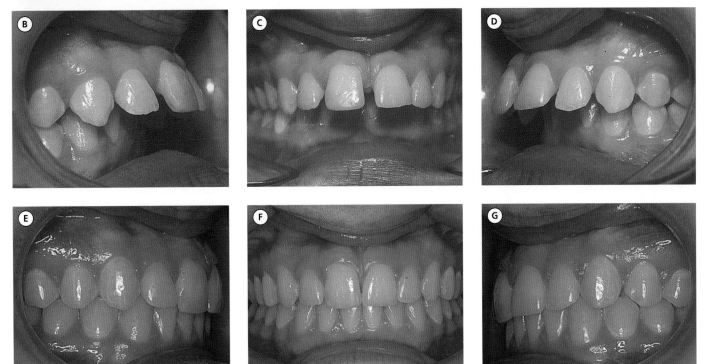

CASE REPORT: T.K. AGED 14 YEARS 9 MONTHS

This girl was a late starter and was approaching 15 years old when Twin Blocks were fitted. It may be tempting to consider surgery to assist correction for a girl who is past the pubertal growth phase and whose growth is virtually complete, especially as the pre-treatment profile is poor. The convexity of 3 mm is due to maxillary protrusion as the mandible is well developed and exhibits a brachyfacial growth pattern. This gives the appearance of overclosure, resulting from reduced lower facial height. The upper incisors are severely proclined, with the lower lip trapped in an overjet of 13 mm. The lower incisors are retroclined and biting into the palate with an excessive overbite, and are positioned 3 mm lingual to the A–Po line as a result of lower alveolar retrusion.

In this type of malocclusion the vertical correction is as important as sagittal correction. The profile improves with anterior repositioning of the mandible and adjustment of the blocks to allow vertical development of lower molars.

CASE REPORT: T.K.

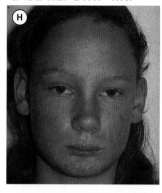

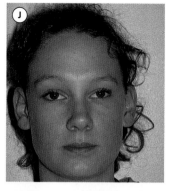

Fig. 15.2 Progress during treatment of this severe malocclusion (cont.):
H Facial appearance before treatment.
J Facial appearance after treatment.
K–M Occlusion out of retention at age 20 years 2 months.

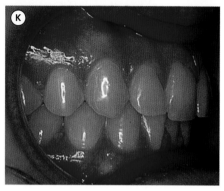

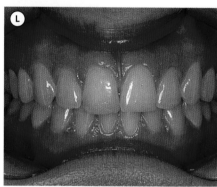

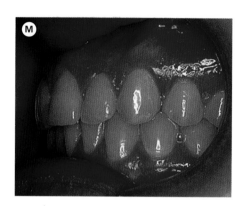

The final orthodontic phase repositions the lower incisors in correct relationship to the anterior limit of the skeletal base (within the range of +1 to +3 to the A–Po line) to improve the contour of the lower lip. Final records show the position out of retention at age 20 years 2 months (Fig. 15.2).

This is an example of forward positioning of the mandible due to an alteration in the angle of growth of the condyle, as clearly shown in the mandibular superimposition.

The distal direction of condylar growth is evident from the increased gonial angle. As a result the mandible rotates forward significantly changing the shape of the lower face in profile and full face views.

Twin Blocks: 15 months
Bite plane: 3 months
Fixed appliances: 12 months
Total treatment time: 2 years 6 months followed by retention.

CASE REPORT: C.M. AGED 11 YEARS 5 MONTHS

by Forbes Leishman

This case presents another severe malocclusion, treated in early permanent dentition, where surgery might have been considered as a possible solution. Altered incisal angulations contribute to an overjet of 15 mm and excessive overbite with the lower incisors 5 mm lingual to the A–Po line in this case. Once again the large overjet can be partly attributed to unfavourable lip posture, as a severely trapped lower lip accentuates the problem.

A brachyfacial growth pattern and 8 mm convexity is due mainly to mandibular retrusion, and at this age the potential for correction with the assistance of growth is favourable. The convexity is reduced to 3 mm with a fully corrected occlusion and the improvement is maintained 3 years after completion of treatment (Fig. 15.3). This case also shows significant distal growth and lengthening of the condyle, resulting in forward positioning of the mandible.

Twin Blocks: 9 months
Bite plane: 5 months
Fixed appliances: 12 months
Total treatment time: 2 years 3 months followed by retention.

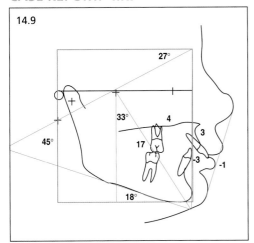

14.9

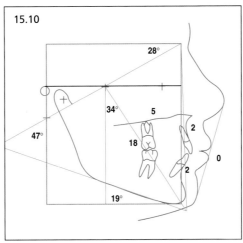

15.10

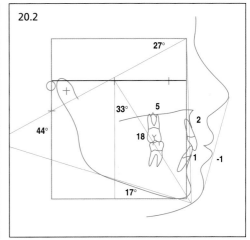

20.2

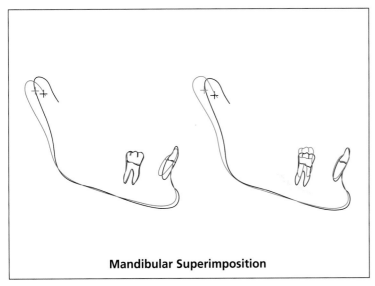

Mandibular Superimposition

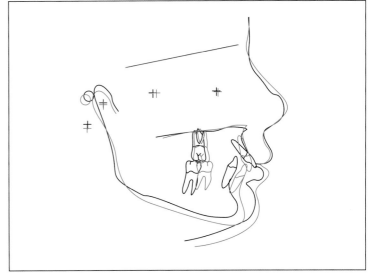

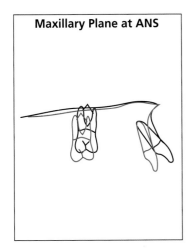

Maxillary Plane at ANS

T.K. Age	14.9	15.10	20.2
Cranial Base Angle	27	28	27
Facial Axis Angle	33	34	33
F/M Plane Angle	18	19	17
Craniomandibular Angle	45	47	44
Maxillary Plane	4	5	5
Convexity	3	2	0
U/Incisor to Vertical	37	20	18
L/Incisor to Vertical	26	35	27
L/Incisor to A/Po	−3	2	1
L/Lip to Aesthetic Plane	−1	0	−1
6 to Pterygoid vertical	17	18	18

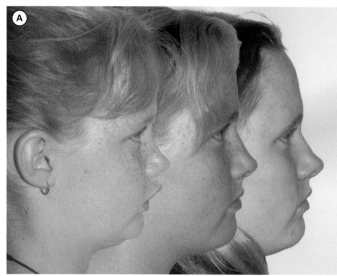

Fig. 15.3 Progress during treatment of this severe malocclusion:
A Profiles at ages 11 years 5 months (before treatment),
13 years 9 months (after treatment) and 17 years (out of
retention).
B Facial appearance before treatment.
C Facial appearance after treatment.
D Facial appearance out of retention.
E–G Occlusion before treatment.
H–K Occlusion out of retention. The incisal edges of 1|1 were
trimmed to improve the appearance in the end result.

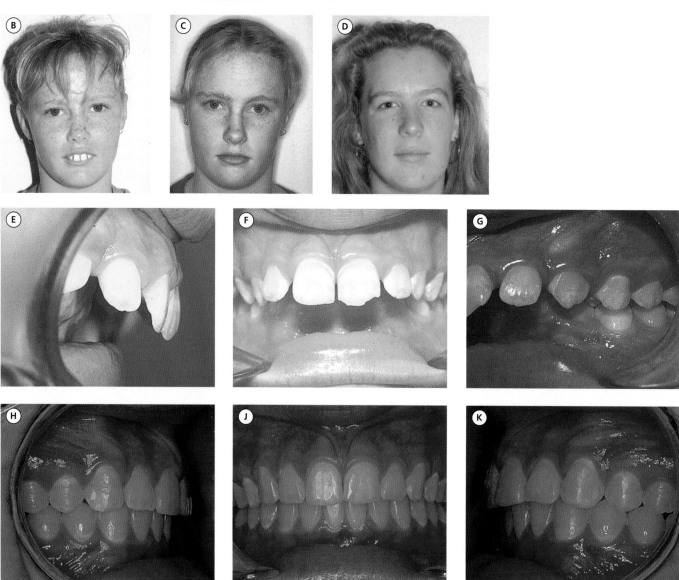

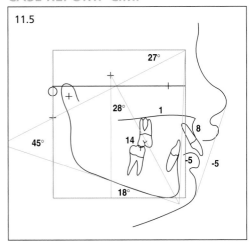

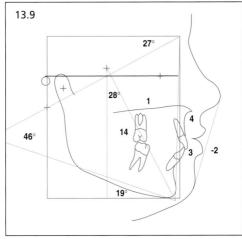

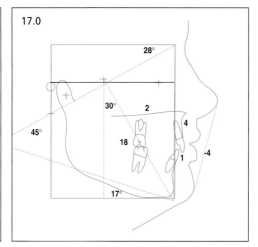

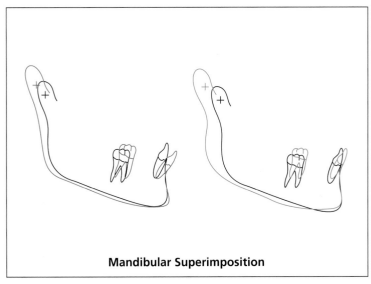

Mandibular Superimposition

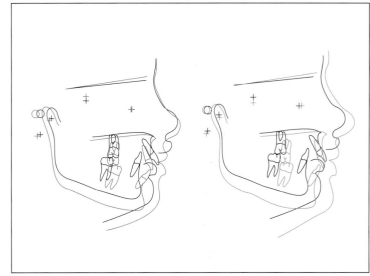

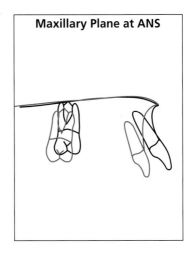

Maxillary Plane at ANS

C.M. Age	11.5	13.9	17.0
Cranial Base Angle	27	27	28
Facial Axis Angle	28	28	30
F/M Plane Angle	18	19	18
Craniomandibular Angle	45	46	45
Maxillary Plane	1	1	2
Convexity	8	4	4
U/Incisor to Vertical	30	21	14
L/Incisor to Vertical	20	40	25
L/Incisor to A/Po	-5	3	1
L/Lip to Aesthetic Plane	-5	-2	-4
6 to Pterygoid vertical	14	14	18

CASE REPORT: A.B.

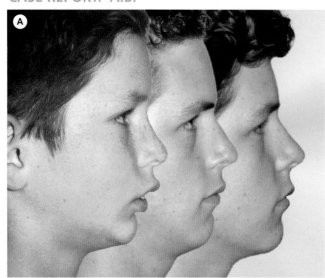

Fig. 15.4 Progress during treatment of this severe malocclusion:
A Profiles at ages 12 years 8 months (before treatment), 14 years 8 months (after treatment) and 16 years 6 months (out of retention).
B, C Occlusion before treatment.
D–F Occlusion after treatment.

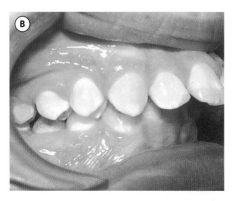

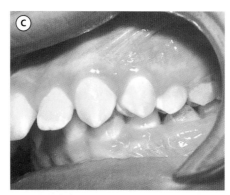

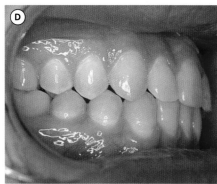

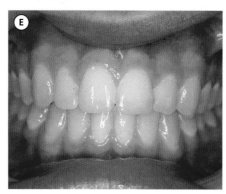

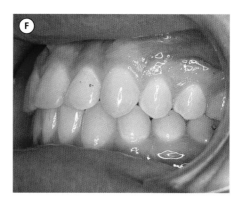

CASE REPORT: A.B. AGED 12 YEARS 8 MONTHS

by Forbes Leishman

This boy has a severe dental Class II malocclusion with buccal occlusion of all the upper premolars in addition to a 12 mm overjet and excessive overbite. The skeletal pattern is mesofacial, with a retrusive mandible, and also slight maxillary retrusion contributing to a retrognathic profile. This malocclusion that requires careful management in view of the severity of the dental malocclusion. Even taking into account the dento-alveolar factors in the aetiology of this malocclusion, correction by orthodontic means alone would be a long and laborious task, to the extent that some practitioners may be tempted to resort to the surgical alternative.

In a combined orthopaedic and orthodontic approach correction of the sagittal relationship by advancing the mandible produces an improvement in the transverse discrepancy, so that the finishing phase with fixed appliances is simplified. Excellent stability and improved facial aesthetics is evident at age 18, 3 years after completion of treatment

CASE REPORT: A.B.

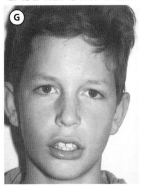

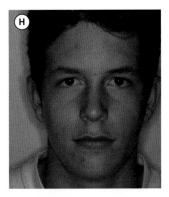

Fig. 15.4 Progress during treatment of this severe malocclusion (cont.):
G Facial appearance before treatment.
H Facial appearance out of retention.
J–L Occlusion out of retention.

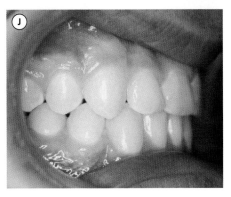

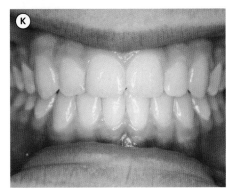

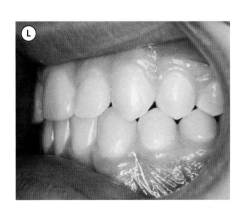

(Fig. 15.4). Once again, the condylar extension is exceptional, presumably taking advantage of the pubertal growth spurt to maximise the orthopaedic response to treatment.

Twin Blocks: 11 months
Bite plane: 3 months
Fixed appliances: 10 months
Total treatment time: 2 years followed by retention.

CASE REPORT: N.M. AGED 11 YEARS

by Forbes Leishman

Severe maxillary protrusion is the main aetiological factor in this case for a girl who presents a brachyfacial pattern with a normal mandible and excessive overjet of 14 mm. The convexity of 6 mm is due entirely to the maxillary protrusion as confirmed by an SNA angle of 90°. This case demonstrates that maxillary protrusion may be treated effectively by

mandibular advancement to produce an excellent balanced profile and good facial aesthetics. It is important to confirm this before treatment by examining the profile with the mandible protruded to register a Class I relationship of the molars. This simple guideline is a preview of the end result, and helps to confirm the diagnosis.

Correction is achieved by advancing the mandible to match the protrusive position of the maxilla. This produces a slightly prognathic straight profile with good facial balance and an aesthetically pleasing result. The maxillary convexity reduced from 6 mm to 2 mm after 1 year of treatment and excellent stability is maintained 3 years after completion of treatment, with a convexity of 1 mm (Fig. 15.5). Condylar extension is again exceptional.

Twin Blocks: 6 months
Harvold activator as retainer: 5 months
Fixed appliances: 21 months
Total treatment time: 2 years 8 months followed by retention.

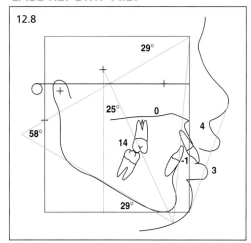

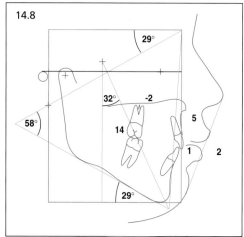

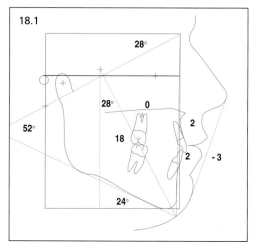

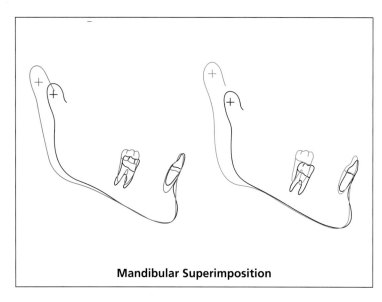

Mandibular Superimposition

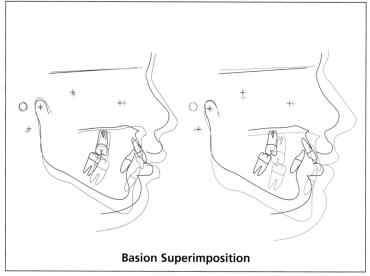

Basion Superimposition

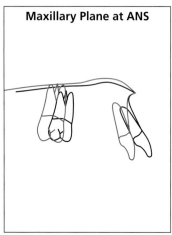

Maxillary Plane at ANS

A.B. Age	12.8	14.8	18.1
Cranial Base Angle	29	29	28
Facial Axis Angle	25	26	28
F/M Plane Angle	29	29	24
Craniomandibular Angle	58	58	52
Maxillary Plane	0	–2	0
Convexity	4	5	2
U/Incisor to Vertical	30	17	19
L/Incisor to Vertical	30	30	20
L/Incisor to A/Po	–1	1	2
L/Lip to Aesthetic Plane	3	2	–3
6 to Pterygoid vertical	14	14	18

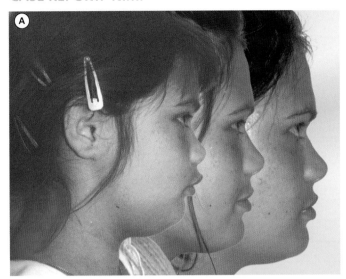

Fig. 15.5 Progress during treatment of this severe malocclusion:
A Profiles at ages 11 years (before treatment), 13 years 10 months (after treatment) and 16 years 6 months (out of retention).
B–D Occlusion before treatment.
E–G Occlusion out of retention.
H Facial appearance before treatment.
J Facial appearance after treatment.
K Facial appearance out of retention.

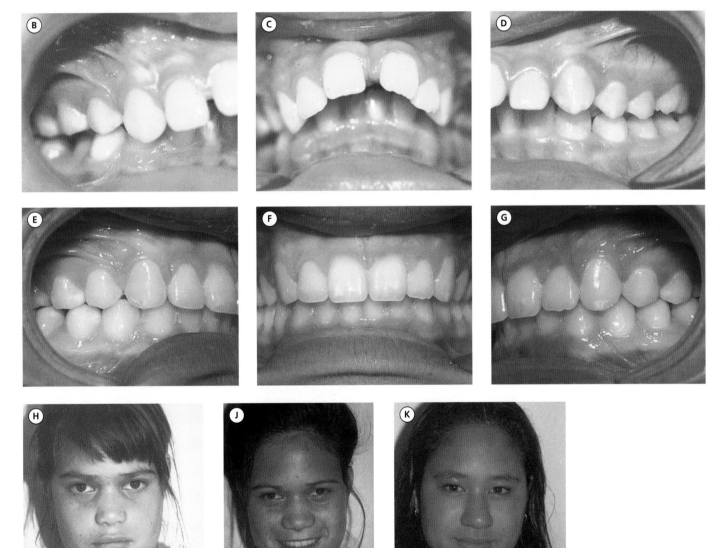

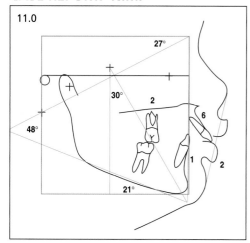

11.0

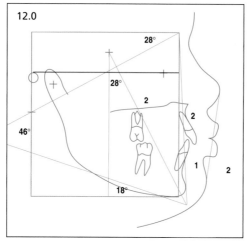

12.0

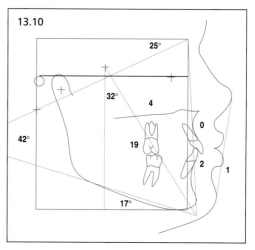

13.10

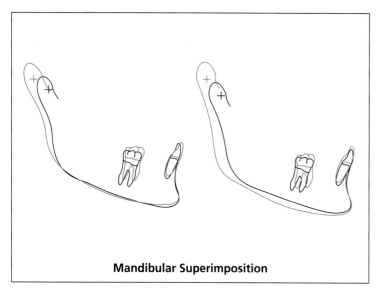

Mandibular Superimposition

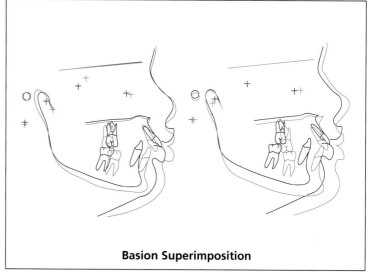

Basion Superimposition

Maxillary Plane at ANS

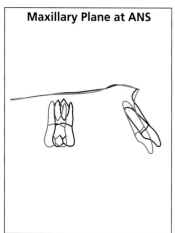

N.M. Age	11.0	12.0	13.10
Cranial Base Angle	27	28	25
Facial Axis Angle	30	32	32
F/M Plane Angle	21	18	17
Craniomandibular Angle	48	46	42
Maxillary Plane	4	4	4
Convexity	6	2	0
U/Incisor to Vertical	43	25	30
L/Incisor to Vertical	21	22	25
L/Incisor to A/Po	–2	2	2
L/Lip to Aesthetic Plane	3	3	1
6 to Pterygoid vertical	18	15	17

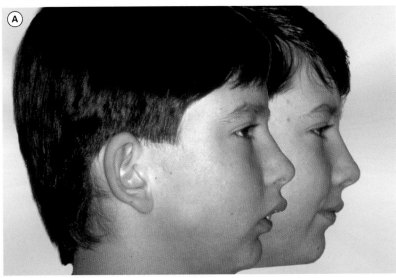

Fig. 15.6 Progress during treatment of this severe malocclusion:
A Profiles at ages 13 years 2 months (before treatment), and 14 years 6 months (after treatment).
B Occlusion before treatment.
C Occlusion after treatment.

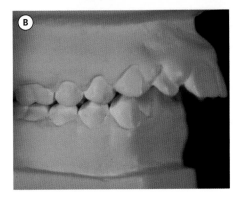

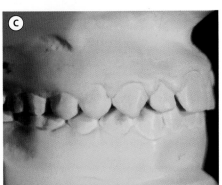

CASE REPORT: G.K. AGED 13 YEARS 2 MONTHS

by Gordon Kluzak

This patient was treated in Calgary by Dr Gordon Kluzak. Prior to consulting Dr Kluzak he had previously attended two orthodontic offices where he was advised to have surgical correction.

A severe malocclusion with a 17 mm overjet and deep overbite was related to a convexity of 11 mm due to maxillary protrusion and mild mandibular retrusion. There was a mild dolichofacial pattern. This boy lacked confidence because he had a disfiguring malocclusion, which resulted in him being teased at school.

His treatment was completed without complications within 16 months using Twin Blocks followed by an anterior inclined plane.

Changes in the temporomandibular joint were recorded by means of an orthophos x-ray unit using a slice technique to record standardised joint x-rays. Films were taken to show the position of the condyle in the glenoid fossa before treatment with the teeth in occlusion, and also with the Twin Blocks in position. A second series of radiographs recorded the position 16 months later after completion of treatment. A cephalometric film was taken at the same visit to show the corrected occlusion.

Joint x-rays recorded the position of the condyles as follows:

1. Before treatment with the teeth in occlusion.
2. At commencement of treatment in occlusion with the Twin Blocks in place.
3. After 16 months of treatment with the teeth in occlusion.

The joint x-rays were examined to measure the distance from the nearest point on the condyle to the nearest point on the bony outline of the auditory canal. These measurements on the x-rays confirmed without doubt that the condyles were repositioned in the glenoid fossa after treatment after correction of the distal occlusion and reduction of the 17 mm overjet to 3 mm (Fig. 15.6).

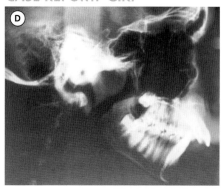

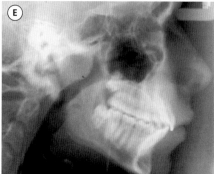

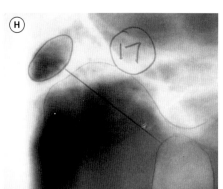

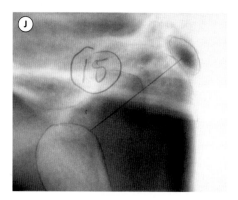

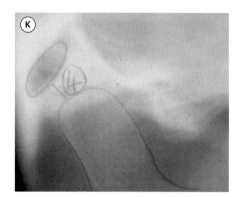

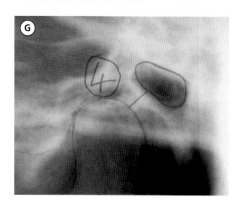

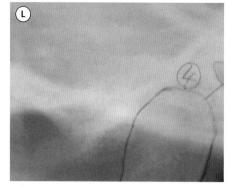

Fig. 15.6 Progress during treatment of this severe malocclusion (cont.):
Cephalometric films and joint x-rays taken before treatment and 16 months later confirm that the occlusion is fully corrected and the condyles are correctly positioned in the glenoid fossae on completion of treatment:
D, E Cephalometric films.
F, G Joint x-rays in occlusion before treatment.
H, J Joint x-rays with Twin Blocks.
K, L Joint x-rays in occlusion after treatment.

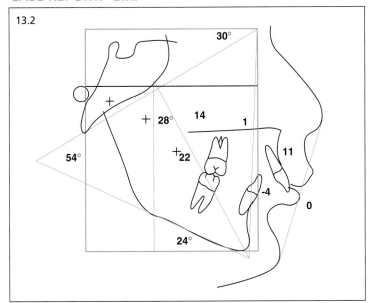

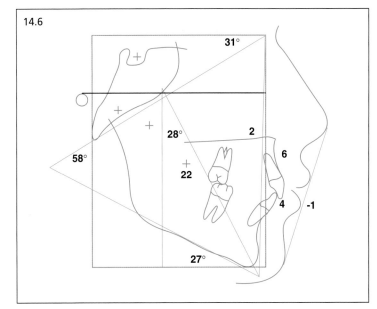

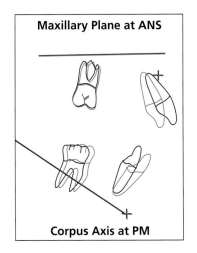

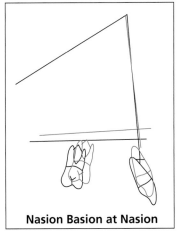

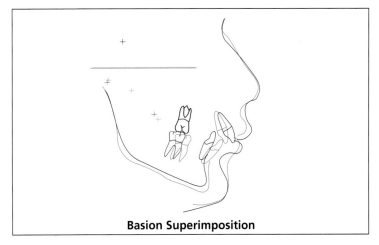

Basion Superimposition

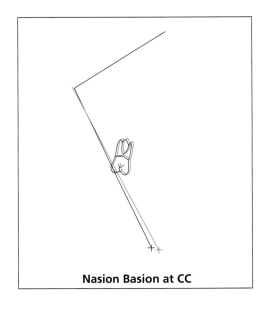

Nasion Basion at CC

G.K.	Age	13.2	14.6
Cranial Base Angle		30	31
Facial Axis Angle		28	28
F/M Plane Angle		24	27
Craniomandibular Angle		54	58
Maxillary Plane		1	2
Convexity		11	6
U/Incisor to Vertical		28	18
L/Incisor to Vertical		29	43
L/Incisor to A/Po		–4	4
L/Lip to Aesthetic Plane		0	–1
6 to Pterygoid vertical		22	22

DISCUSSION

Several of the patients illustrated in this chapter were advised by orthodontists that they required surgical correction. Considering the risks involved, they were not willing to have major surgery. They were subsequently treated to excellent results by an orthopaedic approach, when appropriate, combined with orthodontics.

All of these patients exhibit an exceptional growth response during Twin Block treatment, and it is likely that the treatment is timed to coincide with the pubertal growth spurt, perhaps with the exception of T.K. (pages 235–237). This case illustrates that altering the direction of growth of the condyle is as important as extending condylar length. The resulting forward rotation of the mandible significantly changes the contours of the lower face, both in profile and full face views. It is also evident that increased ramus height significantly alters the facial contours. In suitable cases, orthopaedic correction is a valid alternative to surgery in the growing child or adolescent.

CHAPTER 16

Management of Crowding

NON-EXTRACTION THERAPY

Interceptive treatment
Arch development

Crowding and irregularity of the dental arches may necessitate an interceptive stage of treatment to align the arches and improve the archform as a preliminary to the correction of arch-to-arch relationships. Interceptive treatment should be initiated as early as possible in the mixed dentition to develop correct archform before permanent successors erupt.

Examination of the occlusion prior to treatment establishes the necessity for an interceptive phase of arch development. If significant crowding is present, the upper and lower archform does not match and, as a result, a preliminary stage of interceptive treatment becomes necessary.

Treatment concept

The upper and lower dental arches must be compatible to achieve a stable occlusion. This can be checked before treatment by sliding the lower model forward to eliminate the overjet and correct the buccal segment relationships. If the archform does not match it is not possible to fit the models together correctly. It is then necessary to correct the archform before mandibular translation. A similar clinical guideline is observed by posturing the mandible forward to see if the teeth will interdigitate correctly in good occlusion when the mandible is advanced to correct the distal occlusion. If forward movement of the mandible would result in a poor occlusion it may be necessary to correct the archform first before advancing the mandible by functional therapy.

Integration of Twin Blocks and fixed therapy

Combined orthopaedic and orthodontic treatment may be planned in two phases, depending on the age of the patient at the start of treatment and the degree of severity of the skeletal and dental problems. Arch development and functional therapy in the mixed dentition is frequently followed by a finishing phase of orthodontic treatment at a later stage of development.

In the permanent dentition fixed appliance treatment may precede Twin Block treatment to correct an irregular archform where the irregularity is moderate or severe. Alternatively, in less crowded cases fixed appliances may be integrated with Twin Blocks by the addition of brackets to correct anterior alignment. Further integration with fixed appliances can continue in the lower arch during the support phase, when the lower Twin Block is left out or, alternatively, a transition to full fixed appliances may be made on completion of functional correction. The treatment of patients presenting a combination of crowding, dental irregularity and skeletal discrepancy requires more time compared to the treatment of uncrowded cases with good archform.

ARCH DEVELOPMENT BEFORE FUNCTIONAL THERAPY

Combination fixed/functional therapy

CASE REPORT: K.C. AGED 11 YEARS 2 MONTHS

A severe Class II division 1 malocclusion is complicated by crowding in the lower arch. The position of the lower incisors 4 mm lingual to the A–Po line compensates for the degree of crowding in the lower arch. Each millimetre advancement of the lower incisors results in a gain of 2 mm in arch length, equivalent to 1 mm on each side. This permits the lower incisors to be advanced by 4 mm during arch development to resolve 7 mm of crowding prior to functional therapy. The facial pattern is brachyfacial and retrognathic with mandibular retrusion. The dental relationship is severe Class II with a full unit distal occlusion and an overjet of 13 mm and excessive overbite. A lower canine is excluded from the arch

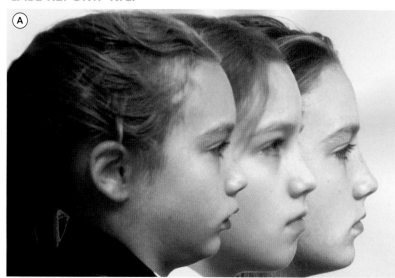

Fig. 16.1 Treatment:
A Profiles at ages 11 years 11 months (before Twin Blocks), 12 years 2 months (after 8 months with Twin Blocks) and 14 years 7 months (18 months out of retention).
B–D Occlusion before treatment.
E, F Bihelix to improve the lower archform at age 11 years 2 months and 11 years 11 months.
G Upper fixed appliance to improve the upper archform.
H, J Tracing and profile before arch development.

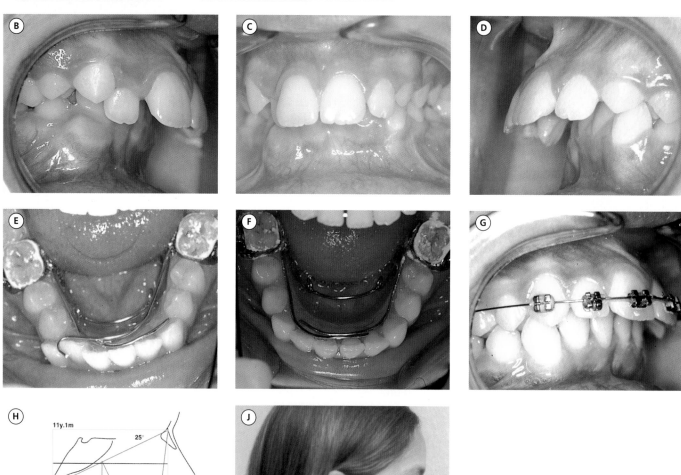

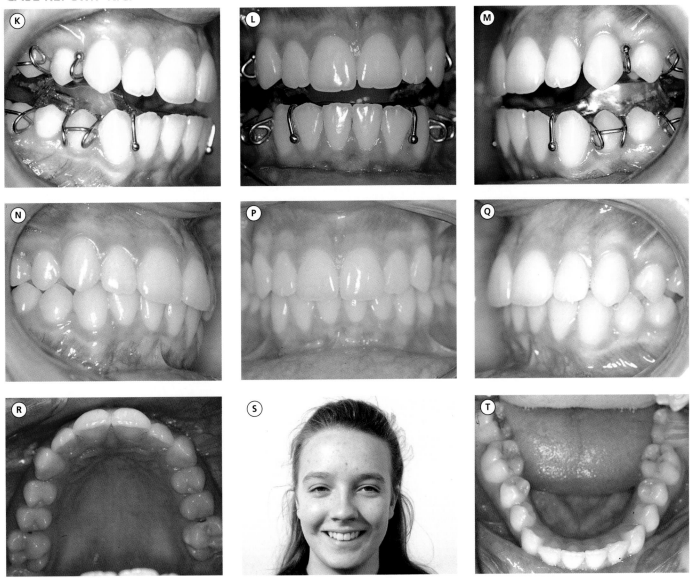

Fig. 16.1 Treatment (cont.):
K–M Twin Blocks in phase 2.
Note the rapid improvement in the profile after 2 1/2 months with Twin Blocks is maintained out of retention.

N–Q Occlusion at age 14 years 7 months.
R, T Upper and lower archform after treatment.
S Facial appearance at age 17 years 3 months.

buccally, with a resulting displacement of the lower centre line.

During an initial phase of arch development a quad helix is used to expand the maxillary arch with brackets on the upper anterior teeth to correct alignment. In the lower arch a bihelix is used to correct the archform with cross-arch anchorage to accommodate the blocked-out canine. The Curve of Spee improves as the lower arch is levelled during arch development.

An overjet of 10 mm and a full unit distal occlusion remains after arch development and is corrected with Twin Blocks. A dramatic change in facial balance is evident after only 8 weeks of treatment with Twin Blocks, and following the rapid response, the improvement proved to be stable 18 months out of retention (Fig. 16.1).

Arch development: 11 months
Twin Blocks: 7 months
Retention: 7 months
Treatment time: 25 months
Final records: 18 months out of retention at age 14 years 9 months.

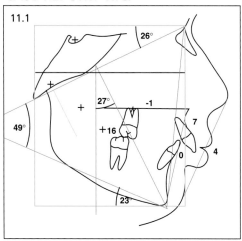

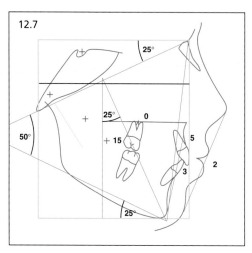

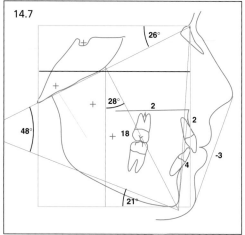

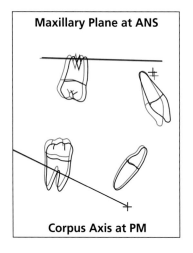

Maxillary Plane at ANS

Corpus Axis at PM

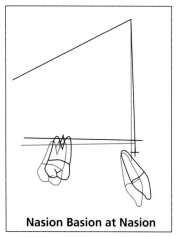

Nasion Basion at Nasion

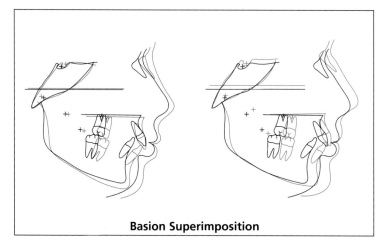

Basion Superimposition

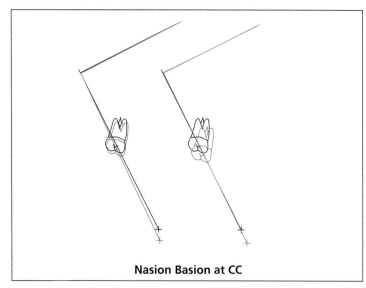

Nasion Basion at CC

K.C.	Age	11.11	12.7	14.7
Cranial Base Angle		26	25	26
Facial Axis Angle		27	25	28
F/M Plane Angle		23	25	21
Craniomandibular Angle		49	50	48
Maxillary Plane		−1	0	2
Convexity		7	5	2
U/Incisor to Vertical		31	22	21
L/Incisor to Vertical		37	42	36
Interincisal Angle		112	116	123
6 to Pterygoid Vertical		16	15	18
L/Incisor to A/Po		0	3	4
L/Lip to Aesthetic Plane		4	2	−3

MANAGEMENT OF CROWDING: NON-EXTRACTION THERAPY

When a Class II division 1 malocclusion is associated with a severe lip trap the conspiring labial muscle imbalance can lead to collapse of the lower labial segment and crowding in the lower arch. The profile determines whether the patient should be treated by extraction or non-extraction therapy, taking into account the degree of crowding in the lower arch, the position of the lower incisors relative to the anterior limit of the skeletal base and the lip contour relative to the aesthetic line (Fig. 16.2).

Premolar extractions are contraindicated when the skeletal growth pattern is severe brachyfacial, with a strong horizontal growth tendency in the mandible. Tight lip musculature with the lower lip trapped in the overjet is the primary causative factor for the crowding in the lower labial segment. The strong lip musculature is an indication that extraction of the premolars would be more likely to damage the profile by loss of support for the lips. Examination of the profile with the mandible postured forward to reduce the overjet confirms that facial balance would be improved by treatment to place the lower lip labial to the upper incisors.

The lower archform must be corrected first, however, to align the lower incisors prior to mandibular advancement. Lower arch crowding of 9 mm can be resolved by advancing the lower incisors from –4 mm behind the A–Po line before treatment to +1 mm to gain 10 mm of arch length. Extraction of the second molars is planned during the course of treatment to accommodate the third molars and to relieve the pressure from distal crowding in the lower arch.

Clinical management

An initial stage of treatment with a bihelix and a lower lip bumper is followed by a bonded lower fixed appliance over a period of 6 months to align the lower arch in preparation for functional correction. During this stage there is little change in the overjet or the profile.

Twin Blocks are fitted after correcting the lower archform. An immediate improvement in profile is observed as the facial balance improves dramatically in the early stages of treatment. Arch relationships are corrected in 6 months and an anterior inclined plane is fitted with a Wilson lower lingual arch to retain the position.

In spite of severe crowding in the lower labial segment before treatment the lower arch proved to be stable out of retention. It is likely that extraction of second molars contributed to the stability of the lower labial segment after treatment by reducing the mesial component of force that is normally associated with the development and eruption of third molars.

Arch development: 6 months
Twin Blocks: 6 months
Support and retention: 14 months.

CASE REPORT: N.K.

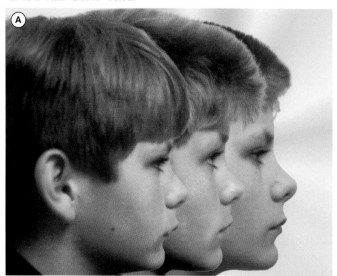

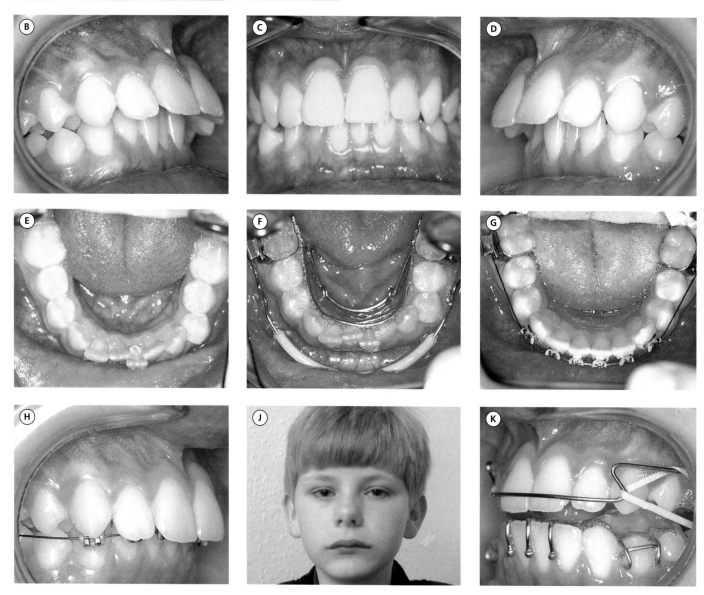

Fig. 16.2 Treatment:
A Profiles at ages 11 years 11 months (before treatment), 13 years (after Twin Blocks) and 15 years 10 months (out of retention).
B–D Occlusion before treatment.
E Lower arch crowding before treatment (ALD = 9 mm).
F Phase 1 arch development – bihelix and lip bumper.
G Detailing with the fixed appliance.
H Occlusion after arch development.
J Appearance before treatment.
K Phase 2 – Twin Blocks.

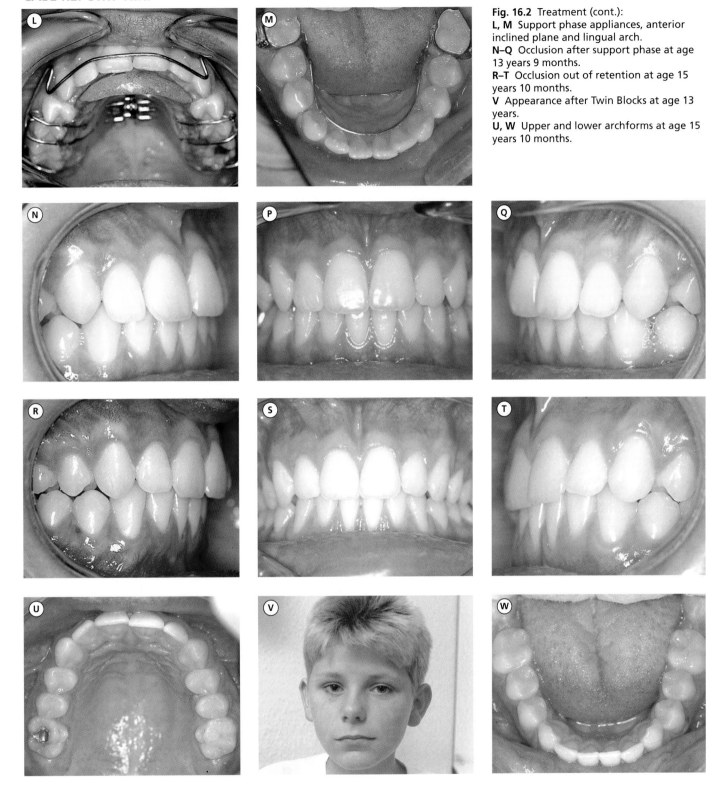

Fig. 16.2 Treatment (cont.):
L, M Support phase appliances, anterior inclined plane and lingual arch.
N–Q Occlusion after support phase at age 13 years 9 months.
R–T Occlusion out of retention at age 15 years 10 months.
V Appearance after Twin Blocks at age 13 years.
U, W Upper and lower archforms at age 15 years 10 months.

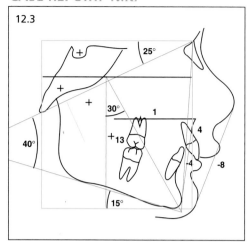

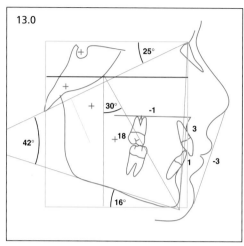

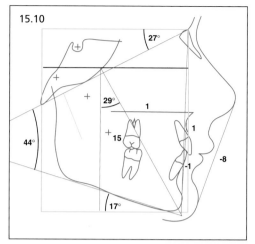

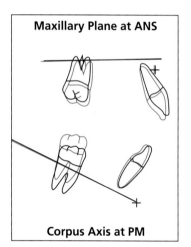

Maxillary Plane at ANS

Corpus Axis at PM

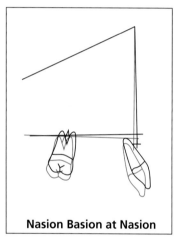

Nasion Basion at Nasion

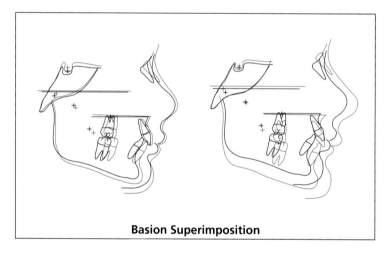

Basion Superimposition

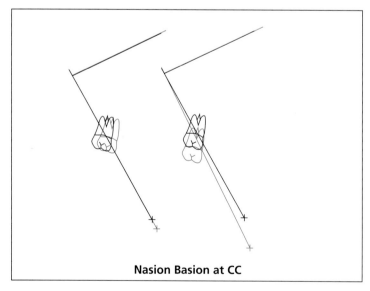

Nasion Basion at CC

N.K.	Age	12.3	13.0	15.10
Cranial Base Angle		25	25	27
Facial Axis Angle		30	30	29
F/M Plane Angle		15	16	17
Craniomandibular Angle		40	42	44
Maxillary Plane		1	−1	1
Convexity		4	3	1
U/Incisor to Vertical		28	23	13
L/Incisor to Vertical		37	25	28
Interincisal Angle		115	132	139
6 to Pterygoid Vertical		13	18	15
L/Incisor to A/Po		0	1	−1
L/Lip to Aesthetic Plane		−8	−3	−8

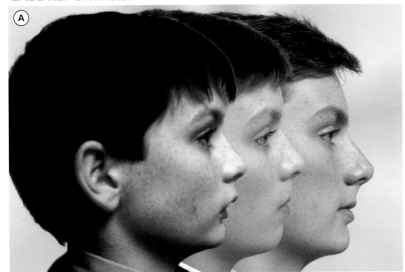

Fig. 16.3 Treatment:
A Profiles at ages 12 years 6 months (before treatment), 13 years 4 months (after 6 months with Twin Blocks) and 15 years 11 months.
B–D Occlusion before treatment.

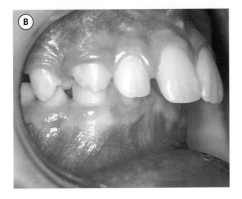

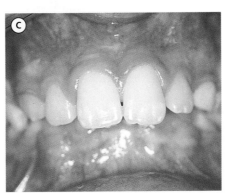

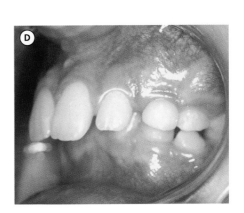

CASE REPORT: J.S. AGED 12 YEARS 6 MONTHS

This boy presents a Class II division 1 malocclusion with mild lower labial crowding. The facial type is severe brachyfacial with mandibular retrusion and a moderate convexity of 5 mm. Severe retrusion of the lower incisors (9 mm lingual to the A–Po line before treatment) is associated with an excessive overbite of 10 mm, and an excessive curve of Spee. The flattening of the lower labial segment is due to an active lower lip that is trapped in a 15 mm overjet. Arch development is indicated followed by functional mandibular advancement. It is difficult to design a satisfactory lower Twin Block until the alignment of the lower arch is improved. The treatment objectives are first to improve the archform, followed by functional correction to Class I occlusion and a final stage with fixed appliances to detail the occlusion (Fig. 16.3).

During treatment the lower incisor is advanced from a position 9 mm behind the A–Po line to its final position with the tip of the incisor on the A–Po line. This correction is by a combination of incisor proclination during initial arch development, and the forward translation of the incisors that accompanies mandibular advancement. Intermaxillary traction is applied in the final stage of treatment to stabilise the incisors and complete the correction. The facial appearance changes significantly as the lower lip moves from its trapped position lingual to the lower incisors. The lip contour improves as the lower incisors move labially to give better support to the lips and these changes have a profound influence on the soft-tissue balance of the lower third of the face.

Arch development: 3 months
Twin Blocks: 9 months
Support phase: 10 months
Fixed appliances: 8 months.

CASE REPORT: J.S.

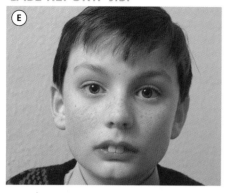

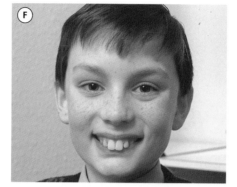

Fig. 16.3 Treatment (cont.):
E, F Appearance before treatment.
G–J Phase 1 – arch development, Wilson quad helix and lingual arch.
K, L Occlusion after 3 months of arch development.
M Occlusion after Twin Blocks.
N Twin Blocks in Phase 2.
P Occlusion after Twin Blocks.

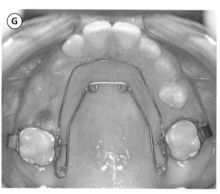

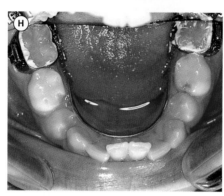

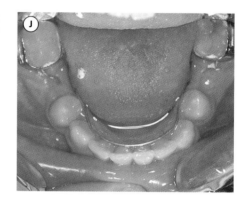

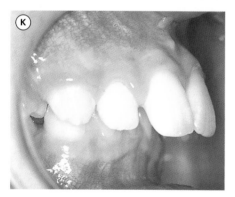

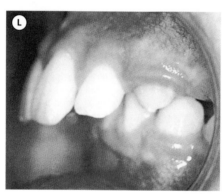

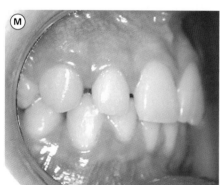

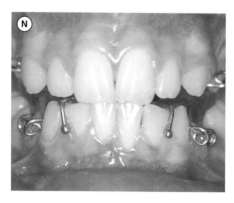

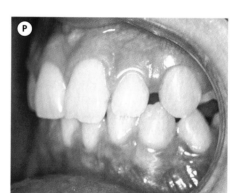

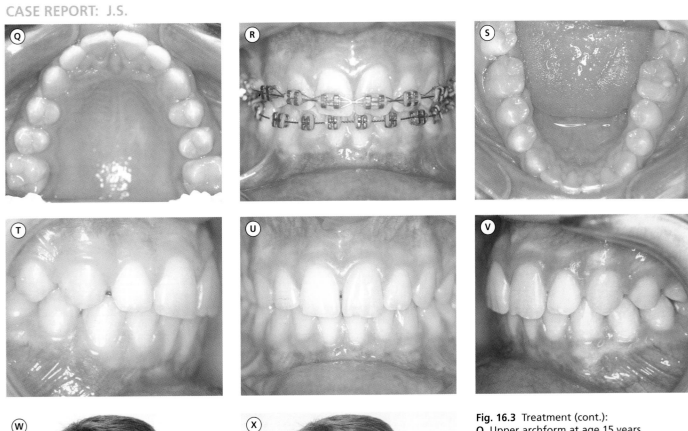

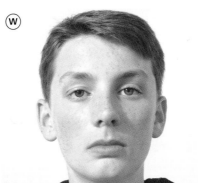

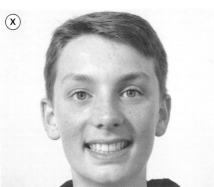

Fig. 16.3 Treatment (cont.):
Q Upper archform at age 15 years 11 months.
R Fixed appliances.
S Lower archform at age 15 years 11 months.
T–V Occlusion at age 15 years 11 months.
W, X Appearance at age 15 years 11 months.

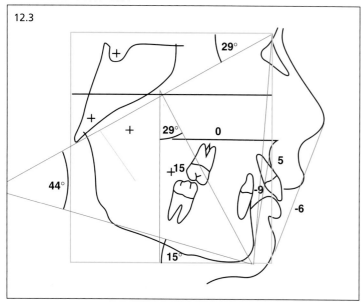

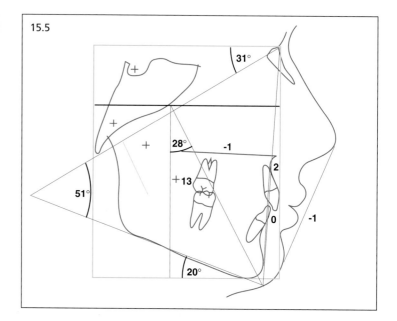

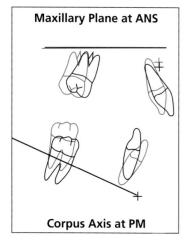

Maxillary Plane at ANS

Corpus Axis at PM

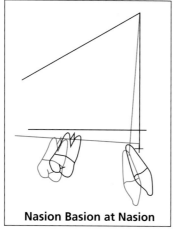

Nasion Basion at Nasion

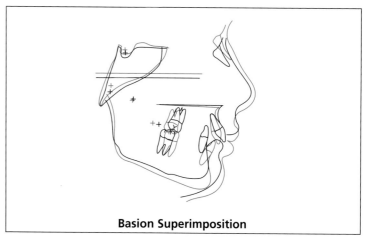

Basion Superimposition

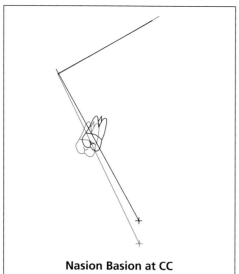

Nasion Basion at CC

J.S.	Age	12.3	15.5
Cranial Base Angle		29	31
Facial Axis Angle		29	28
F/M Plane Angle		15	20
Craniomandibular Angle		44	51
Maxillary Plane		0	-1
Convexity		5	2
U/Incisor to Vertical		27	15
L/Incisor to Vertical		12	33
Interincisal Angle		141	132
6 to Pterygoid Vertical		15	13
L/Incisor to A/Po		–9	0
L/Lip to Aesthetic Plane		–6	–1

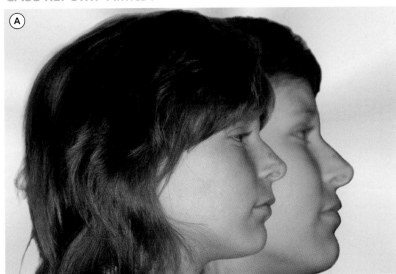

Fig. 16.4 Treatment:
A Profiles at ages 12 years 9 months (before treatment) and 15 years (after treatment).
B, C Occlusion before treatment.

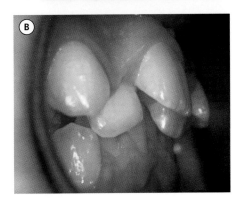

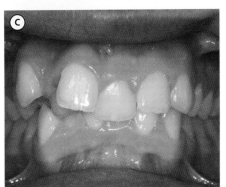

Treatment concept

Avoiding extraction of premolars generally produces a better profile by providing good lip support from well-formed dental arches, thus maintaining better facial balance. Extraction of premolars is seldom required to relieve upper arch crowding, when arch development provides a valid alternative.

This patient was treated by Dr Gordon Kluzak in his paedodontic practice in Calgary.

CASE REPORT: A. McD. AGED 12 YEARS 9 MONTHS

by Gordon Kluzak

Crowding of the upper and lower labial segments is resolved in the first phase of arch development using a partial upper fixed appliance with two molar bands and four incisor brackets. This is combined with the Trombone and Lingual Arch Developer (see Chapter 22) to correct archform in the lower arch. This is followed by 8 months of Twin Block treatment, and treatment is completed in 18 months. The Bergasson occluso-guide is selected as the most appropriate retainer. For the first 3 months the occluso-guide is worn for 2 hours during the day and at nights, before reducing to night-time wear only. This preformed positioner is an excellent functional retainer which can be used successfully to settle and detail the occlusion. Second molars were later extracted to accommodate third molars (Fig. 16.4).

CASE REPORT: A.McD.

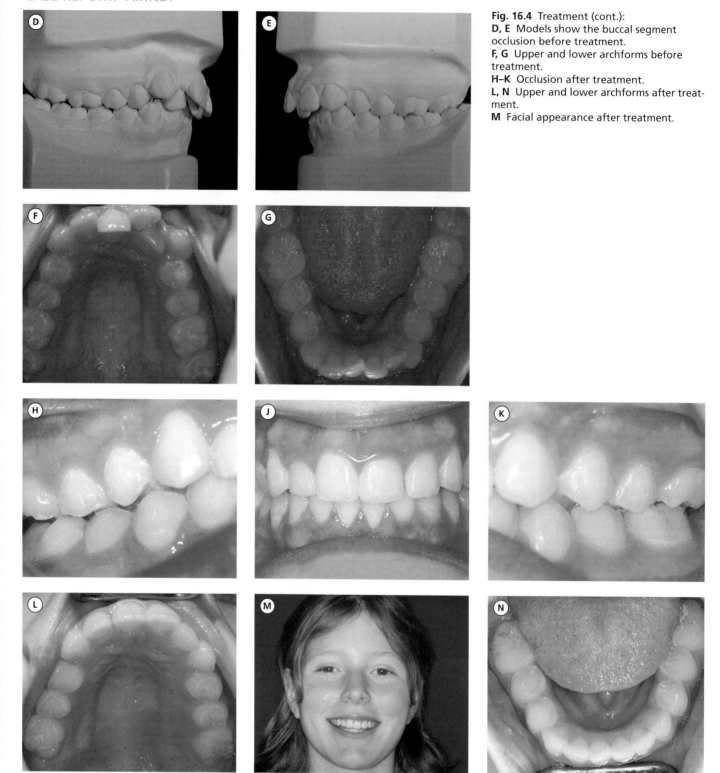

Fig. 16.4 Treatment (cont.):
D, E Models show the buccal segment occlusion before treatment.
F, G Upper and lower archforms before treatment.
H–K Occlusion after treatment.
L, N Upper and lower archforms after treatment.
M Facial appearance after treatment.

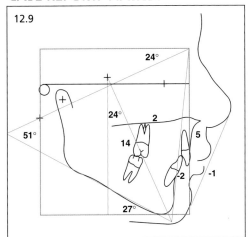

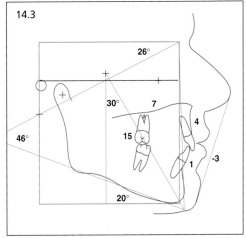

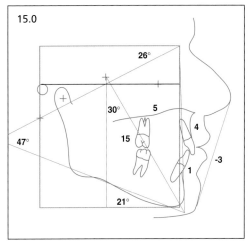

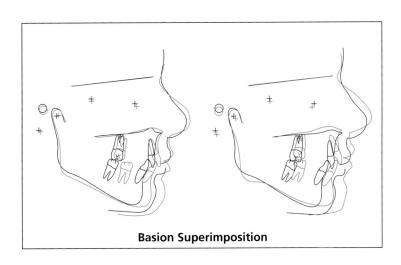

Basion Superimposition

A.McD. Age	12.9	14.3	15.0
Cranial Base Angle	24	26	26
Facial Axis Angle	24	30	30
F/M Plane Angle	27	20	21
Craniomandibular Angle	51	46	47
Maxillary Plane	2	7	5
Convexity	5	4	4
U/Incisor to Vertical	5	19	19
L/Incisor to Vertical	26	32	30
L/Incisor to A/Po	–2	1	1
L/Lip to Aesthetic Plane	–1	–3	–3
6 to Pterygoid vertical	12	13	13

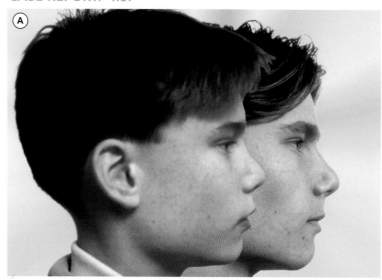

Fig. 16.5 Treatment:
A Profiles at ages 14 years 2 months (before treatment) and 16 years 7 months (1 year out of retention).
B–D Occlusion before treatment.
E–G Archform corrected by sagittal Twin Blocks after 9 months.

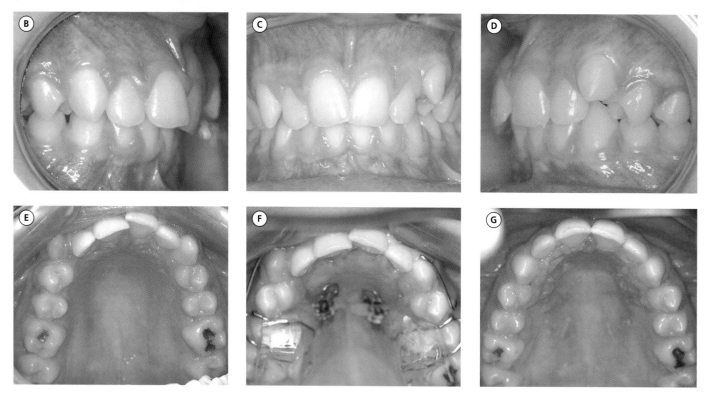

CLASS II DIVISION 1 MALOCCLUSION WITH CROWDED CANINES

Combination therapy by Twin Blocks and fixed appliances

CASE REPORT: T.S. AGED 14 YEARS 2 MONTHS

There are many examples of Class II malocclusion with crowding in the upper labial segment, resulting in displacement and irregularity of the incisors, or alternatively the upper canines may be crowded buccally out of the arch. The Twin Block sagittal appliance can be used to treat upper labial segment crowding and, at the same time, will correct distal occlusion and reduce overjet (Fig. 16.5).

A moderate Class II skeletal pattern with a convexity of 5 mm is due to maxillary protrusion, but the profile improves when the mandible is advanced, therefore functional correction is preferred to maxillary retraction. This allows the crowded canines to be accommodated in the upper arch by advancing the retroclined upper incisors.

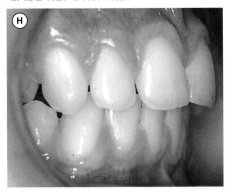

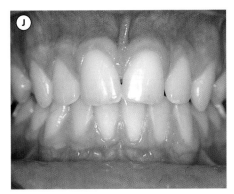

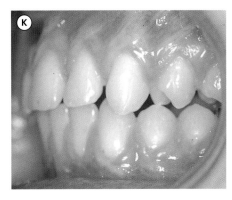

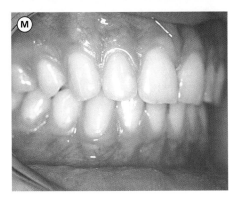

Fig. 16.5 Treatment (cont.):
H–K Occlusion after 1 year at age 15 years 2 months.
L Fixed appliances.
M–P Occlusion 1 year out of retention at age 16 years 7 months.

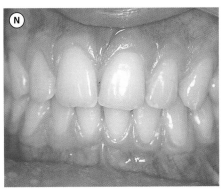

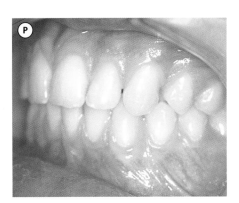

Clinical management

The palatal screws in the sagittal Twin Block are turned two quarter-turns per week to align the upper incisors. The appliance is trimmed clear of the single proclined incisor, so that the activation of the screws advances only the retroclined upper incisors. The palatal acrylic on the upper appliance is trimmed to relieve the pressure on the palatal gingivae lingual to 21/12 during treatment which is incidental to screw expansion. It is important to maintain appliance contact on the lingual surfaces of the teeth that are being advanced, and therefore no trimming is done where the appliance contacts these teeth.

In this case the transition to fixed appliances was made after a short support phase when the buccal teeth settled into Class I occlusion, during which period a lower lingual arch corrected the lower archform. Subsequent detailing of the occlusion was simple after achieving the major correction during the Twin Block phase of treatment.

Twin Blocks: 8 months
Support phase: 6 months
Fixed appliances: 9 months
Retention: 1 year.

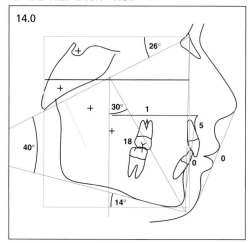

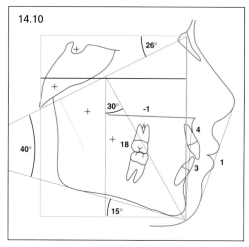

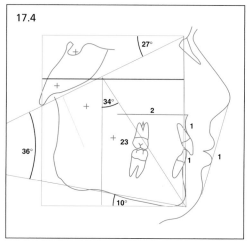

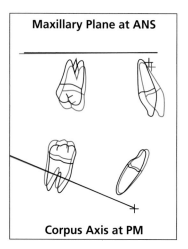

Maxillary Plane at ANS

Corpus Axis at PM

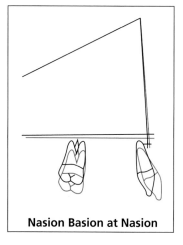

Nasion Basion at Nasion

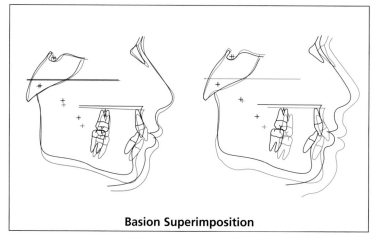

Basion Superimposition

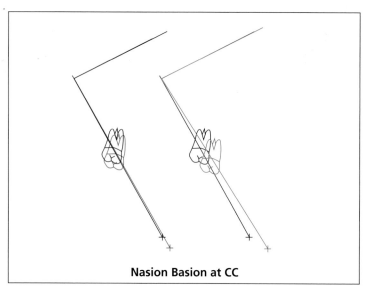

Nasion Basion at CC

T.S.	Age	14.0	14.10	17.4
Cranial Base Angle		26	26	27
Facial Axis Angle		30	30	34
F/M Plane Angle		14	15	10
Craniomandibular Angle		40	40	37
Maxillary Plane		1	−1	2
Convexity		5	4	1
U/Incisor to Vertical		11	22	26
L/Incisor to Vertical		33	33	23
Interincisal Angle		136	125	131
6 to Pterygoid Vertical		18	18	23
L/Incisor to A/Po		0	3	1
L/Lip to Aesthetic Plane		0	1	1

CASE REPORT: R.G.

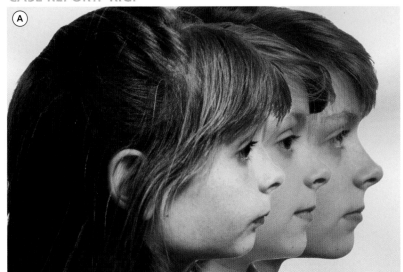

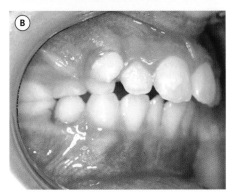

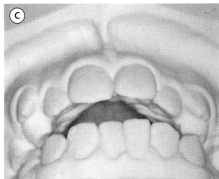

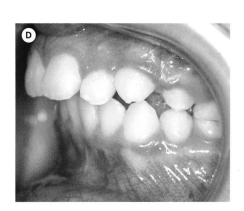

Fig. 16.6 Treatment:
A Profiles at ages 11 years 6 months (before treatment), 11 years 11 months (after 5 months' treatment with Twin Blocks) and 15 years 0 months (out of retention).
B–D Occlusion before treatment.

MANAGEMENT OF CROWDING WITH AN ANTERIOR OPEN BITE

CASE REPORT: R.G. AGED 11 YEARS 6 MONTHS

A girl with an anterior open bite and mild lower labial crowding presents a brachyfacial growth pattern which is favourable for correction by a combination of an initial functional phase to improve the profile followed by fixed appliances to detail the occlusion. The prognosis for correction of the anterior open bite is good as the primary cause was a thumb sucking habit which has now stopped. A moderate maxillary protrusion and mild mandibular retrusion contribute to a convexity of 10 mm and an overjet of 9 mm. Mild crowding in the lower labial segment is treated when second deciduous molars are still present by holding the lower molar position to gain lee-way space. The lower Twin Block should incorporate a midline screw to assist in alignment of the lower incisors.

Twin Blocks: 9 months
Support appliance: 4 months
Fixed appliances: 18 months (Fig. 16.6).

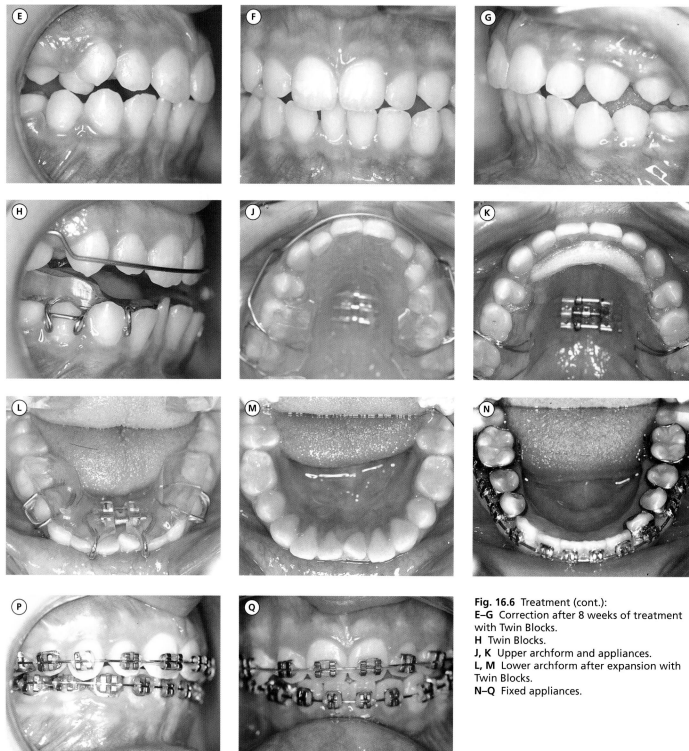

Fig. 16.6 Treatment (cont.):
E–G Correction after 8 weeks of treatment with Twin Blocks.
H Twin Blocks.
J, K Upper archform and appliances.
L, M Lower archform after expansion with Twin Blocks.
N–Q Fixed appliances.

CASE REPORT: R.G.

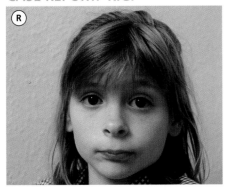

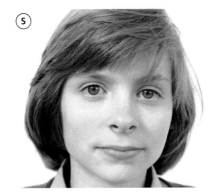

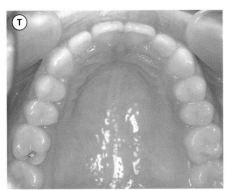

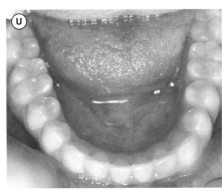

Fig. 16.6 Treatment (cont.):
R Appearance before treatment.
S Appearance after treatment at age 14 years.
T, U Upper and lower archforms at age 16 years.
V–X Occlusion 1 year out of retention at age 16 years.

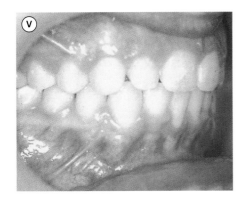

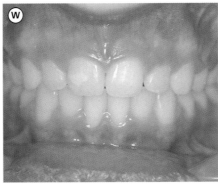

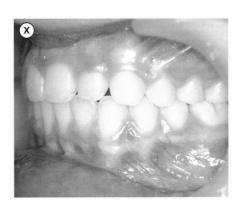

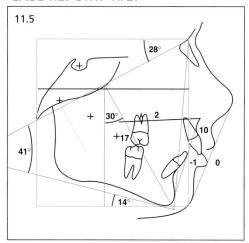

11.5

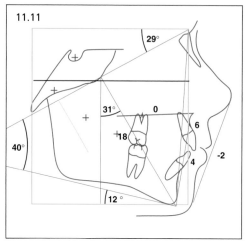

11.11

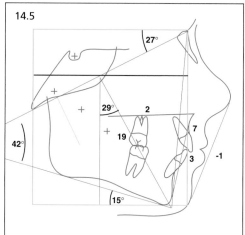

14.5

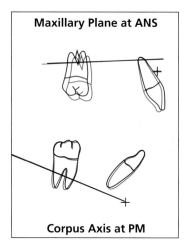

Maxillary Plane at ANS

Corpus Axis at PM

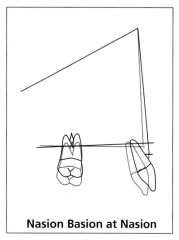

Nasion Basion at Nasion

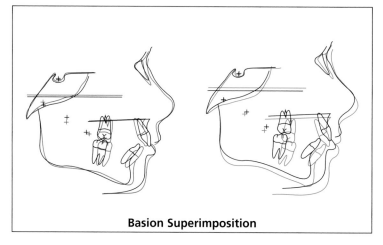

Basion Superimposition

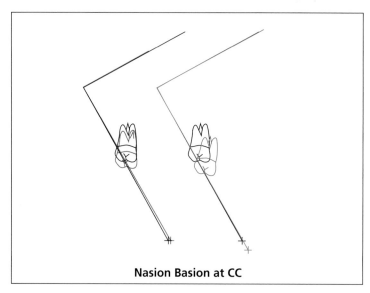

Nasion Basion at CC

R.G.	Age	11.5	11.11	14.5
Cranial Base Angle		28	29	27
Facial Axis Angle		30	31	29
F/M Plane Angle		14	12	15
Craniomandibular Angle		41	40	42
Maxillary Plane		2	0	2
Convexity		10	6	7
U/Incisor to Vertical		26	19	30
L/Incisor to Vertical		47	40	40
Interincisal Angle		107	121	110
6 to Pterygoid Vertical		17	18	19
L/Incisor to A/Po		−1	4	3
L/Lip to Aesthetic Plane		0	−2	−1

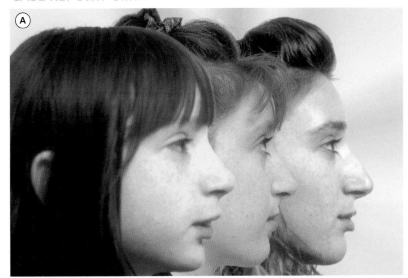

Fig. 16.7 Treatment:
A Profiles at ages 12 years 5 months (before treatment), 13 years (after 7 months' treatment with Twin Blocks) and at 19 years 8 months.
B–D Occlusion before treatment.

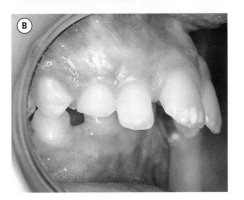

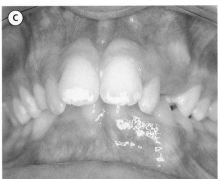

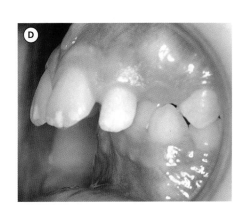

TREATMENT OF CONTRACTED ARCHFORM

CASE REPORT: S.M. AGED 12 YEARS 5 MONTHS

This is an example of treatment in a girl who has passed the pubertal growth spurt. Although growth slows significantly in females at this stage, it is still possible to correct severe distal occlusion, and to reduce an excessive overjet by functional correction.

The upper arch is V shaped in this severe Class II division 1 malocclusion and the lower arch is constricted within the narrow upper arch with a crowded lower labial segment. An overjet of 13 mm and excessive overbite are caused by the lower lip being trapped in the overjet, with severe protrusion of upper central incisors while the lower incisors are retroclined and positioned 5 mm lingual to the A–Po line. The

skeletal base relationship is a mild retrognathic pattern with convexity of 6 mm and a vertical growth tendency. The approach to treatment is by a combination of Twin Blocks, arch development and fixed appliances.

The upper incisors are vulnerable to damage due to their exposed position. On account of this a decision was made to correct the overjet and distal occlusion with Twin Blocks in the first stage. This is followed by arch development during the support phase, and a final stage with fixed appliances (Fig. 16.7).

Twin Blocks: 9 months
Arch development: 6 months
Fixed appliances: 2 years.

Treatment may sometimes extend over a longer period at this age, especially if combination therapy is required.

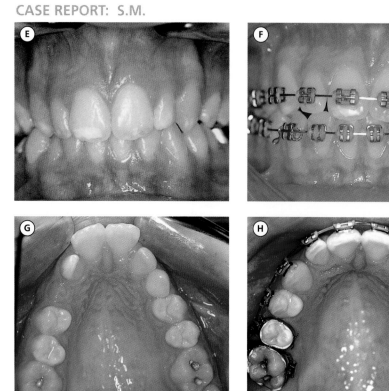

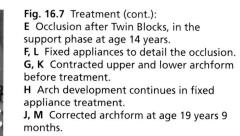

Fig. 16.7 Treatment (cont.):
E Occlusion after Twin Blocks, in the support phase at age 14 years.
F, L Fixed appliances to detail the occlusion.
G, K Contracted upper and lower archform before treatment.
H Arch development continues in fixed appliance treatment.
J, M Corrected archform at age 19 years 9 months.

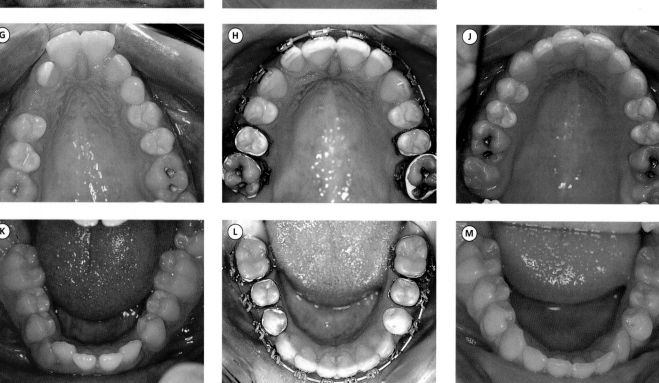

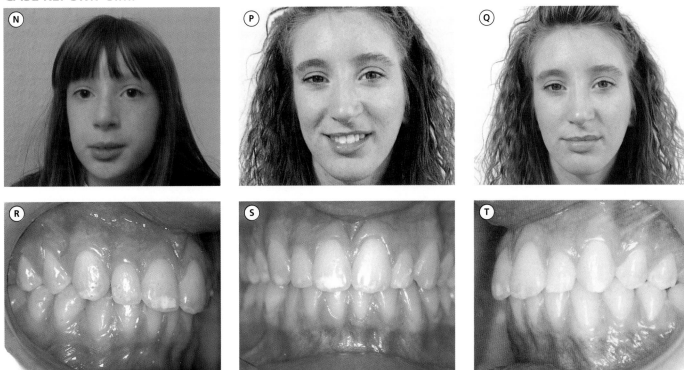

Fig. 16.7 Treatment (cont.):
N Appearance before treatment.
P, Q Appearance at age 19 years 8 months.
R–T Occlusion out of retention at age 19 years 8 months.

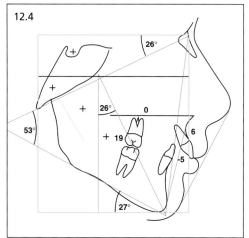

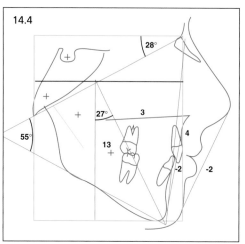

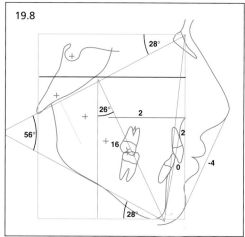

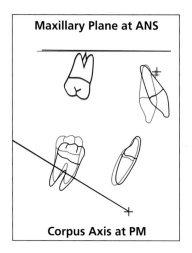

Maxillary Plane at ANS

Corpus Axis at PM

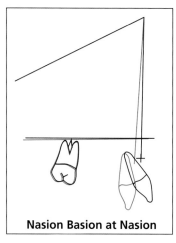

Nasion Basion at Nasion

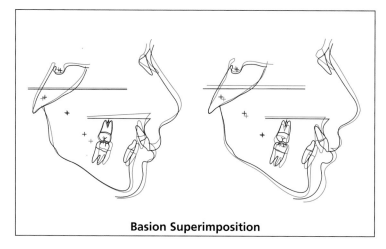

Basion Superimposition

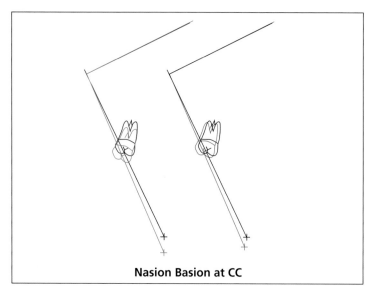

Nasion Basion at CC

S.M.	Age	11.7	12.3	18.10
Cranial Base Angle		26	29	28
Facial Axis Angle		27	28	24
F/M Plane Angle		22	22	24
Craniomandibular Angle		48	51	51
Maxillary Plane		0	1	-1
Convexity		6	3	3
U/Incisor to Vertical		26	17	16
L/Incisor to Vertical		30	39	34
Interincisal Angle		124	124	130
6 to Pterygoid Vertical		20	20	23
L/Incisor to A/Po		-4	1	0
L/Lip to Aesthetic Plane		-6	-5	-7

CHAPTER 17

Extraction Therapy

It is unusual to combine extraction of premolars with functional therapy. With certain exceptions, premolar extraction therapy and functional appliance therapy are almost contradictory terms. In a minority of cases, the degree of crowding mesial to the first permanent molars may be so severe that premolar extractions are inevitable, although the patient may still benefit from functional correction. In other cases, the patient may present too late to control crowding by interceptive treatment and arch development, but may still require functional mandibular protrusion. In these circumstances, fixed and functional therapy is required to correct archform, close spaces and correct arch relationships.

The protocol for combination of fixed and functional therapy is illustrated in Chapter 10 with an example of a treated case following extraction of premolars. (Case report: M.Z., pages 148–150). It is possible to relieve crowding and correct archform with space closure using fixed appliances in the first stage of treatment, followed by mandibular advancement in an integrated fixed/functional approach to treatment.

Patients presenting with vertical growth patterns and a high mandibular plane angle cannot be expected to grow favourably during treatment. In such cases, when significant crowding is present in the lower arch, it may only be resolved by premolar extractions.

Examples of extraction therapy are illustrated to demonstrate the management of these problems, which are exceptional rather than typical in Twin Block therapy.

CASE REPORT: K.M. AGED 11 YEARS 9 MONTHS

This is an example of Twin Block treatment for a girl who presented a Class II division 1 malocclusion in the permanent dentition with severe crowding in the lower buccal segments with second premolars blocked out of the arch and impacted. Twin Blocks were used to correct the distal occlusion and reduce the overjet, followed by extraction of premolars to relieve crowding. Sectional upper fixed appliances were used to close extraction spaces. In the lower arch $\overline{4|4}$ were extracted to provide space for $\overline{5|5}$ to erupt (Fig. 17.1).

A dramatic change in facial appearance is again observed during the early stages of treatment with Twin Blocks as the large overjet and distal occlusion are corrected.

The improvement in facial balance is maintained as shown in the final records 5 years out of retention:

Twin Blocks: 10 months
Support phase: 4 months
Sectional fixed appliance: 6 months.

CASE REPORT: K.M.

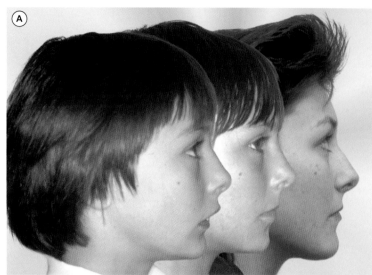

Fig. 17.1 Treatment:
A Profiles at ages 11 years 9 months (before treatment), 12 years 3 months (after 6 months' treatment) and 18 years 10 months.
B Appearance before treatment.
C Appearance after 6 months treatment.
E–G Occlusion before treatment.
H, K Occlusion 6 months after treatment.
D, J Appearance at age 18 years 10 months.

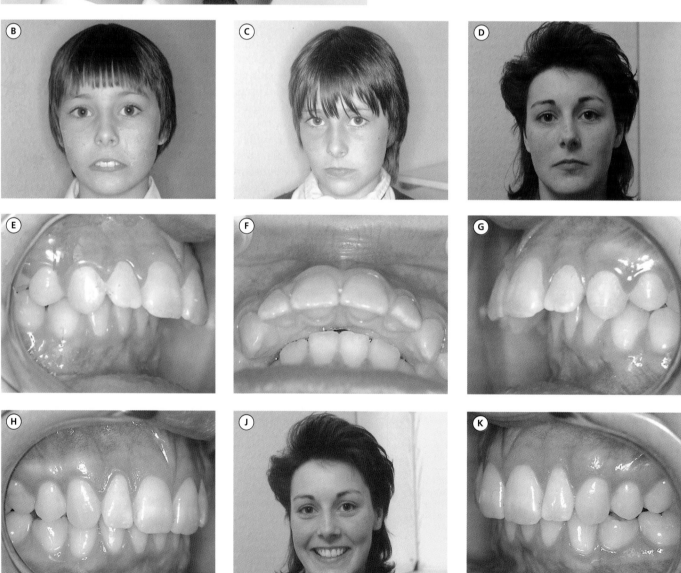

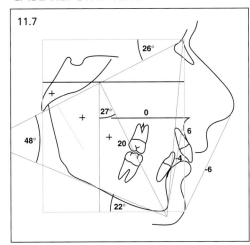

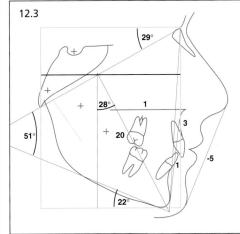

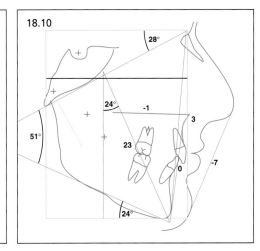

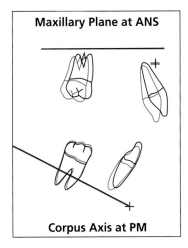

Maxillary Plane at ANS

Corpus Axis at PM

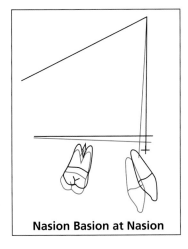

Nasion Basion at Nasion

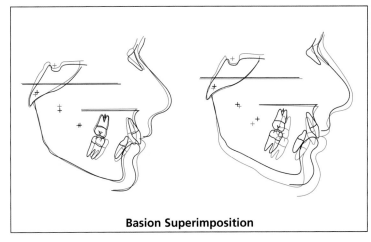

Basion Superimposition

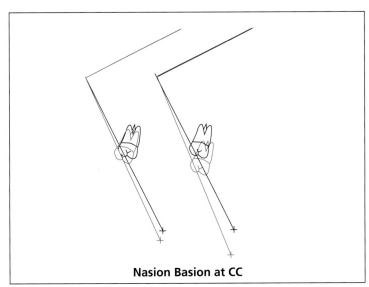

Nasion Basion at CC

K.M. Age	11.7	12.3	18.10
Cranial Base Angle	26	29	28
Facial Axis Angle	27	28	24
F/M Plane Angle	22	22	24
Craniomandibular Angle	48	51	51
Maxillary Plane	0	1	−1
Convexity	6	3	3
U/Incisor to Vertical	26	17	16
L/Incisor to Vertical	30	39	34
Interincisal Angle	124	124	130
6 to Pterygoid Vertical	20	20	23
L/Incisor to A/Po	−4	1	0
L/Lip to Aesthetic Plane	−6	−5	−7

TREATMENT OF PATIENTS WITH UNFAVOURABLE SKELETAL AND DENTAL FACTORS

CASE REPORT: G.McD. AGED 12 YEARS 1 MONTH

This patient presents a difficult problem with a severe Class II skeletal relationship, mandibular retrusion, a vertical growth pattern, severe lower labial crowding and deep overbite. Because of the vertical growth pattern, the profile does not significantly improve when the mandible postures forwards. Extraction of the premolars is indicated to improve the profile (Fig. 17.2).

The combination of a high mandibular plane angle and deep overbite is a warning sign that facial height will increase if the mandible is translated forwards. This is confirmed in the profile change observed when the patient postures forwards before treatment. In such cases, an alternative approach is to intrude the incisors with fixed appliances, for example using utility arches, before the functional phase of treatment. The mandible may then be translated forwards without increasing the facial height.

The degree of crowding in the lower arch and the position of the lower dentition relative to the basal bone are the factors which determine whether or not extractions are required, and influence the choice of extraction. If the lower dentition is crowded and significantly protrusive beyond the anterior limit of basal bone, extraction therapy is indicated. The normal position of the tip of the lower incisor relative to the A–Po line is +1 mm to +3 mm.

Several unfavourable factors contribute to this malocclusion. Maxillary protrusion and severe mandibular retrusion combine to produce a convexity of 10 mm with increased lower facial height and a moderate dolichofacial growth pattern. The lower incisors are severely crowded and are already positioned at + 3 mm to the A–Po line. The overjet and overbite are increased, while the occlusion of the buccal teeth registers a Class I relationship before treatment, due to mesial drift of the lower buccal segments, with lower canines crowded labially.

It is evident when the lower model is advanced to reduce the overjet that the resulting occlusion would be unsatisfactory, as the teeth would not interdigitate correctly. In an effort to improve the profile an attempt was made to advance the mandible in the first stage of treatment, followed by the extraction of four premolars to relieve crowding and the use of bonded fixed appliances to close the spaces and reduce the prominence of the lips.

The overjet reduced from 8 mm to 2 mm in 4 months with Twin Blocks. On this occasion the profile did not improve due to lengthening of the lower facial height. The position was retrieved after the extraction of four premolars, when a Wilson lower lingual arch was fitted to maintain arch length and align the lower labial segment. After closing buccal segment spaces and establishing a Class I occlusion, the upper and lower incisors were retracted by space closing mechanics, allowing the profile to improve as the lips were retracted.

Orthopaedic phase: 4 months
Orthodontic phase: 2 years
Retention: 1 year
Total treatment time: 1 year 6 months.

CASE REPORT: G.McD.

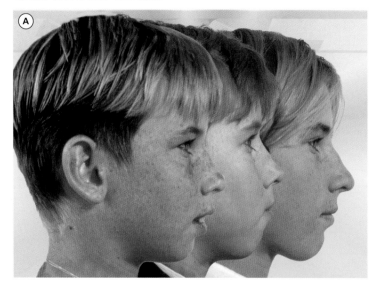

Fig. 17.2 Treatment:
A Profiles at ages 12 years 4 months (before treatment), 13 years 2 months (10 months after treatment with Twin Blocks), and 15 years 2 months (after treatment).

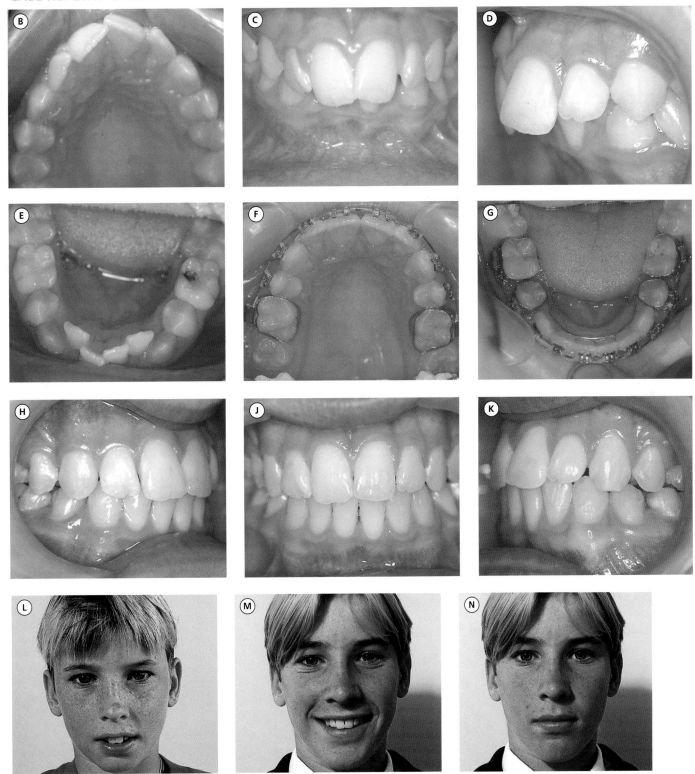

Fig. 17.2 Treatment (cont.):
B–E Contracted upper and lower archform and occlusion before treatment.
F, G Upper and lower archform after extractions and space closure in phase 2.
H–K Occlusion after treatment.
L Facial appearance before treatment.
M–N Facial appearance after treatment.

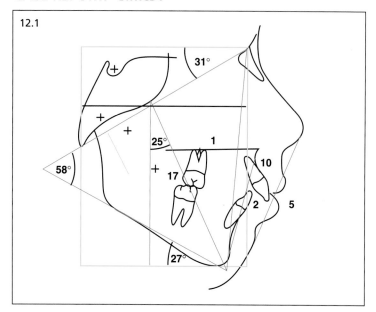

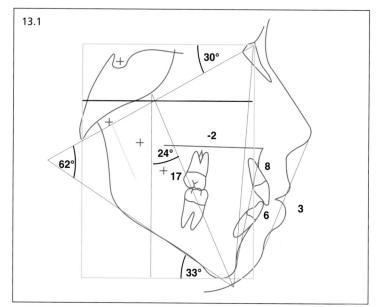

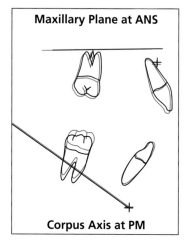

Corpus Axis at PM

Maxillary Plane at ANS

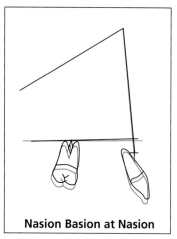

Nasion Basion at Nasion

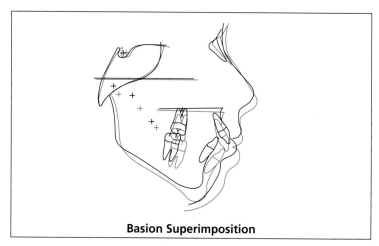

Basion Superimposition

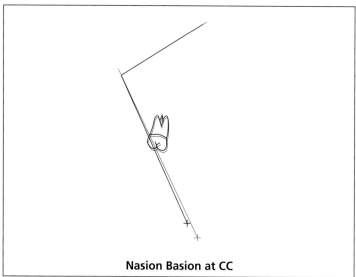

Nasion Basion at CC

G.McD.	Age	12.1	13.1
Cranial Base Angle		31	28
Facial Axis Angle		25	24
F/M Plane Angle		27	33
Craniomandibular Angle		58	62
Maxillary Plane		1	−2
Convexity		10	8
U/Incisor to Vertical		28	22
L/Incisor to Vertical		36	40
Interincisal Angle		116	118
6 to Pterygoid Vertical		17	17
L/Incisor to A/Po		2	6
L/Lip to Aesthetic Plane		5	3

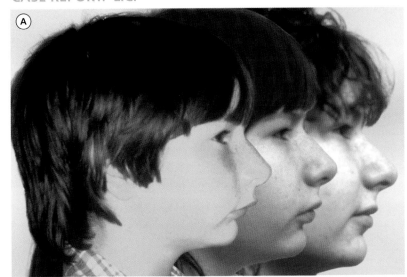

Fig. 17.3 Treatment:
A Profiles at ages 10 years 9 months (before treatment), 12 years 3 months (after the Twin Block phase) and 16 years 7 months.
B–D Occlusion before treatment.

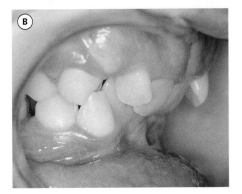

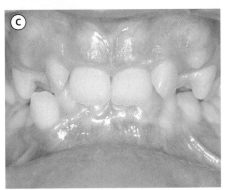

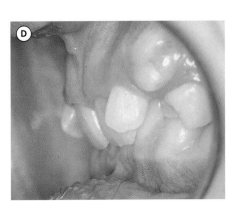

CASE REPORT: L.C. AGED 10 YEARS 9 MONTHS

This girl presented a severe Class II division 2 malocclusion with a typical brachyfacial growth pattern and reduced lower facial height. A convexity of 10 mm is due to a combination of maxillary protrusion and mandibular retrusion. Severe retroclination of upper and lower incisors is reflected in an interincisal angle of 175°, and the lower incisors are 7 mm behind the A–Po line, with an excessive overbite of 10 mm. It is very unusual to extract premolars in Class II division 2 malocclusion; this case is an exception due to the severity of lower arch crowding in permanent dentition (ALD = 19 mm). Combination therapy used Twin Blocks to correct arch relationships and fixed appliances to close extraction spaces and detail the occlusion (Fig. 17.3).

Clinical management

The construction bite registered an edge-to-edge incisor occlusion. In view of the excessive overbite no additional interincisal clearance was necessary in this case. Twin Blocks were worn for 16 months to advance the mandible and procline the upper incisors. During this period $\frac{4|4}{2|4}$ were extracted

to relieve crowding. Towards the end of the Twin Block stage, brackets were fitted on the upper anterior teeth to improve alignment. An anterior inclined plane was worn for 2 months to allow the occlusion to settle before fitting the fixed appliances to complete the treatment. The finishing stage was slow and extended over a period of 3 years. Final records show the position at age 18 and confirm the stability of the result.

Orthopaedic phase: 16 months
Orthodontic phase: 3 years
Retention: 1 year.

It is never ideal to resolve a Class II division 2 malocclusion by premolar extractions, but this was an exception to the general rule. In this case the severe lower arch crowding resulted from extraction of lower deciduous molars, allowing the first molars to drift mesially and causing impaction of the lower second premolars. Arch development at an earlier stage might have allowed treatment to be completed without extractions, with a better improvement in the profile.

CASE REPORT: L.C.

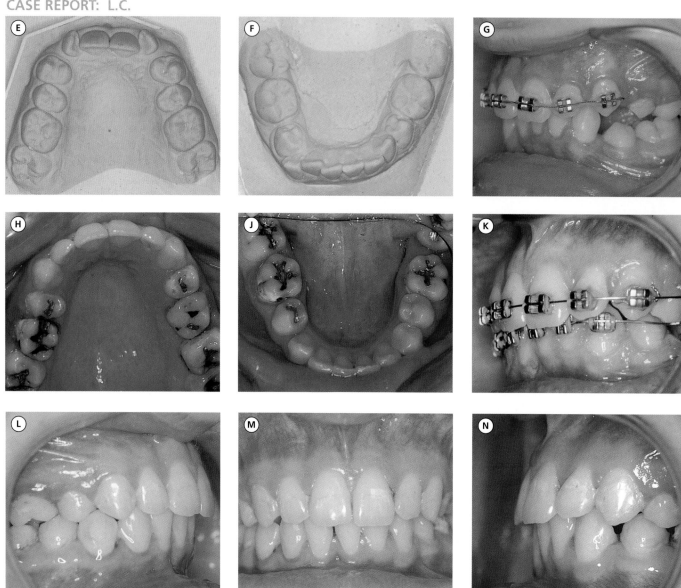

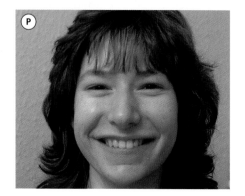

Fig. 17.3 Treatment (cont.):
E, F Archform before treatment, 19 mm crowding in the lower arch.
G Brackets on the upper anterior teeth during the Twin Block phase.
H, J Archform at age 18 years 3 months.
K Phase 2 – fixed appliances.
L–M Occlusion at age 18 years 3 months.
P Appearance after treatment at age 16 years 7 months.

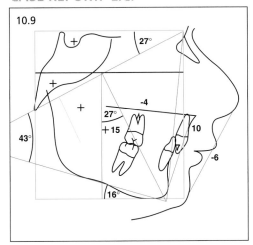

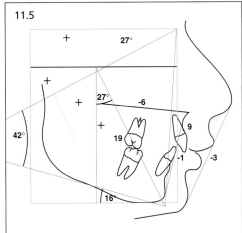

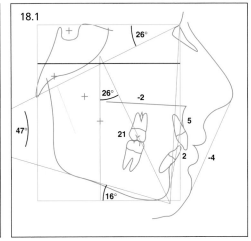

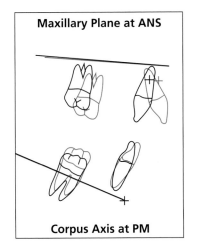

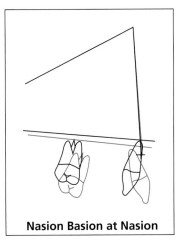

Maxillary Plane at ANS

Corpus Axis at PM

Nasion Basion at Nasion

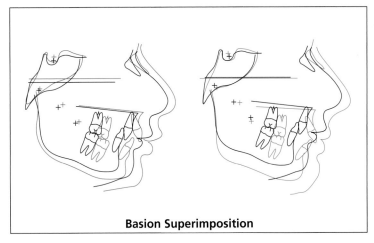

Basion Superimposition

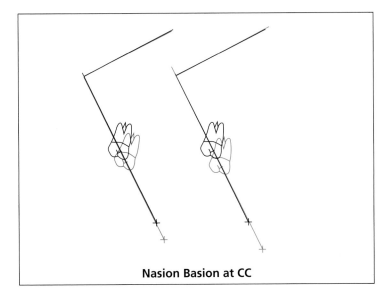

Nasion Basion at CC

L.C.	Age	10.9	11.5	18.1
Cranial Base Angle		27	27	26
Facial Axis Angle		27	27	26
F/M Plane Angle		16	16	16
Craniomandibular Angle		43	42	42
Maxillary Plane		−4	−6	−2
Convexity		10	9	5
U/Incisor to Vertical		−17	16	21
L/Incisor to Vertical		22	35	40
Interincisal Angle		175	129	119
6 to Pterygoid Vertical		15	19	21
L/Incisor to A/Po		−7	−1	2
L/Lip to Aesthetic Plane		−6	−3	−4

CHAPTER 18

Treatment of Facial Asymmetry

The occlusal inclined plane is an ideal functional mechanism for unilateral activation, and Twin Blocks are extremely effective in the correction of facial and dental asymmetry. The sagittal Twin Block is the appliance of choice for correction of asymmetry because the sagittal design allows unilateral activation to restore symmetry in buccal and labial segments.

This girl presented facial and dental asymmetry with the lower centre line displaced to the right. In the anterior facial view the chin point was displaced to the right in open and closed position, confirming a true skeletal asymmetry. The skeletal pattern shows a moderate Class II discrepancy with 6 mm convexity due to mandibular retrusion. The distal occlusion is more marked on the right side. Combination therapy is the treatment of choice with Twin Blocks to improve the asymmetry, followed by an orthodontic phase of detailed finishing with fixed appliances.

Bite registration

Correction of asymmetry in the construction bite ensures that the occlusal forces activate the appliance to restore symmetry. The construction bite is registered with the incisors edge-to-edge with 2 mm vertical clearance, and the centre lines correct. The objective is to improve the facial asymmetry and correct the mandibular retrusion at the same time.

Appliance design

An upper Twin Block sagittal appliance with two palatal screws is designed to advance retroclined upper incisors and drive upper molars distally. The screw is turned more frequently on the side that requires more distal movement. The mechanical action of the palatal screws is reinforced by occlusal forces on the inclined planes, favouring the working side to correct the midline displacement (Fig. 18.1).

Clinical management

The initial response to treatment resulted in rapid correction of the asymmetry and reduction of the overjet. After 7 weeks

of treatment, at the second visit for adjustment, the centre lines were corrected and the overjet was fully reduced. A new muscle balance position was established whereby it was not possible for the patient to retract the mandible into its former retruded asymmetrical position. The rapid improvement in muscle balance is evident in the facial photographs at this

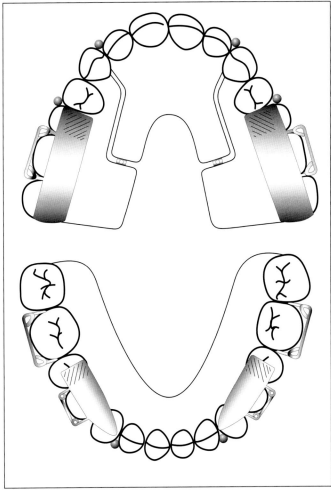

Fig. 18.1 Sagittal Twin Blocks give better control for correction of dental or facial asymmetry. Good fixation is necessary in the lower arch.

CASE REPORT: M.McK.

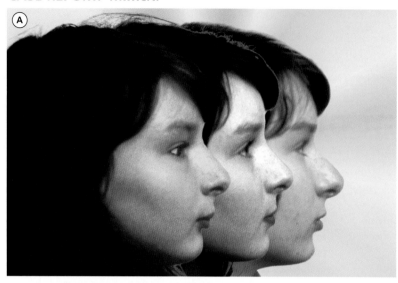

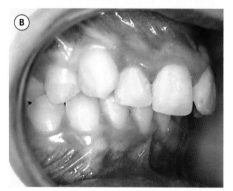

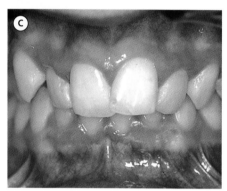

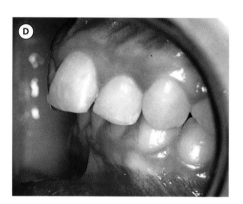

Fig. 18.2 Treatment:
A Profiles at ages 10 years 4 months (before treatment), 10 years 6 months (after 6 weeks' treatment) and 15 years 4 months (1 year out of retention).
B–D Asymmetrical occlusion before treatment.

stage and there is already a marked improvement in the facial asymmetry and profile.

At the start of treatment the upper bite block was trimmed occlusodistally to encourage lower molar eruption. At the second visit the inclined planes on the left side were trimmed out of contact in order to reinforce the corrective occlusal forces on the active right side.

At this stage the lateral open bite is increased on the right side. Asymmetry is normally associated with a vertical discrepancy, which can be identified when the centre lines are corrected in the construction bite. The vertical space between the posterior teeth is more marked on the side to which the mandible is displaced. The height of the occlusal blocks in the premolar region on the right side was slightly reduced over a period of 2 months to encourage vertical correction.

After 6 months of treatment the buccal segment occlusion was corrected to Class I with the overjet and overbite reduced. The centre lines were now correct, and the lateral open bite was closed sufficiently to proceed to the next stage.

The lower Twin Block was replaced by a lower fixed appliance to commence orthodontic correction in the lower arch. An upper appliance with an anterior inclined plane was fitted to support the corrected incisor relationship, leaving the posterior teeth free to erupt fully into occlusion.

Brackets were placed on the upper anterior teeth to improve alignment during the support phase. A full transition to fixed appliances was made after 10 months of treatment, when the distal occlusion and dental asymmetry corrected, and there was considerable improvement in the facial asymmetry. Treatment continued in an orthodontic phase with full-bonded fixed appliances, followed by retention (Fig. 18.2).

The rapid improvement in facial and dental asymmetry in this case was achieved by unilateral activation of the occlusal inclined planes. This improvement was maintained out of retention.

Twin Blocks: 6 months
Support phase: 5 months
Fixed appliances: 1 year
Retention: 1 year.

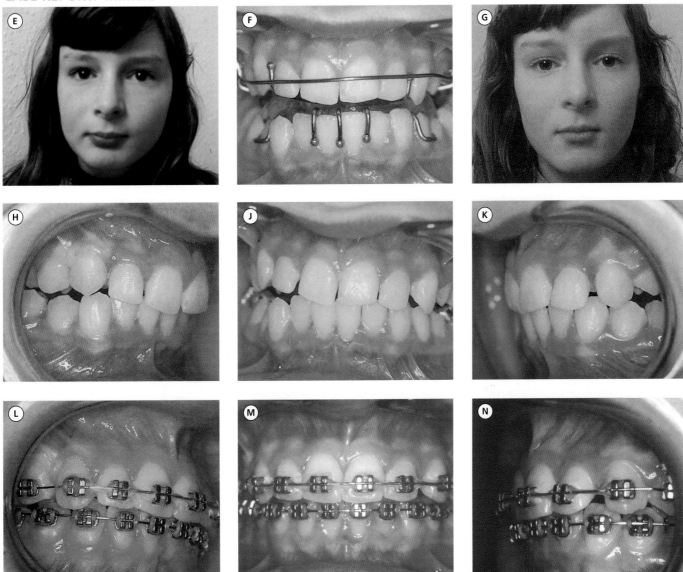

Fig. 18.2 Treatment (cont.):
E Appearance before treatment at age 10 years 4 months.
F Construction bite corrects the asymmetry.
G Improvement in asymmetry after 10 weeks at age 10 years 6 months.
H–K Correction of occlusion at age 10 years 7 months.
L–N Fixed appliances to detail the occlusion.

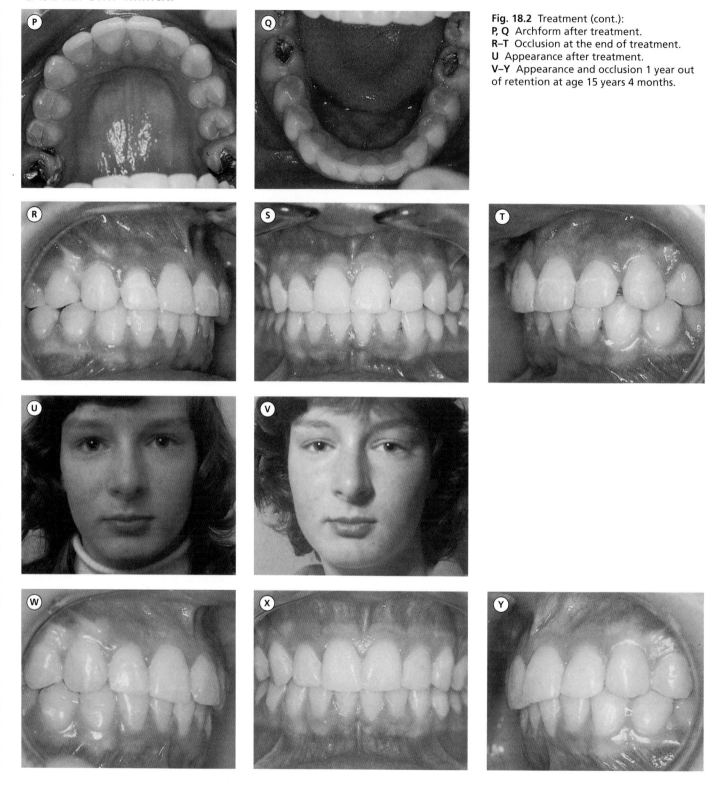

Fig. 18.2 Treatment (cont.):
P, Q Archform after treatment.
R–T Occlusion at the end of treatment.
U Appearance after treatment.
V–Y Appearance and occlusion 1 year out of retention at age 15 years 4 months.

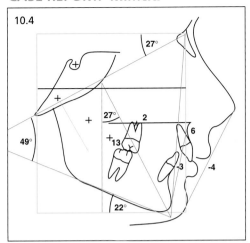

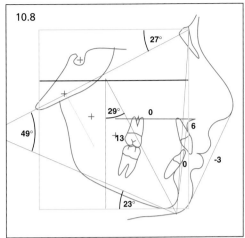

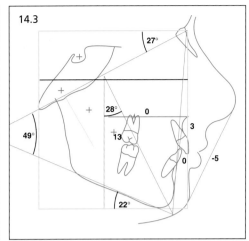

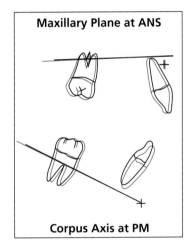

Maxillary Plane at ANS

Corpus Axis at PM

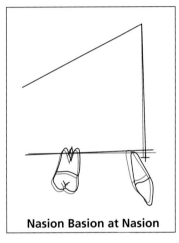

Nasion Basion at Nasion

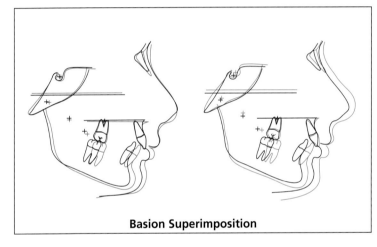

Basion Superimposition

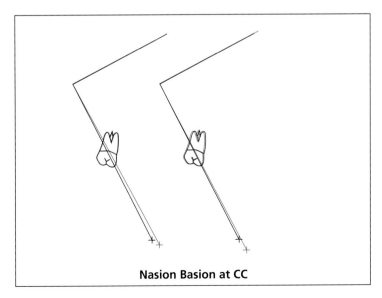

Nasion Basion at CC

M.McK.	Age	10.4	10.8	14.3
Cranial Base Angle		27	27	27
Facial Axis Angle		27	29	28
F/M Plane Angle		22	23	22
Craniomandibular Angle		49	49	49
Maxillary Plane		2	0	0
Convexity		6	6	3
U/Incisor to Vertical		19	22	27
L/Incisor to Vertical		24	36	35
Interincisal Angle		137	122	118
6 to Pterygoid Vertical		13	13	13
L/Incisor to A/Po		−3	0	0
L/Lip to Aesthetic Plane		−4	−3	−5

CHAPTER 19

Magnetic Twin Blocks

The role of magnets in Twin Block therapy is specifically to accelerate correction of arch relationships. The purpose of the magnets is to encourage increased occlusal contact on the bite blocks to maximise the favourable functional forces applied to correct the malocclusion.

Two types of rare earth magnet (samarium cobalt and neodynium boron) have been used to examine the response to attracting magnetic forces in Twin Block treatment. Both are effective, but neodynium boron delivers a greater force from a smaller magnet. At this stage no statistical comparison has been made by the author to evaluate the response to magnetic and non-magnetic appliances, and the following observations are based on clinical evaluation.

Attracting magnets incorporated in occlusal inclined planes may be effective in maintaining forward mandibular posture when the patient is asleep. Patients who have magnets added to Twin Blocks during treatment report increased occlusal contact by day and observe also that the blocks are in contact on waking.

MAGNETIC FORCE

Magnetic force is a new factor under investigation as an activating mechanism in orthodontic and orthopaedic treatment. Animal experiments in mandibular advancement (Vardimon *et al.*, 1989, 1990) indicate an improved mandibular growth response to magnetic functional appliances compared to non-magnetic appliances of similar design.

Similar experiments using a magnetic appliance with an adjustable screw for maxillary advancement showed midfacial protraction with horizontal maxillary displacement and antero-superior premaxillary rotation (Vardimon *et al.*, 1989, 1990).

Clinical investigations are now proceeding to develop new appliance systems to utilise magnetic forces. The author has modified Twin Blocks by the addition of attracting magnets to occlusal inclined planes, using magnetic force as an activating mechanism to maximise the orthopaedic response to treatment. Darendeliler & Joho (1993) have described similar appliances which are essentially based on the magnetic Twin Block.

ATTRACTING OR REPELLING MAGNETS

The first consideration on the use of magnets in inclined planes is whether the opposing poles should attract or repel. There are logical reasons to support the use of both systems. The advantages of both methods may be summarised as follows, with examples of current clinical research.

Attracting magnets

In favour of attracting magnets it may be said that increased activation can be built into the initial construction bite for the appliances. The attracting magnetic force pulls the appliances together and encourages the patient to occlude actively and consistently in a forward position. The functional mechanism of Twin Blocks stimulates a proprioceptive response by repeated contact on the occlusal inclined planes. Attracting magnets may accelerate progress by increasing the frequency and the force of contact on the inclined planes, thus enhancing the adaptive response to functional correction.

The author has used rare earth attracting magnets in five different clinical situations, described below.

Class II division 1 malocclusion with a large overjet
This resulted in more rapid correction of distal occlusion than would normally be expected without magnets. After 1 month of treatment, the overjet reduced from 10 mm to 6 mm, and after 2 months of treatment, a further reduction to 2 mm was observed (Fig. 19.1).

Mild residual Class II buccal segment relationship
This was proving difficult to resolve and was mainly a unilateral problem. Magnetic inclined planes were used to accelerate correction of the buccal segment relationship to a 'super Class I' relationship, which was quickly achieved (Fig. 6.13, p.72).

Mild Class II division 1 malocclusion with an overjet of 7 mm
The patient was failing to posture forwards consistently with conventional Twin Blocks and, as a result, was making slow

progress. The addition of attracting magnets noticeably improved occlusal contact on the bite blocks, and progress improved as a consequence. Patients with weak musculature fail to respond to functional therapy because they do not make the muscular effort required to engage the appliance actively by occluding on the inclined planes. It appears that attracting magnets will benefit this type of patient by increasing the frequency of favourable occlusal contacts.

Unilateral Class II adult patient with temporomandibular joint pain

Magnets were fitted unilaterally to correct the mandibular displacement to the affected side. This was immediately effective in resolving the symptoms, and occlusal correction is proceeding to produce a long-term resolution of the problem.

Skeletal Class III malocclusion with persistent crossbite, failed to resolve with conventional mechanics

Class III magnetic Twin Blocks were used to apply orthopaedic forces to correct mandibular displacement and to advance the maxilla, with an additional sagittal expansion component. This was effective in resolving quickly the mandibular displacement. The initial response to Class III correction is excellent.

Treatment of facial asymmetry

Magnetic force may be used to counteract asymmetrical muscle action in the development of facial asymmetry. Mandibular displacement responds rapidly to correction with attracting magnets in the occlusal inclined planes on the working side. The non-active side may be activated to a lesser degree to encourage centre line correction.

Repelling magnets

Repelling magnets may be used in Twin Blocks with less mechanical activation built into the occlusal inclined planes. The repelling magnetic force is intended to apply additional stimulus to forward posture as the patient closes into occlusion.

In 1990 Moss & Shaw reported at the European Orthodontic Congress on a controlled study of 12 patients with repelling magnets placed in occlusal inclines of Twin Block appliances. The results indicated a 50% increase in the rate of correction of overjet compared to a similar group of patients where magnets were not used, although an improved growth response was not established. The repelling magnets were intended to induce additional forward mandibular posture without reactivation of the blocks.

The appliances used in this study were not designed to allow vertical development in the buccal segments and, therefore, produced a large posterior open bite which subsequently had to be closed by fixed appliances. These appliances did not conform to the basic principles of Twin Block design for control of the vertical dimension.

After a short period of investigation it appears that magnetic Twin Blocks may help to resolve some of the problems encountered in the management of difficult cases. It is still to be established whether attracting or repelling magnets are more effective, although attracting magnets would appear to have an advantage by increasing contact on the inclined planes.

Magnets should be used only where speed of treatment is an important consideration, or where the response to non-magnetic appliances is limited. Similar results may be achieved by the addition of vertical elastics, as described in chapter 12.

CASE REPORT: F.H. AGED 14 YEARS 11 MONTHS

This boy attended for treatment in his mid-teens and presented labial segment crowding and irregularity in both arches. A traumatic occlusion was related to gingival recession of a lower central incisor with an overjet of 10 mm and an excessive overbite.

Although cephalometric analysis indicated mild maxillary protrusion and a normal mandible, the profile improved significantly when the patient postured the mandible forwards to reduce the overjet and correct the distal occlusion. This clinical guideline always takes precedence over cephalometric evaluation in assessing suitability for functional therapy.

An initial stage of arch development with a Wilson quad helix and lower lingual arch was combined with brackets on the upper anterior teeth. This was followed by Twin Blocks with attracting magnets to accelerate the orthopaedic stage of treatment. Rapid progress was observed as the overjet reduced from 10 mm to 2 mm in 2 months. The Twin Blocks were worn for a further 3 months to stabilise the corrected occlusion before discarding the lower appliance and fitting an upper appliance with an anterior inclined plane. There was a short period of passive retention at this stage, during which the lower labial fraenum was resected to improve the gingival recession on the lower central incisor.

Detailing of the occlusion was carried out with bonded fixed appliances. Lingual root torque was applied to position the root of the central incisor in alveolar bone in order to stabilise the incisor relationship and improve the gingival attachment of this tooth (Fig. 19.1).

Arch development: 6 months
Twin Blocks: 5 months
Fixed appliances: 20 months
Retention: 1 year.

CASE REPORT: F.H.

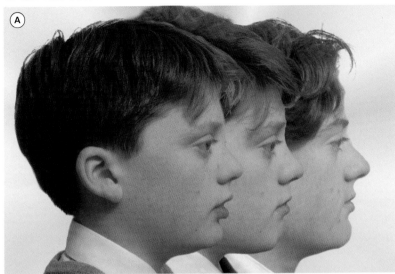

Fig. 19.1 Treatment:
A Profiles at ages 14 years 7 months (before treatment), 15 years 9 months (after Twin Blocks) and 19 years 4 months (out of retention).
B–D Occlusion before treatment – note the gingival recession of 1̲.
E, F Phase 1 – arch development (quad helix and Wilson lingual arch).
G Improved lower archform after arch development.
H Occlusion before Twin Blocks.
J Phase 2 – magnetic Twin Blocks in edge-to-edge occlusion.
K, Q Correction of the overjet and distal occlusion after 2 months.

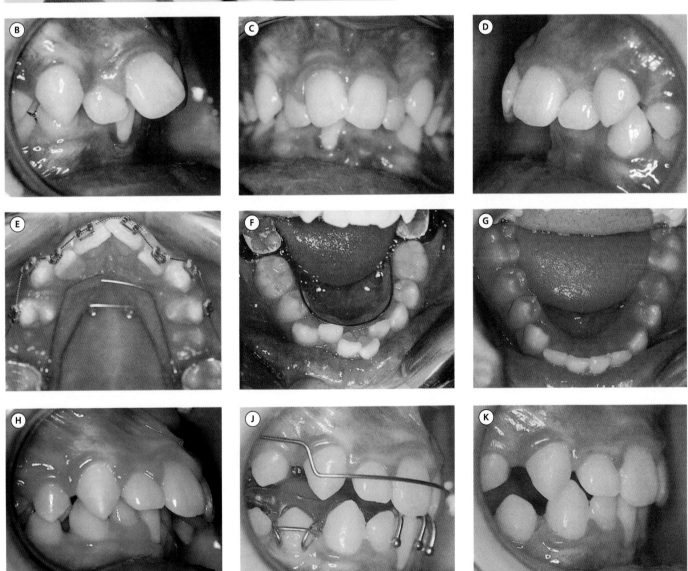

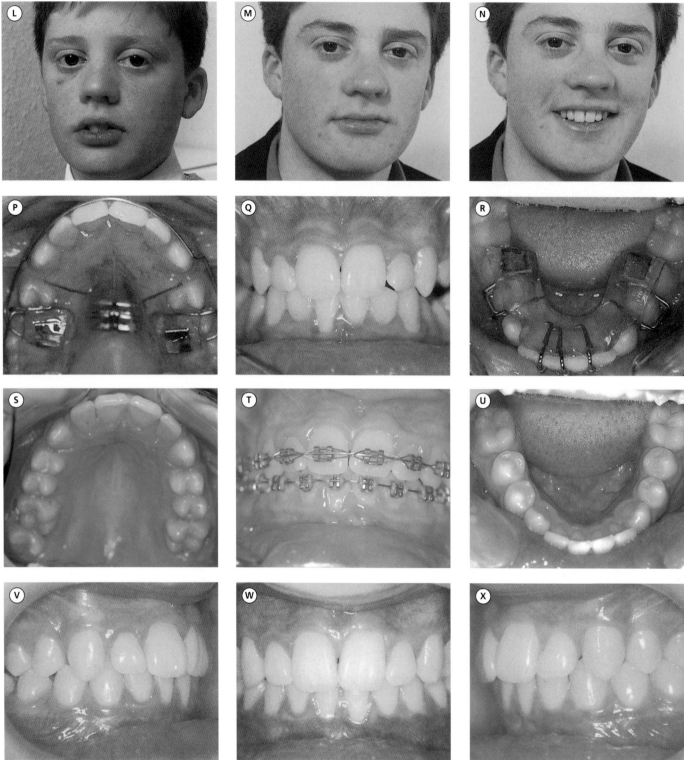

Fig. 19.1 Treatment (cont.):
L Appearance before treatment.
M, N Appearance at age 19 years 4 months.
P, R Occlusal view of magnetic Twin Blocks.
S, U Corrected archform at age 19 years 4 months.
T Fixed appliances to detail the occlusion.
V–X Occlusion 1 year out of retention at age 19 years 4 months.

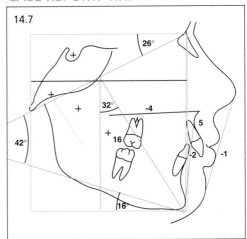

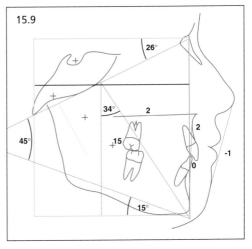

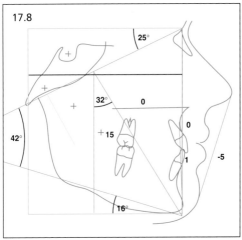

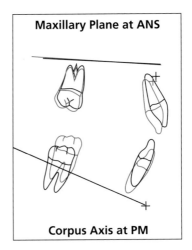

Maxillary Plane at ANS

Corpus Axis at PM

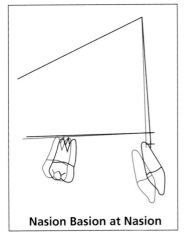

Nasion Basion at Nasion

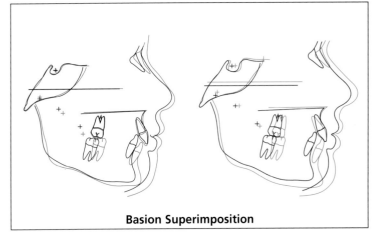

Basion Superimposition

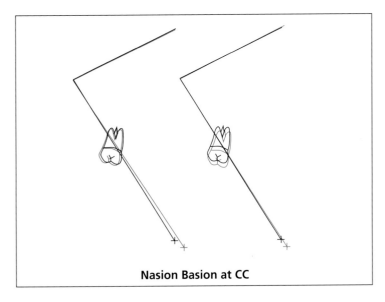

Nasion Basion at CC

F.H.	Age 14.7	15.9	17.8
Cranial Base Angle	26	26	25
Facial Axis Angle	32	34	32
F/M Plane Angle	16	15	16
Craniomandibular Angle	42	45	43
Maxillary Plane	–4	2	0
Convexity	5	2	0
U/Incisor to Vertical	21	21	27
L/Incisor to Vertical	24	31	29
Interincisal Angle	135	128	126
6 to Pterygoid Vertical	16	15	15
L/Incisor to A/Po	–2	0	1
L/Lip to Aesthetic Plane	–1	–1	–5

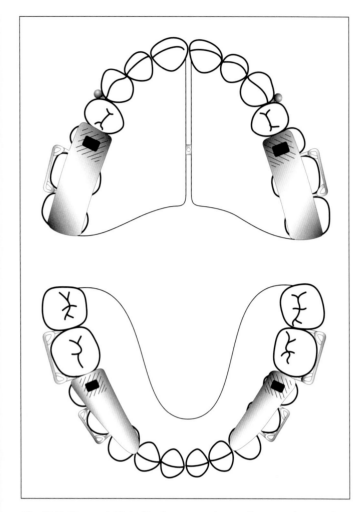

Fig. 19.2 Magnetic Twin Blocks can accelerate the rate of correction.

MAGNETIC FORCE IN THE CORRECTION OF FACIAL ASYMMETRY

Inclined planes with attracting magnets provide an excellent training mechanism to improve facial balance by controlling muscle action. Magnetic Twin Blocks have the potential to accelerate the rate of correction achieved by conventional functional appliances (Fig. 19.2).

REFERENCES

Darendeliler, M.A. & Joho, J.P. (1993). Magnetic activator device II (MAD) for correction of Class II Division I malocclusions. *Am. J. Orthod. Dentofac. Orthop.*, **103:** 223–39.

Vardimon, A.D., Stutzmann, J.J., Graber, T.M., Voss, L.R. & Petrovic, A.G. (1989). Functional Orthopedic Magnetic Appliance (FOMA) II – modus operandi. *Am. J. Orthod. Dentofac. Orthop.*, **95:** 371–87.

Vardimon, A.D., Graber, T.M., Voss, L.R. & Muller, T.M. (1990). Functional Orthopedic Magnetic Appliance (FOMA) III – modus operandi. *Am. J. Orthod. Dentofac. Orthop.*, **97:** 135–48.

CHAPTER 20

Adult Treatment

Tooth movements are slower in older patients, and the skeletal response diminishes with the patient's age. In adult orthodontic treatment we should anticipate a dentoalveolar response with limited skeletal adaptation. This still leaves scope for significant facial change, but only when the skeletal discrepancy is not severe. Surgical correction should be considered for cases of severe skeletal discrepancies in adults.

CASE REPORT: H.C. AGED 42 YEARS 8 MONTHS

This patient attended for treatment at the age of 42 because her upper incisors were migrating labially due to loss of bony support. This case shows a typical dentoalveolar response in adult treatment where periodontally compromised teeth are the weakest link in the biological chain of reaction due to lack of bony support. Combined extraoral and intermaxillary traction were applied at night during the orthopaedic phase of treatment, using the Concorde facebow to accelerate tooth movements. This was followed by an orthodontic phase with fixed appliances. Finally, upper and lower Rochette splints were fitted as fixed lingual retainers. These served the dual purpose of orthodontic retainer and splint to stabilise the anterior teeth for periodontal support (Fig. 20.1 A–P).

Twin Blocks: 4 months
Support phase: 3 months
Fixed appliance: 8 months.

Superimposed x-rays confirm that the correction was due to dentoalveolar compensation, with no skeletal change. The upper dentition was retracted and the lower dentition moved mesially. Significant growth changes should not be anticipated in the treatment of adults who are beyond the growth stage. The response to treatment is likely to be dentoalveolar, especially where there is a loss of periodontal support.

CASE REPORT: H.C.

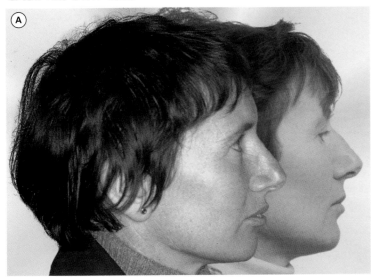

Fig. 20.1 Treatment:
A Profiles at ages 42 years 8 months (before treatment) and 44 years 8 months (after treatment).

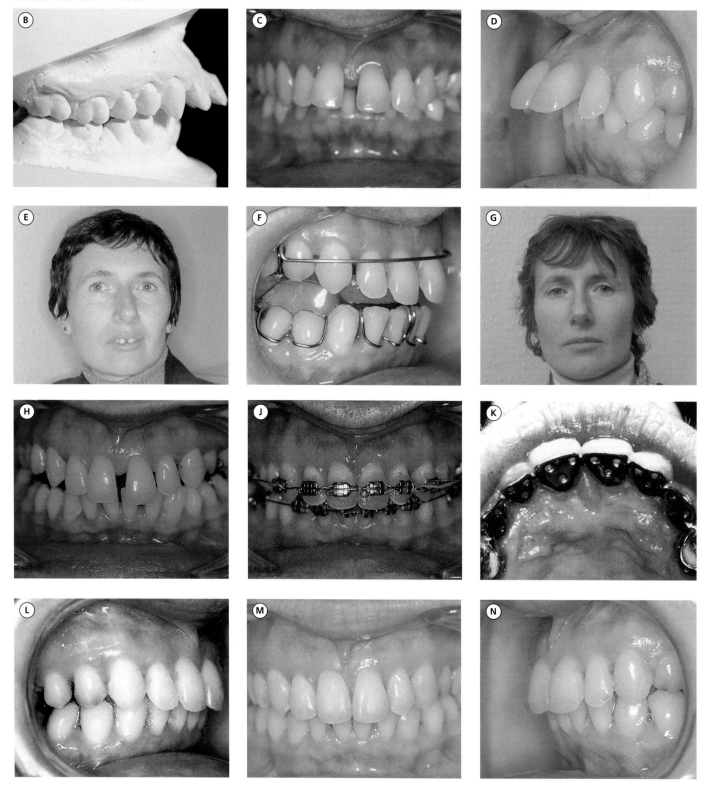

Fig. 20.1 Treatment (cont.):

B–D Occlusion before treatment – note the gingival recession.
E Appearance before treatment at age 42 years 8 months.
F Twin Block appliances.
G Appearance after treatment.

H Phase I – Twin Blocks – change after 4 months.
J Phase 2 – fixed appliances.
K Fixed lingual retainer (Rochette splint).
L–N Occlusion after treatment at age 44 years 8 months.

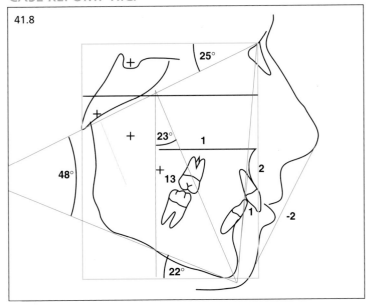

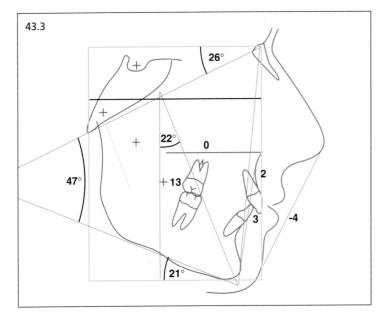

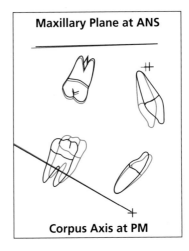

Corpus Axis at PM

Nasion Basion at Nasion

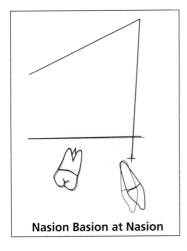

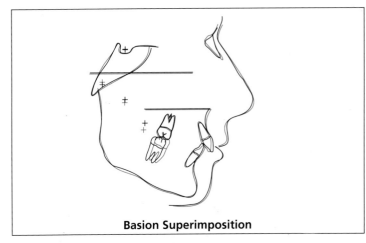

Basion Superimposition

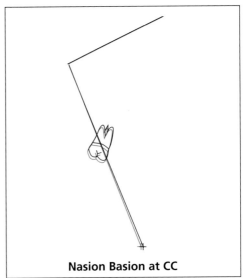

Nasion Basion at CC

H.C. Age	41.8	43.3
Cranial Base Angle	25	26
Facial Axis Angle	23	22
F/M Plane Angle	22	21
Craniomandibular Angle	48	47
Maxillary Plane	1	0
Convexity	2	2
U/Incisor to Vertical	26	21
L/Incisor to Vertical	39	45
Interincisal Angle	115	114
6 to Pterygoid Vertical	13	13
L/Incisor to A/Po	1	3
L/Lip to Aesthetic Plane	−2	−4

CASE REPORT: P.W.

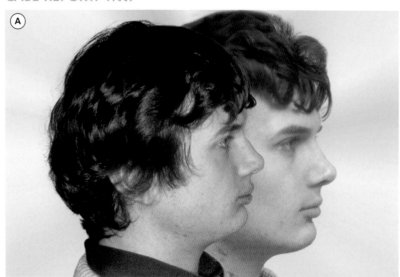

Fig. 20.2 Treatment:
A Profiles at ages 17 years 4 months (before treatment) and 18 years 4 months (after treatment).
B Occlusion before treatment.
C Occlusion after 6 weeks of treatment.
D Occlusion after 18 months of treatment.
E Occlusion after 3 years, at age 20 years 4 months, 18 months out of retention.

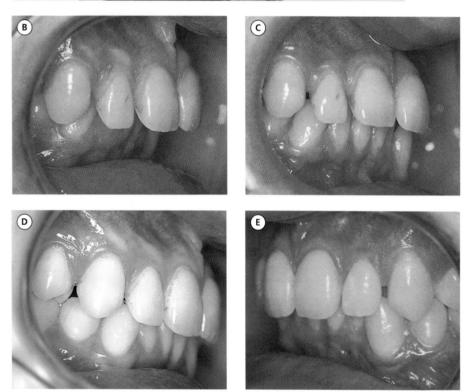

TREATMENT OF A YOUNG ADULT

CASE REPORT: P.W. AGED 17 YEARS 4 MONTHS

This is an example of a young adult who was treated in his late teens by Twin Blocks after the pubertal growth spurt. He presented a severe dental Class II division I malocclusion with a Class I skeletal base and a strong brachyfacial growth pattern. In this case dental correction only was required, and there was a rapid response to treatment as the overjet reduced from 10 mm to 6 mm within the first 6 weeks, and to 4 mm after 4 months of treatment. The patient declined a final stage of treatment to detail the occlusion with fixed appliances. The result proved to be stable although no significant growth changes are recorded at this age.

Growth continues into middle and late teens in boys and Twin Block treatment can be very successful in this age group provided the appliances are worn full time (Fig. 20.2 A–F).

Twin Blocks: 9 months
Support and retention: 9 months.

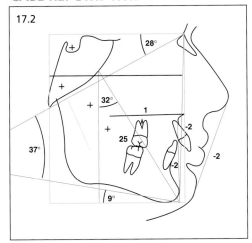

17.2

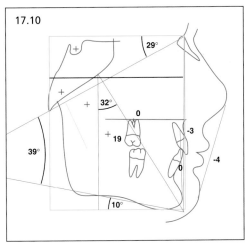

17.10

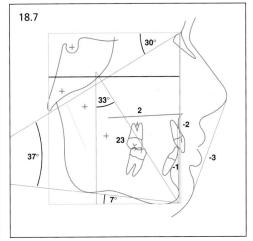

18.7

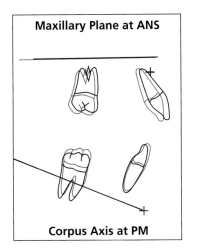

Maxillary Plane at ANS

Corpus Axis at PM

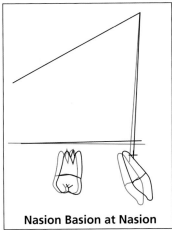

Nasion Basion at Nasion

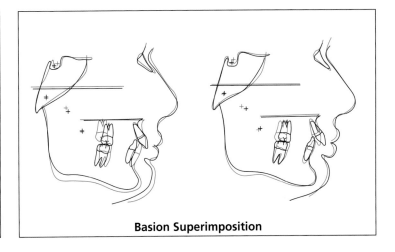

Basion Superimposition

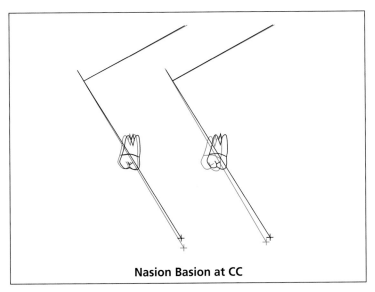

Nasion Basion at CC

P.W.	Age	17.2	17.10	18.7
Cranial Base Angle		28	29	30
Facial Axis Angle		32	32	33
F/M Plane Angle		9	10	7
Craniomandibular Angle		37	39	37
Maxillary Plane		1	0	2
Convexity		−2	−3	−2
U/Incisor to Vertical		31	25	20
L/Incisor to Vertical		23	24	26
Interincisal Angle		126	131	134
6 to Pterygoid Vertical		25	19	23
L/Incisor to A/Po		−2	0	−1
L/Lip to Aesthetic Plane		−2	−4	−3

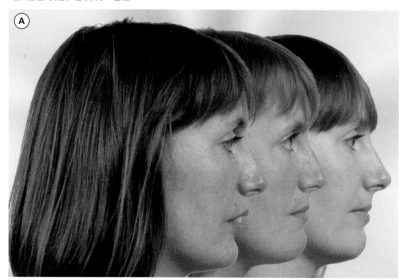

Fig. 20.3 Treatment:
A Profiles at ages 27 years 6 months (before treatment), 27 years 6 months (immediate change in profile when appliance is fitted) and 28 years 8 months.
B, C Occlusion before treatment and with Twin Blocks.
D Occlusion after 6 months of treatment.
E Appearance before treatment.
F Improved smile after treatment.

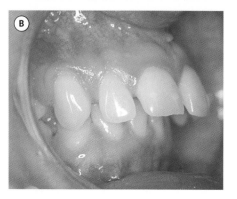

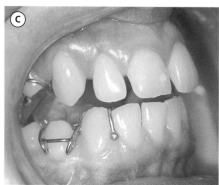

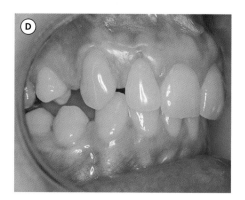

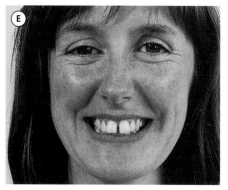

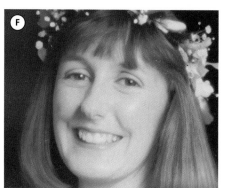

CASE REPORT: G.J. AGED 27 YEARS 6 MONTHS

When this patient attended for examination she asked if treatment to improve her smile could be completed before her wedding in 7 months time. Twin Blocks were fitted and sufficient progress was made to meet her request. An overjet of 10 mm was due to proclined upper incisors and the skeletal base relationship was Class I, so that only dental correction was required (Fig. 20.3 A–H).

Twin Blocks: 9 months
Support phase: 5 months, followed by retention.

CHAPTER 21

Temporomandibular Joint Pain and Dysfunction Syndrome

Occlusion is inevitably related to the health and function of the temporomandibular (TM) joint. No dental condition is more distressing for a patient than chronic TM joint pain. A rationale of treatment is therefore important in dental and orthodontic practice. This is a litigious area of dental practice and second opinions should be sought before embarking on any treatment which may worsen an already established pathological condition.

The dental profession is increasingly aware of a multi-disciplinary approach, recognising the role of chiropractors and craniosacral osteopaths in the diagnosis and resolution of TM joint dysfunction. Muscle spasm and joint pathology cannot be considered in isolation from a holistic examination of other possible causes in body posture and alignment of the vertebral column. Cooperation should be encouraged in interdisciplinary programmes of diagnosis and management.

THE IMPORTANCE OF OCCLUSION

From a dental perspective an excellent functional occlusion is the cornerstone of treatment for TMD (Temporo Mandibular Dysfunction). Ramfjord & Ash (1983) documented the relief of pain and related its timing with the return to symmetrical muscle activity when occlusal interferences were removed in patients with pain and muscle dysfunction.

Krogh-Poulsen & Olsson (1968) demonstrated the relationship between specific interferences and functional muscle abnormalities. Beyron (1954) also related occlusal interferences to asymmetrical abrasion of the tooth surfaces. Graf (1975) showed that occlusal interferences altered the deglutition reflex and concluded that a stable occlusal contact relationship in maximum intercuspation seems to be essential for adequate masticatory function.

Bakke & Moller (1980) have documented significant changes in muscular activity from induced occlusal interferences as thin as 50 μm. The alteration of even one tooth incline has the potential for disrupting the balance and thus the stability of the entire system. Such minute incline interferences often occur in occlusions that appear to have ideal intercuspation. Therefore it is necessary to take mounted casts to identify these small occlusal interferences. Following orthodontic treatment it is important to check the functional occlusion with articulating paper and to examine cuspal guidance in anterior and lateral excursions.

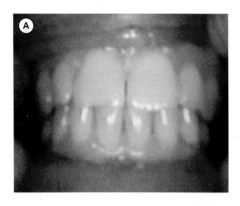

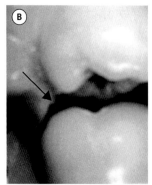

Fig. 21.1 Treatment:
A The occlusion appeared to be normal.
B Interference at a single occlusal contact caused chronic pain.

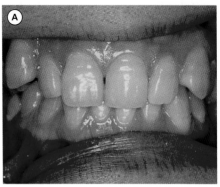

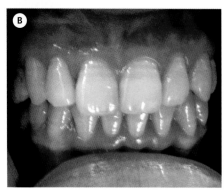

Fig. 21.2 Treatment:
A Retroclined upper incisors caused over-closure and distal condylar displacement.
B TMD pain was relieved by advancing the incisors and leveling the occlusal plane to improve the vertical dimension.

CASE REPORT: J.K. AGED 43 YEARS

by Mel Taskey

This female was referred for examination of severe headaches that resulted from a motor vehicle accident. Professionals had told her that nothing could be done for her because all of her pain existed in her head, and that she should seek psychiatric care.

Upon examination the patient was able to open just enough to determine that the problem was occlusal. She could open a total of 12 mm.

A major deflection from the contact of 1.8 and 4.7 moved the mandible off the disk. The deflection on the mesial lingual cusp of 1.8 was removed. Within 2 minutes the patient was able to open a total of 22 mm. This illustrates the importance of occlusion in the dental equation. This facilitated the taking of impressions to make splints, and to manage the patient's chronic pain by resting the muscles (Fig. 21.1).

CASE REPORT: K.W. AGED 26 YEARS

by Mel Taskey

This female was referred regarding the anterior crowding of her teeth and accompanying TMD pain. Retroclined upper incisors are frequently related to these symptoms in adult dentitions. Twin block appliances were used for a period of 2 years to advance the upper incisors and to level the occlusal plane to improve the vertical relationship. During this time she was completely pain free (Fig. 21.2).

RELIEF OF PAIN

Clinical experience has proved that it is necessary to treat the patient to a comfort zone.

Relief of pain requires that the patient is treated to a 'comfort zone', whereby a functional occlusion provides adequate support for traumatised joint tissues. The fundamentals of treatment are as follows:

- Balanced occlusal support to relieve muscle spasm in the initial stage of treatment. The patient should be pain free before adjusting the occlusion
- Removal of cuspal interferences causing mandibular displacement on closure
- Good vertical support for the joints to function freely without compression of the articular disc
- Freedom of movement with cuspid guidance and incisal guidance when the mandible moves from centric occlusion
- Tripoding of occlusal contacts in the final balanced occlusion

Detailing of the occlusion following orthodontic treatment does not always achieve all of these goals. In the past orthodontic results have been assessed on the basis of a static view of the finished occlusion, with insufficient attention to balancing the occlusion to remove interferences and achieve ideal function. Occlusal prematurities or cross arch interferences in the finished case perpetuate disruption by steering the TM joint. This promotes the tongue to act as a physiological protector and re-enter the occlusal equation. This potentially results in a regression of therapy as it undoes the previously established tooth relationships. It may be argued that after orthodontic treatment the occlusion should be examined and balanced to achieve ideal function.

The abbreviation for temporomandibular joint, TMJ, might equally refer to teeth, muscles and joints, and successful orthodontic treatment depends on achieving balanced function of all the components of the stomato-gnathic system.

The treatment of adult patients is often undertaken by a prosthodontist, or a practitioner who specialises in the management of temporomandibular discomfort. In adult treatment the occlusion is often already compromised, and it may not be feasible to achieve an ideal occlusion. The primary objective of treatment is relief of pain, and to resolve occlusal interference to an acceptable position where the teeth, muscles and joints can work in synergy.

CASE HISTORY AND DIAGNOSIS

Excellent record taking is an essential part of clinical management and treatment. A full case history is necessary to establish any cause-and-effect relationship of occlusal disharmony and mandibular displacement to pain and restriction of mandibular movement. This includes an assessment of any injury, headache, neck and back pain, neuromuscular tension, and tenderness to palpation.

Clinical and radiographic examinations of the TM joint are used to identify the position of the condyle in the glenoid fossae in the closed position, at rest and in the open position. Any radiographic evidence of flattening or irregularity in the shape of the condyle is a sign of pathological change, and patients with signs of osteoarthritic change in the joint should be referred for comprehensive investigation, and expert advice and treatment.

Some of the major signs and clinical symptoms of TM joint dysfunction of a functionally induced nature are diagnosed as pain, muscle tension, joint sounds and limitation of movement. A displaced disc is often associated with clicks and limited opening. In unilateral disc displacement there is displacement of the mandible to the affected side, and limited transverse movement. It is sometimes possible to manipulate the mandible downwards and forwards to recapture the disc. If successful, this would have the immediate response of increased opening. However, manipulation to recapture the disc does not eliminate the cause of disc displacement, which may then recur. Limited opening is also a sign of disc displacement.

Freedom of mandibular movement

It is essential to diagnose any limitation of movement relative to the normal range of movement:

- Normal opening is 48 mm (the three-finger test).
- Transverse movement is 12 mm to each side, measuring the lower midline displacement in maximum lateral movement.

The reciprocal click

A clicking joint is symptomatic of displacement of the articular disc off the head of the condyle. A reciprocal click describes the condition where a click is heard when the disc is recaptured by the head of the condyle on forward translation, and a reciprocal click is heard when the condyle is again displaced off the articular disc on closing. The opening click is louder than the closing click. Although the clicking joint may be otherwise asymptomatic, it is nevertheless already compromised internally and liable to present pathology at a later date due to the chronic displacement of the articular disc.

The timing of a click on opening is significant in the prognosis for resolution:

- Early opening clicks: up to 22 mm opening are usually easy to resolve.
- Mid opening clicks: 22–35 mm opening are moderate to resolve.
- Late opening clicks: over 35 mm opening are difficult to resolve.

Case selection for anterior repositioning of the mandible to relieve TM joint dysfunction is based on the severity of symptoms and condylar position at full occlusion. The prognosis is better for recapturing the disc for an early opening click. It becomes progressively more difficult for the mid and late opening click, when pathological osteoarthritic change is likely to have occurred in the joint.

Spahl (1993) stresses that, nevertheless, disc recapture is not the main goal of treatment for patients with functionally induced TM joint pain dysfunction problems. The true goal is reduction of symptoms via condylar decompression procedures involving muscular advancement of the mandible followed by reconstruction of the occlusion in some manner to support the mandible/condyle in that advanced position.

The closed lock

Limitation of movement on opening is diagnostic of a disc which is displaced, usually anteromedially to the condyle, and is not recaptured on opening. In the initial stages, the patient may be pain free and may complain only of restriction of movement. This may be an episodic experience, where the disc is displaced from time to time and the patient may be able periodically to recapture the disc until the displacement becomes more severe. If not detected and treated, the disc may gradually become folded forwards and not recapturable, leading eventually to painful function and restricted opening due to osteoarthritis. A 'closed lock' should be diagnosed early from restricted movement and should be treated by anterior or vertical repositioning to recapture the disc. Treatment should then be effected to create vertical space in the joint by positioning the condyles downwards and forwards in the glenoid fossae, and to establish balanced occlusal support.

Internal derangement

The three stages of TM internal derangement are:

- Stage 1: painless clicking caused when an anteriorly displaced disc is recaptured on the condyle during opening translation.
- Stage 2: locking – persistent displacement of the disc which arrests condyle motion at mid opening.
- Stage 3: disc displacement through all phases of jaw function. The anteromedially displaced disc becomes distorted and folded on opening, with chronic pain and signs of osteoarthritis. The disc remains permanently unrecapturable.

Stages 1 and 2 respond to splint therapy and anterior repositioning to recapture the disc, subject to correct case selection (Solberg, 1989) (Fig. 21.3).

Treatment rationale

Hawthorn & Flatau (1990) summarise the approach to joint dysfunction as described below.

Conservative clinical treatment of joint dysfunction is based on the concept of the need to reduce loading within the joint itself in order to achieve satisfactory long-term results, and to maintain the relationship of the meniscus to the condylar head.

Conservative management of joint conditions ranging from arthritic degeneration to internal joint derangement is directed towards:

1. The reduction of functional loads exerted on the TM joint by restoration of interarch support.

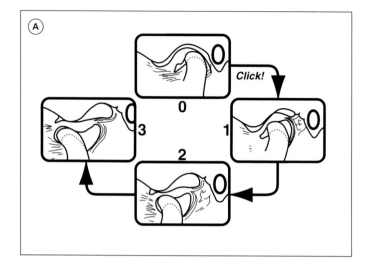

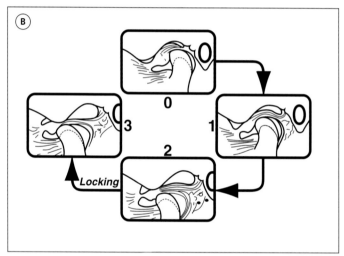

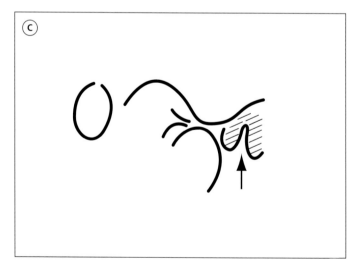

Fig. 21.3 A A clicking joint: the sequence of opening and closing. **B, C** The closed lock with a folded articular disc.
Reproduced from *Temporomandibular Disorders*, William K. Solberg, 1986, pp. 91, 92 and 93. Courtesy of the *British Dental Journal*, London.

2. The correction of the closing pathway as determined by tooth contacts. The constraints imposed on jaw movement in a sagittal plane by tooth contacts have a major effect on the movement of both the condyle and the meniscus during mandibular closure.

TM joint pain and dysfunction are frequently related to occlusal disharmony with premature occlusal contact, causing posterior or lateral shift of the mandible from centric relation and distal displacement of the condyles in the joint. Distal displacement of the condyle in occlusion is associated with anterior displacement of the articular disc.

The management of treatment in the past has been in three phases:

1. Sagittal expansion to advance the upper incisors, with occlusal cover to take the mandible out of occlusion and relieve pain.
2. Functional therapy to advance the mandible with a one-piece functional appliance.
3. Vertical development of the posterior teeth using vertical elastic forces provided by appliances such as the Spahl vertical corrector or the biofinisher (Lynn, 1985), with occlusal reconstruction if required to increase the vertical dimension and to stabilise and balance the occlusion.

TEMPOROMANDIBULAR JOINT THERAPY

Our efforts in treatment must not move the mandible back, or restrict the joint space. If occlusal imbalance is present, the muscles are the prime movers in causing mandibular displacement to avoid unfavourable premature occlusal contacts. Disc displacement and muscle spasm are secondary features of chronic occlusal imbalance, which cause the condyle to be displaced distally.

The goals of therapy are:

- Relieve the pain caused by distal displacement of the condyle.
- Retrain the muscles to a healthy pattern.
- Recapture the disc when possible by advancing the displaced condyle.
- Move the teeth that are causing occlusal imbalance and mandibular misguidance.
- Increase the vertical dimension to reduce deep overbite.

Splint therapy

The occlusal splint is a valuable diagnostic tool that can deal effectively with most patient pain problems. Splints that are carefully monitored in approximately 4-week intervals provide valuable information. Judicious adjustment on the splint can determine the vertical dimension that will be comfortable for the patient, also all muscles of mastication can be assessed as they lose their varied spasm. Patient compliance and attention to their problems can be ascertained before any major work is undertaken.

Subsequent to diagnostic splint therapy, with the muscles of mastication relaxed, there usually remains a significant difference between centric relation (the relationship of the mandible and maxilla when the condyle-disc assemblies are in their most superior position against the eminentia irrespective of tooth position or vertical dimension), and centric occlusion (the maxilla and mandible relationship when the teeth are in maximum intercuspation). Mandibular deflection upon closure, and the lack of posterior tooth support to protect the jaw during trauma, only compounds the occlusal instability and perpetuation of myalgia. The importance of cuspid guidance cannot be overstated. Composite dental material may be placed to restore cuspid guidance or group function, thus reinforcing posterior support for the joints.

Anterior guidance can be likened to the steering wheel of a car as it provides direction for the mandible throughout all movements of the jaw, including deglutition and mastication. When the teeth are considered in the stomatognathic system there is a unique influence on the entire interbalance of the occlusion and temporomandibular joints. If the intercuspation is not in harmony with the joint-ligament muscle balance, a stressed and exhausting protective role is forced onto the muscles. Therefore it is important to ensure posterior occlusal support, anterior guidance and proper group function while maintaining the temporomandibular joints in their most comfortable physiological position.

Twin Blocks in temporomandibular joint therapy

Case selection

A full diagnosis and case history is essential before proceeding to corrective treatment in TM joint therapy. If any signs of joint pathology are detected, expert advice should be sought. If in doubt, a diagnostic splint should first be supplied to resolve the pain and rest the joint before proceeding to more active therapy.

Twin Blocks are most likely to be indicated to resolve an early click when the condyle is displaced distal to the disc and the disc is recaptured at an early stage in the opening movement. Twin Blocks then achieve the following objectives in the first phase of treatment:

- Pain is relieved immediately when Twin Blocks are fitted or, in more difficult cases, within 4–7 days.
- The muscles are retrained automatically to a healthy pattern. A consistent feature of Twin Block therapy is the

rapid improvement in facial balance. Muscle spasm is relieved when Twin Blocks are fitted, by changing the pattern of muscle activity to achieve a new position of equilibrium in muscle balance.

- The disc is recaptured by posturing the mandible downwards and forwards to advance the condyles.
- Rather than act as a passive splint, Twin Blocks are designed to move the teeth that are causing occlusal imbalance.
- The upper block may be trimmed selectively over the lower first molars only, using molar bands with vertical elastics to accelerate eruption of the first molars. To continue to rest the joint, a posterior occlusal stop is maintained by occlusal contact of the blocks with the second or third molars to support the vertical dimension.

The Twin Block sagittal appliance is usually appropriate to achieve all these objectives (Fig. 21.4). In bite registration the Exactobite is used to guide the mandible downwards and forwards to a comfortable position. It is important to recognise that if pain is not relieved by forward posture, and the disc does not appear to be recaptured, there may be internal derangement, or folding of the disc, which will not respond to Twin Block therapy.

A common cause of unilateral condylar displacement is occlusal interference causing a mandibular displacement and sideways shift, with the condyle displaced distally on the affected side, often associated with a unilateral distal occlusion. Unilateral sagittal activation to drive upper molars distally and advance the mandible simultaneously to correct the centre line and restore symmetry may help to resolve this type of occlusal imbalance.

APPLIANCE DESIGN

The sagittal Twin Block is used to relieve compression on the joint by posturing the mandible downwards and forwards and advancing retroclined upper incisors. In sagittal appliance design, the further forwards the screws, the more anterior the movement; the further back the screws, the more posterior the movement.

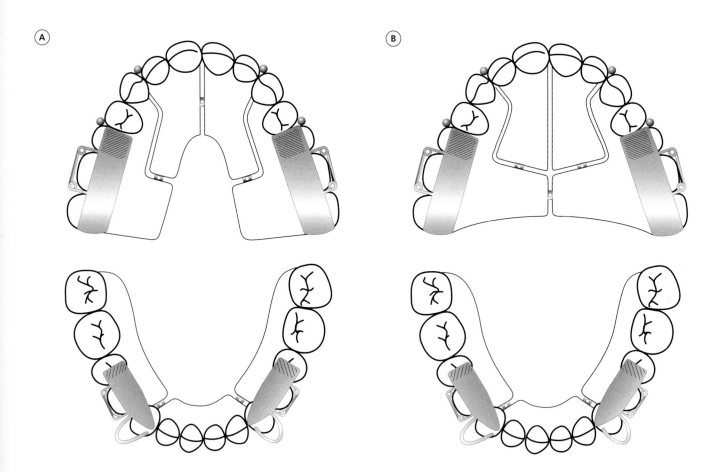

Fig. 21.4 A, B The three-screw sagittal Twin Block to develop archform.

CLINICAL MANAGEMENT

In the management of deep overbite, the occlusal cover is trimmed progressively over the first molars only to allow the eruption of posterior teeth, without creating enough vertical clearance to allow the tongue to spread laterally between the teeth. Only after the first molars have erupted fully into occlusion may the blocks be trimmed selectively to encourage eruption of premolars or second or third molars as required.

It is especially important in the treatment of TM joint dysfunction to maintain posterior occlusal support at all times in order to relieve compression in the joint. A transition may be made to an anterior inclined plane to support the corrected occlusion after good posterior occlusal support is restored. This approach can be usefully combined with the Spahl vertical corrector in the support phase to accelerate correction of the vertical dimension.

Traction to open the bite

Vertical elastics may be used to accelerate the bite opening by stretching elastics from the upper appliance to hooks bonded to the lower posterior teeth, having first relieved occlusal acrylic to encourage selective eruption. This is not generally required in the treatment of the growing child, where eruption occurs naturally to close a posterior open bite. The addition of elastics is especially useful in adult treatment to accelerate eruption in patients who are no longer actively growing. Vertical traction assumes an increasingly important role as an effective method of increasing the vertical dimension in the treatment of patients who have TM joint dysfunction due to overclosure.

Stages of treatment

Treatment may be divided into three separate objectives of sagittal development, functional repositioning and vertical development. Sagittal Twin Blocks are designed to allow all three corrective phases to proceed simultaneously to relieve a distally displaced condyle. Progressive trimming to encourage vertical development is crucial to the success of the treatment.

Detailed finishing of the occlusion to achieve a functional balance is necessary for long-term stability of joint symptoms. A finishing stage of treatment with bonded fixed appliances is frequently required to achieve this objective. When this is not possible, the alternative of occlusal rehabilitation by restorative means may be preferred if the occlusion is compromised by loss of teeth.

Round tripping

In the care of injured joints it is never effective to wear crutches part time and sometimes discard them – this results in relapse. This principle applies equally in TM joint therapy, whether a splint or a more active appliance is being used to rest the joint. Intermittent appliance wear only relieves the pain temporarily, and under certain circumstances may worsen it!

Pain is relieved when the appliance is worn and the condyle is positioned downwards and forwards in the joint. If the patient takes the appliance out for eating, or for any other reason, the condyle is again displaced up and back in the glenoid fossa and the pain returns.

It is important not to introduce splint dependency, but to endeavour to resolve the occlusal imbalance related to TM disorders. Successful TM joint treatment requires a full-time commitment from the patient to see the treatment through until the occlusion is reconstructed with the condyles positioned correctly in the glenoid fossae. Depending on the aetiology of the condition this may involve orthopaedic repositioning, orthodontic balancing of the occlusion, occlusal reconstruction or a combination of these disciplines.

CASE REPORT: R.D.

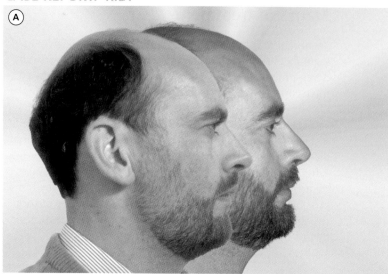

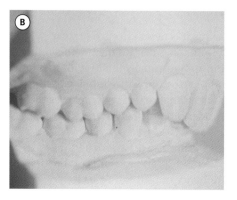

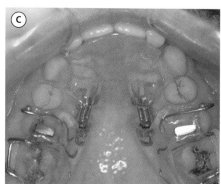

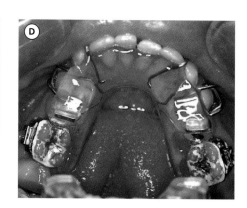

Fig. 21.5 Treatment:
A Profiles at ages 36 ages 0 months (before treatment) and 38 years 3 months (after treatment).
B Occlusion before treatment.
C Magnetic sagittal Twin Block.
D Lower magnetic Twin Block with lower molar bands.

CASE REPORT: R.D. AGED 36 YEARS

This patient presented a severe Class II division 2 malocclusion and a history of chronic headaches three or four times a week for as long as he could remember. He had come to accept this as part of normal life until he learned that the headaches might be related to his dental occlusion, at which stage he presented for treatment.

Upper and lower incisors were severely retroclined with an interincisal angle of 180°, while the incisal edges of the lower incisors were 10 mm behind the A–Po line, resulting in a traumatic deep overbite lingual to the upper incisors.

The aim of treatment was to relieve the compression in the TM joint by releasing the mandible from its trapped position in distal occlusion. This required upper anterior arch development followed by functional correction to advance the mandible. The objective was then to build the vertical dimension and position the condyles downwards and forwards in the glenoid fossae. Vertical elastics were used to accelerate eruption of the molars and premolars during the Twin Block and support phases of treatment. A final restorative stage of treatment was anticipated to increase the width of the upper incisors to correct the Bolton relationship after correcting the canines to a Class I occlusion. A fixed lingual retainer was fitted in the lower arch (Fig. 21.5).

The patient quickly experienced a remission of headaches during the first stage of treatment as the upper incisors advanced. The improvement continued throughout the treatment and the headaches did not return.

Twin Blocks: 9 months
Support phase: 9 months
Fixed appliances: 1 year.

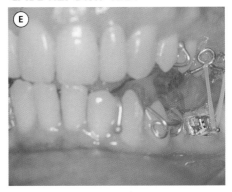

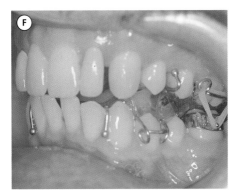

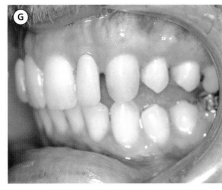

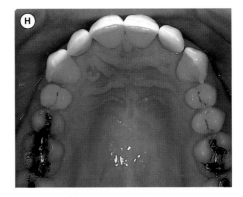

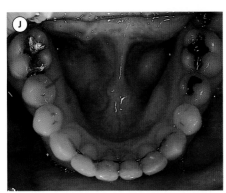

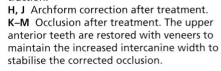

Fig. 21.5 Treatment (cont.):
E, F Vertical traction to elevate the molars.
G Molars in occlusion after 4 months of traction.
H, J Archform correction after treatment.
K–M Occlusion after treatment. The upper anterior teeth are restored with veneers to maintain the increased intercanine width to stabilise the corrected occlusion.

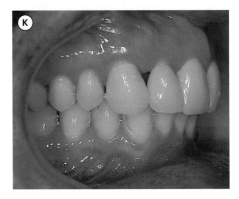

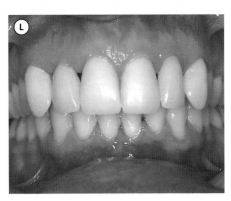

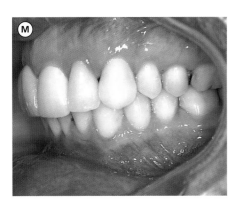

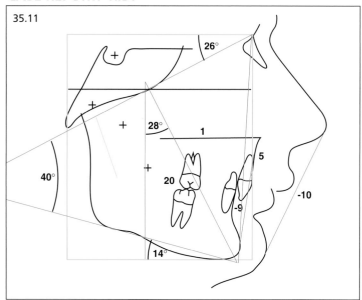

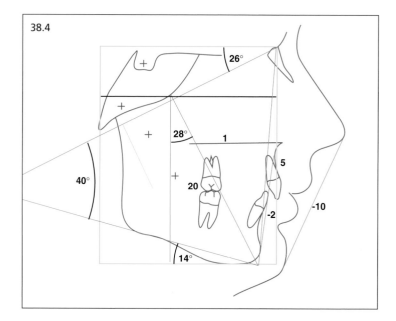

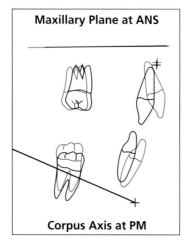

Maxillary Plane at ANS

Corpus Axis at PM

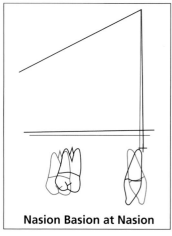

Nasion Basion at Nasion

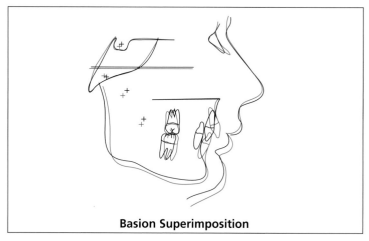

Basion Superimposition

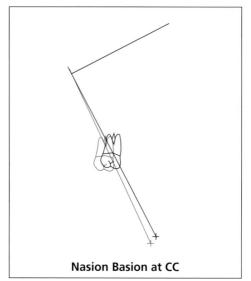

Nasion Basion at CC

R.D.	Age	35.11	38.4
Cranial Base Angle		26	26
Facial Axis Angle		28	28
F/M Plane Angle		14	14
Craniomandibular Angle		40	40
Maxillary Plane		1	1
Convexity		5	5
U/Incisor to Vertical		−11	14
L/Incisor to Vertical		14	28
Interincisal Angle		177	138
6 to Pterygoid Vertical		20	16
L/Incisor to A/Po		−5	−2
L/Lip to Aesthetic Plane		−10	−10

CASE REPORT: M.L.

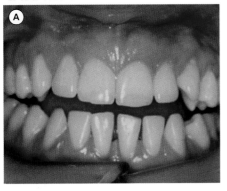
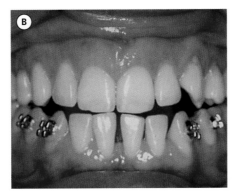
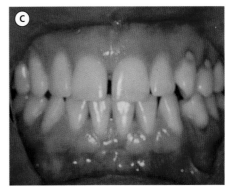

Fig. 21.6 Treatment:
A Anterior open bite contracting only on posterior molars.
B Brackets on 43|34 for vertical elastics.
C The open bite closed after 6 months of treatment and is stable 5 years out of retention.

ANTERIOR OPEN BITE TEMPORO-MANDIBULAR JOINT DYSFUNCTION

CASE REPORT: M.L. AGED 38 YEARS

by Mel Taskey

This 38-year-old female suffered from constant headaches and could not chew her food because of the anterior open bite. Joint symptoms in anterior open bite relate to the lack of anterior and cuspal guidance, placing more strain on the muscles to maintain the occlusal relationship of the teeth during normal function. It is necessary to restore incisal and cuspal guidance to resolve the cycle of chronic pain.

Twin Blocks were inserted to mitigate the patient's pain and align the arches. Vertical elastics were passed from the labial bow on the upper Twin Block to brackets on the lower canines and premolars to close the open bite, while the occlusal blocks applied an intrusive force to the posterior teeth. In 6 months the open bite was closed. Finished casts illustrate good posterior cusp fossa/relationship, giving good joint support. The patient has been comfortable without retention for 5 years. The position is stable because the posterior teeth are in a cusp–fossa relationship and group function exists in the bicuspids (Fig. 21.6).

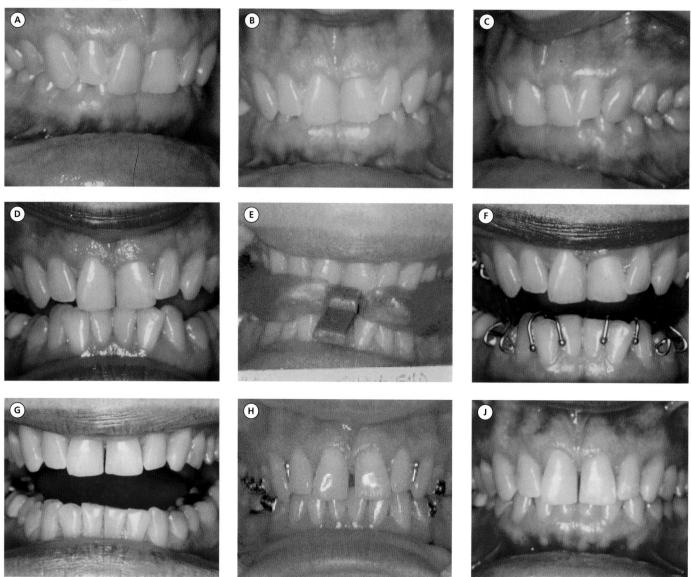

Fig. 21.7 Treatment:
A–C Occlusion before treatment.
D Deep overbite with excessive curve of Spee in the lower arch.
E Registering the construction bite.
F Twin Blocks fitted.
G Curve of Spee levelled after treatment.
H, J Occlusion settles after retention.

CASE REPORT: L.J. AGED 44 YEARS

by Mel Taskey

This 44-year-old female presented suffering from severe headaches following whiplash injury in a motor vehicle accident. After 5 years she had no definitive diagnosis to this point. A diagnostic mandibular splint was inserted and this reduced her severe headaches. The use of Twin Blocks was explained to the patient and treatment was initiated. The patient was pain free after 1 week, and continued to wear Twin Blocks for 18 months. In phase 2 a Spahl vertical corrector was selected to increase the vertical dimension and restore posterior support. Brackets were placed on all posterior teeth with vertical elastics to increase the vertical dimension. The posterior teeth were in occlusion after 10 months and posterior support with brackets and elastics continued to be used for the next 10 months. Finally an elastodent finishing appliance was worn for 1 year. No retention appliance has been worn for 3 years.

Treatment has resulted in levelling of the curve of Spee, with correction of the vertical dimension and reduction of the excessive overbite. The distal occlusion has been corrected and, most importantly, the chronic pain has been eliminated. In treatment of temporomandibular joint dysfunction the results are not based on the standard of orthodontic finishing, but on successfully getting the patient free of pain. Compromise is often necessary in the treatment of adult patients, as ideal occlusion is often not a feasible objective (Fig. 21.7).

ACKNOWLEDGEMENTS

The sections on 'The Importance of Occlusion' and 'Splint Therapy' are contributed by Dr Mel Taskey, who has 40 years' experience in practice in Edmonton, Alberta, specialising in the treatment of temporomandibular joint dysfunction, and the management of traumatic injuries. Dr Taskey also supplied examples of treatment for four patients, K.W., J.K., L.J. and M.L.

REFERENCES

Bakke, M. & Moller, E. (1980). Distortion of maximal elevator activity by unilateral premature tooth contact. *Scand. J. Dent. Res.*, **88**: 67.

Beyron, H. (1954). Occlusal changes in adult dentition. *J. Am. Dent. Assoc.*, **48**: 674.

Graf, H. (1975). Occlusal forces during function. In *Occlusion Research in Form and Function*, ed. N.H. Rowe. Ann Arbor, Michigan, University of Michigan Press.

Hawthorn, R. & Flatau, A. (1990). In *A Textbook And Colour Atlas of the Temporomandibular Joint Diseases, Disorders, Surgery*, eds J.E.deB. Norman & P. Bramley. London, Wolfe Medical Publications.

Krough-Poulson, W.G., & Olsson A. (1968) Management of the occlusion of the teeth, background, definitions, rationale. In *Facial Pain and Mandibular Dysfunction*, eds L. Schwarz & C. Chayes. Philadelphia, W.B. Saunders.

Lynn, J.M. (1985). "Biofinisher". *Functional Orthod.*, **2**: 36–41.

Ramfjord, S. & Ash, M.M. (1983). *Occlusion*, 3rd edn. Philadelphia, W.B. Saunders.

Solberg, W.K. (1989). *Temporomandibular Disorders*, 2nd edn. London, British Dental Journal, pp. 91–92.

Spahl, T.J. (1993). The Spahl split vertical eruption acceleration appliance system. *Functional Orthod.*, **10**: 10–24.

FURTHER READING

Riise, C. & Sheikholeslam, A. (1984). Influence of experimental interfering occlusal contacts on the activity of the anterior temporal and masseter muscles during mastication. *J.Oral Rehabil.*, **11**: 325.

CHAPTER 22

New Horizons in Orthodontics

In research the horizon recedes as we advance . . . and research is always incomplete (Mark Pattison 1813–1884)

The rate of technological change in contemporary society is accelerating, and orthodontics is not exempt from this process. In a highly developed speciality it is only human to be comfortable with familiar concepts, as with familiar techniques, and to resist progress. The danger of complacency can apply equally in the academic or clinical environment. In challenging the status quo, the burden of proof rests with the innovator, and understandably there is a time lag between the development of new clinical techniques and their acceptance by the profession as a whole. It is encouraging to note that, with increasingly sophisticated methods of investigation, current research is providing consistent evidence to support the benefits of full-time appliances for functional therapy.

After a century of inconclusive evidence in the examination of orthopaedic techniques, the question of whether or not we can modify craniofacial growth by functional orthopaedic techniques still remains to be resolved. A new paradigm for successful treatment presents a philosophical challenge to combine the benefits of orthodontic and orthopaedic techniques in the treatment of malocclusions which require a combination of dental and skeletal correction.

The question is fundamental to the organisation and delivery of treatment in the specialty of orthodontics. Past generations of orthodontists have based their treatment on the premise that we could not assist the mandible to grow beyond its genetic potential. On the basis of the early cephalometric studies of growth and development, this view was undoubtedly correct, until such time as new clinical and research techniques were developed to prove otherwise. Interpretation of the genetic paradigm is largely a matter of perspective. If the mandible is locked in a distal occlusion, it cannot necessarily fulfil its full genetic potential of forward growth, because it is trapped by an unfavourable functional environment. Unlocking the malocclusion may either help the mandible to grow or, by adjusting the direction of growth, allow the mandible to adopt a more forward position. New methods of research now confirm that full-time functional appliances are unquestionably more efficient in the correction of skeletal discrepancies than conventional fixed appliances.

Charting the course of orthodontics in the next century presents a challenge to consider alternatives to the techniques of the present day. While orthodontic practice is well equipped and organised to deliver comprehensive treatment in the permanent dentition, the same cannot be said for interceptive techniques, which do not receive the attention they deserve. Two thirds of facial growth occurs by the age of 8 years. It is important to identify the benefits of early treatment to improve the form of the dental arches. Abnormal developmental factors, if allowed to persist, are detrimental to both general and dental health in the longer term. The importance of increasing the airway has been stressed in relation to Twin Block treatment, whereby advancing the mandible has the beneficial effect of advancing the tongue, thereby increasing the airway.

Consideration of the transverse dimension is no less important in relationship to the efficiency of orofacial functions. The airway may be restricted either in the anteroposterior or transverse dimensions. A contracted maxilla is of particular significance, in view of its relationship to constriction of the nasal passages, with direct implications for the essential function of breathing, and fundamental effects on general health. Patients with restricted airway are subject to nasopharyngeal infection and allergies, and their general health may be adversely affected (Timms, 1968, 1976).

Successful treatment of these conditions is firmly related to early interceptive treatment and is often associated with tooth-size/arch-size discrepancies. (McNamara & Brudon, 1983). In many respects this is contrary to the present philosophy of a regimen for orthodontic practice based on treatment in the permanent dentition. By the time the permanent teeth have erupted the mid-palatal suture is closed, together with other sutures in the craniofacial complex, and the scope for effective maxillary expansion is reduced. Straightwire technique is based on treatment in permanent dentition, and is the most common fixed appliance technique of the present day. Unfortunately that does not cater for the needs of many orthodontic patients who require interceptive treatment in mixed dentition. All too often under present regulations their treatment is delayed to conform with the organisation of orthodontic practice, or to meet the restrictive requirements of insurance companies or government health schemes.

Based on histological studies, the prognosis for the treatment of labial segment crowding is better in mixed dentition than in permanent dentition. Melsen (1972) carried out an investigation to determine the histological effect of rapid expansion of the mid-palatal suture in children of various ages. A true stimulation of sutural growth was found only in children who had not attained maximum pubertal growth. In older individuals, expansion was attended by numerous micro-fractures in the sutural region. The post-traumatic reaction around these fractures was of significance for the course of healing, preventing further growth in the suture from taking place.

Interceptive treatment is related to functional development, and will assume greater importance in orthodontic and orthopaedic treatment in future generations. Interception and prevention may prove to be one of the most significant factors of change in orthodontics in the next century.

ARCH DEVELOPMENT

Maxillary contraction is a common feature in all classes of malocclusion, which is frequently the primary aetiological factor, with secondary effects on the development of the mandible and the lower dental arch. In functional therapy arch development is often indicated as a preliminary to mandibular advancement in cases exhibiting crowding and irregularity in the dental arches.

Development of the maxilla to correct the archform is frequently the first step in treatment to unlock the malocclusion. The maxilla may be contracted anteroposteriorly or transversely, and frequently in both dimensions, when three-way expansion is indicated. Anteroposterior contraction is characterised by retroclined incisors, as commonly found in Class I bimaxillary retrusion, Class II division 2 and Class III malocclusion. Even in some Class II division 1 malocclusions the incisors must first be proclined to allow the mandible to be advanced fully into a Class I relationship.

In planning treatment of a Class II malocclusion the upper and lower models should be viewed in occlusion with the lower model advanced to a Class I molar relationship. If crowding or irregulaity is present the teeth do not articulate correctly, and it is evident that the archform should be corrected first. After a preliminary phase of arch development the functional correction is then achieved more simply and efficiently.

The most natural method of arch development is by gentle pressure from the lingual aspect by the tongue. Lingual appliances for arch development simulate this natural process by applying gentle controlled forces to the lingual surfaces of the teeth, causing the teeth to migrate through the alveolar bone toward ideal archform position. Lingual arch development is well established as a method of correcting archform in interceptive treatment as a first phase of treatment prior to detailed orthodontic finishing.

There are significant advantages in directing corrective forces from the lingual aspect. The management of malocclusion in mixed dentition is improved by an efficient first phase appliance system, which can be used consistently to control a developing malocclusion at a stage when parents seek interceptive orthodontic treatment. Lingual appliances are used to uncrowd, gain arch length, and correct archform prior to functional therapy or fixed appliance finishing.

Arch development techniques are effective in the correction of all classes of malocclusion, and may be indicated from early mixed dentition to adult treatment. Invisible lingual appliances are 'patient friendly', and therefore acceptable to patients who might otherwise be reluctant to wear orthodontic appliances.

During the past 6 years the author has been involved in designing a new series of active lingual appliances to achieve these objectives. An active lingual arch is used to align the labial segment and improve arch shape in the sagittal and transverse dimensions. Arch width and arch length are controlled simultaneously by gentle spring-driven activation, combining ease of control, and a long range of activation in a simple appliance. The appliances are fixed/removable, and are designed to correct both upper and lower arches. Fixed/removable appliances are removable by the doctor for adjustment, but cannot be removed by the patient, thus eliminating the problem of patient compliance.

Initial designs were based on a modified double lingual tube and post assembly as a means of attachment of the lingual appliance. More recently the same principle has been adapted for use with horizontal lingual tubes. Both methods are effective, irrespective of the method of attachment to the lingual surface of the molar bands.

Spring-driven forces, applied from the lingual aspect, are used to activate a preformed lingual arch to extend archform by applying gentle pressure to the lingual surfaces of the teeth, similar to the forces applied by the tongue. Several designs are available specifically to control archform in the sagittal and transverse dimensions.

APPLIANCE DESIGN

The Trombone and Lingual Arch Developer

This appliance was initially designed with a coil spring as the activating mechanism. Appliance design is based on the slide principle, whereby an inner tube slides freely in an outer tube with the facility to extend or contract the length of the appliance. The mechanism is similar to the slide trombone, from which this appliance derives its name (Fig. 22.1).

The molar section is retained by a double lingual post and tube attachment with a vertical insertion. A distally extending occlusal wire is recurved distal to the molar to pass mesially as a horizontal tube at gingival level. The gingival tube is 12 mm long, offering a range of active extension measuring 10 mm, thus allowing the same appliance to be used to treat a short arch or a long arch, depending on the length of the coil spring. The first version of the appliance was pre-activated with the appropriate length of coil spring to correct the archform.

The design of this appliance was subsequently improved by using a length of silicone tubing as the activating mechanism. In addition to activating the appliance, the silicone serves to link the molar section (the trombone section) securely to the lingual arch. The silicone tubing is replaced at each visit after 4–6 weeks. After selecting the correct length of silicone for initial activation (typically to achieve 2 mm extension of arch length), subsequent activation is by extending the length of the tubing to reactivate as required until the archform is corrected. The absence of frictional forces allows rapid tooth movement using gentle controlled lingual forces.

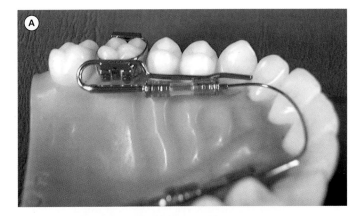

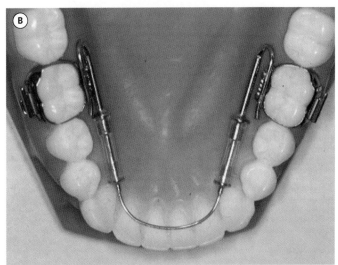

Fig. 22.1 A, B

CASE REPORT: C.S.

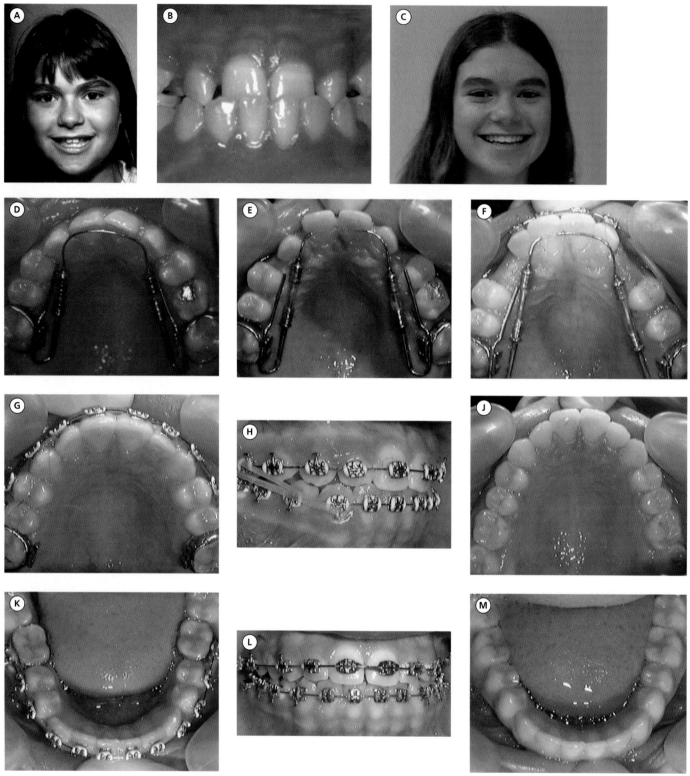

Fig. 22.2 Treatment:
A, B Before treatment.
C After treatment.
D–F Arch development is completed after 9 months to accommodate the canines.
G–M Fixed appliances to complete treatment after 14 months.

CASE REPORT: C.S. AGED 10 YEARS 1 MONTH

An example of maxillary arch development in a Class III malocclusion with upper canines completely blocked out of the arch. After 9 months of treatment the lingual arch developer created adequate space for the canines, allowing them to erupt in good position, and to be accommodated in the corrected archform after 14 months of treatment (Fig. 22.2).

CASE REPORT: L.M. AGED 8 YEARS

Interceptive treatment was used to improve a Class II division 2 malocclusion in early mixed dentition using upper and lower lingual arch developers. It is important first to establish from intra-oral radiographs that the upper canines are clear of the roots of the lateral incisors before fitting a 2 × 4 sectional upper fixed appliance to correct the upper lateral incisor rotations. Appliances were removed after 7 months of treatment. Stable correction of archform is confirmed out of retention after the eruption of premolars and canines (Fig. 22.3).

CASE REPORT: L.M.

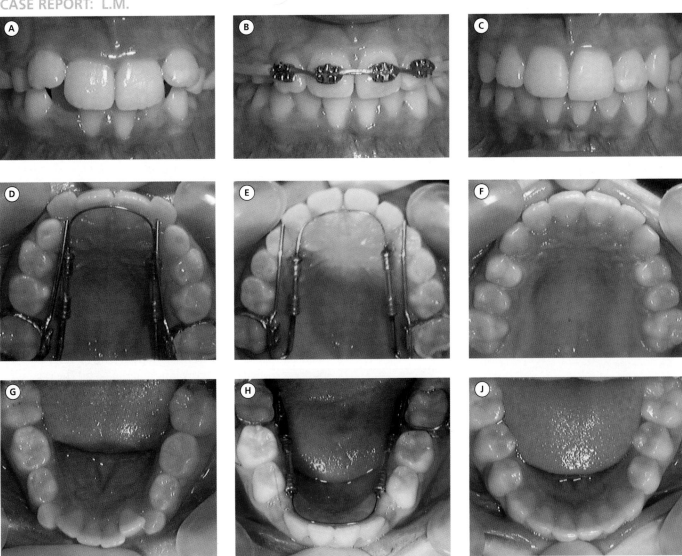

Fig. 22.3 Lingual appliances for arch development in mixed dentition with a simple upper fixed appliance. **C, F, J** show the occlusion and archform out of retention.

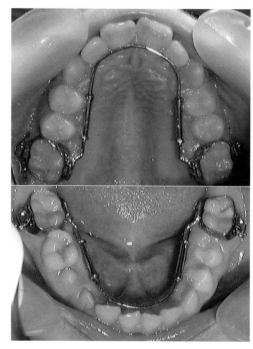

Fig. 22.4 Trans-Force Sagittal appliances are activated by an enclosed coil spring (in cooperation with Ortho Organizers).

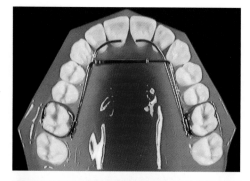

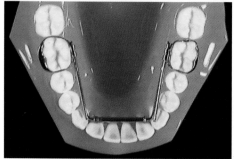

Fig. 22.6 Trans-Force Lingual Appliance for transverse arch development in upper and lower arches is activated by an enclosed coil spring.

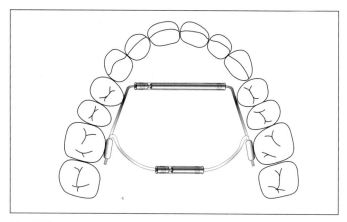

Fig. 22.5

TRANS FORCE LINGUAL APPLIANCES

The following section illustrates a new series of palatal and lingual appliances for insertion in horizontal lingual tubes in molar bands. These also operate on the slide principle, but the design is modified to accommodate a horizontal insertion in the molar tube, which is more commonly used than the vertical means of attachment.

The essential difference compared to the Trombone system is that the appliances are preactivated by a coil spring enclosed in a tube to deliver a smooth continuous force. The force is calibrated according to the requirements of arch development for sagittal or transverse activation. No activation is required after the appliance is fitted, and this principle is extended to a series of appliances for sagittal and transverse arch development.

The Trans Force Sagittal Appliance

The Trans Force Sagittal appliance is specifically designed for anteroposterior arch development in upper or lower arches, and is often indicated to be used simultaneously in both arches. This may be used unilaterally or bilaterally to extend arch length. It incorporates bilateral expansion modules activated by a coil spring enclosed in a stainless steel tube, and extends mesially from the molar tube at gingival level to engage the lingual surfaces of the anterior teeth. The expansion module is activated to lengthen the arch by reciprocal forces on molars and incisors, and as the module expands it also achieves expansion of the intermolar width. The Trans-Force Sagittal appliance is preactivated to achieve the amount of expansion required (Fig. 22.4).

The Trans Force Palatal Expander

The Trans-Force Palatal appliance is for transverse expansion in the upper arch, with twin palatal expanders placed mesially and distally to expand the arch across the molar region, extending to the premolar or deciduous molar region. The Trans-Force mechanism delivers appropriate forces to achieve

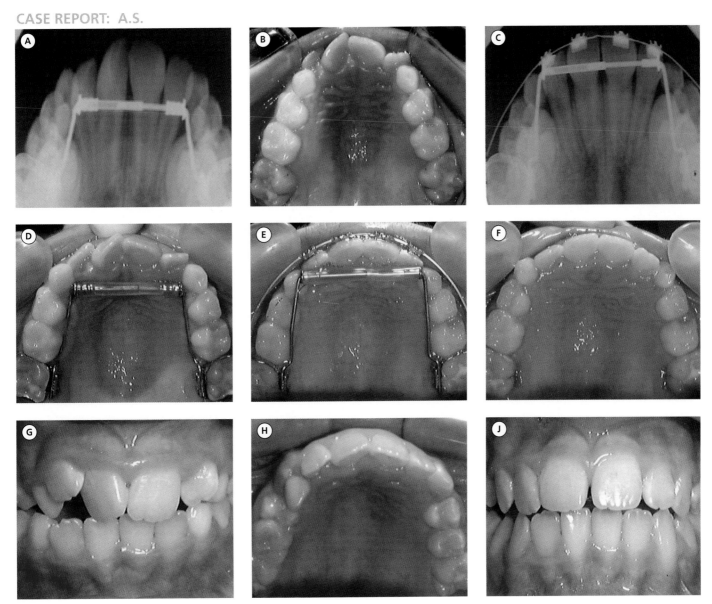

Fig. 22.7 Transverse arch development to correct a unilateral crossbite and resolve anterior crowding.

palatal expansion without resorting to excessive forces beyond physiological limits, thus reducing the discomfort experienced by the application of heavier forces (Fig. 22.5).

The Trans Force Lingual Appliance

The Trans Force Lingual appliance has an expansion module to increase the intercanine width, and may be used in upper or lower arches when expansion is required to accommodate crowding in the labial segments. This is an ideal replacement for the upper or lower Schwarz plate, by achieving a similar effect with a fixed/removable appliance, thus eliminating problems with the non-compliant patient (Fig. 22.6).

CASE REPORT: A.S. AGED 7 YEARS 7 MONTHS

A patient with severe upper labial crowding and rotation of all four upper incisors presented for treatment in early mixed dentition. A prototype appliance for transverse arch development was used to create space by anterior expansion to accommodate the crowded upper incisors. This was combined with an upper sectional fixed appliance to align the rotated incisors. The radiographs show the anterior expansion after 2 months of treatment. Forces of 600 g were applied to achieve 10 mm expansion between the upper deciduous canines after 5 months of arch development. The upper intermolar width also increased (Fig. 22.7).

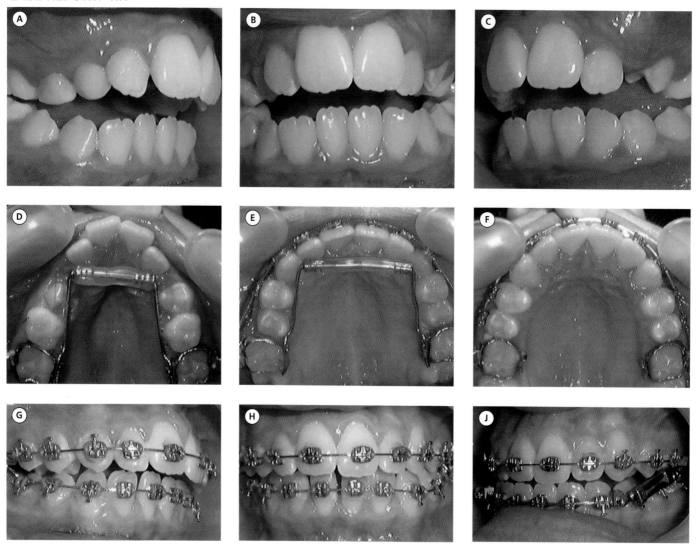

Fig. 22.8 Treatment of a thumb-sucker:
A–C Before treatment.
D–E Transverse expansion of the upper arch.
F–H Fixed appliances.
J Twin Force appliance to correct the distal occlusion.

CASE REPORT: F.P.

Persistent thumb sucking was a major aetiological factor in this Class II division 1 malocclusion, causing contraction of the maxilla with an anterior open bite. The transverse arch developer was used to control thumb sucking, and to correct the maxillary arch width prior to correction of the distal occlusion, and finishing with fixed appliances. In the final stage a Twin Force appliance is used to advance the mandible to complete correction of the distal occlusion and reduce the overjet (Fig. 22.8).

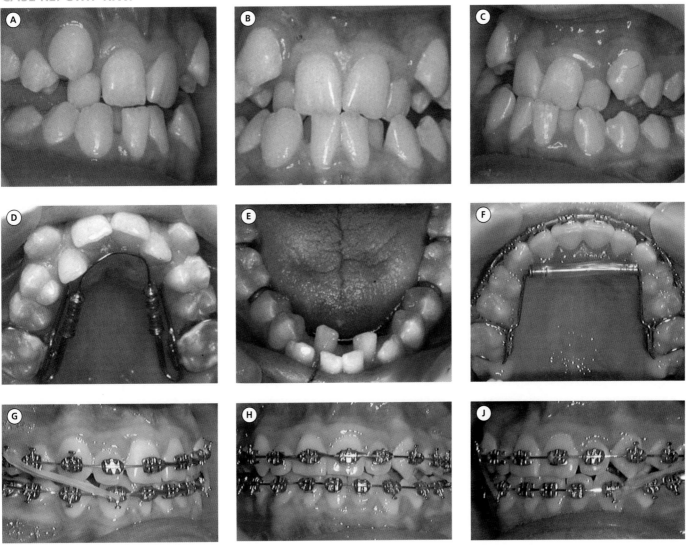

Fig. 22.9 Treatment of a severe Class III malocclusion by upper arch development followed by fixed appliances.

CASE REPORT: R.W. AGED 11 YEARS

Severe maxillary contraction with bilateral crossbite was associated with a Class III malocclusion with a bilateral posterior open bite. The only occlusal contact was between the upper and lower central incisors. Upper lateral incisors were displaced lingual to the upper central incisors, which were already in lingual occlusion to the lower incisors. There was insufficient space for the upper canines, causing them to be displaced mesially and buccally. Severe crowding in the lower labial segment was reduced by extraction of one lower incisor.

The lingual arch developer was used first to make space to accommodate the upper canines, followed by a transverse arch developer to expand the upper arch and correct the bilateral crossbite. Nine months of sagittal arch development was followed by fixed appliances combined with transverse arch development, and treatment in this severe malocclusion was completed after 2 years (Fig. 22.9).

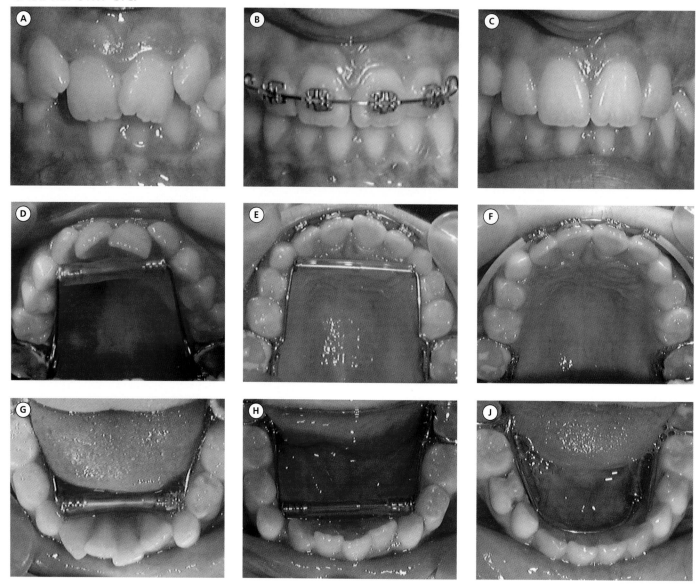

Fig. 22.10 Treatment of Class II division 2 malocclusion in mixed dentition by upper and lower arch development followed by a 2 × 4 sectional fixed appliance.

CASE REPORT: S.C. AGED

Labial segment crowding in both arches is associated with narrow archform, resulting in rotated incisors and a Class II division 2 malocclusion. The first step in treatment was to improve arch width with upper and lower anterior arch developers. This was followed by a 2 × 4 sectional upper fixed appliance and a lower lingual arch developer to complete the alignment of the labial segments (Fig. 22.10).

The Trans-Force Palatal Appliance

The Trans-Force Palatal appliance introduces a new concept in arch development, using preactivated spring components

to achieve simultaneous correction in the sagittal and transverse dimensions. The three-way palatal expander efficiently combines sagittal and transverse components by incorporating three expansion modules to give three-dimensional control of arch development. This approach is indicated for treatment of patients with maxillary contraction involving both anteroposterior and transverse dimensions (Fig. 22.11).

FIXED TWIN BLOCKS

Any orthodontic or orthopaedic appliance system requires sufficient versatility to treat a wide range of malocclusions, and the facility to adapt to meet differing clinical require-

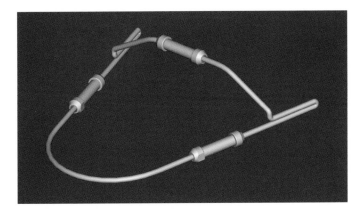

Fig. 22.11 Trans Force Palatal Appliance.

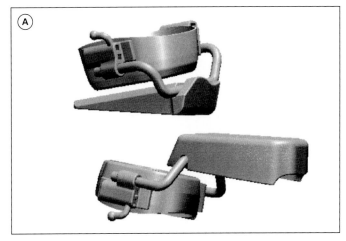

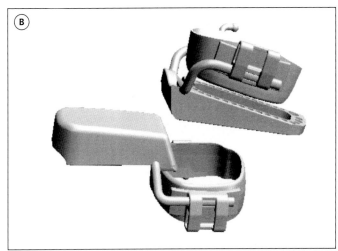

Fig. 22.12 A, B Prototype Fixed Twin Blocks are undergoing clinical testing.

ments. Unlike removable appliances, fixed appliances do not rely on patient compliance, thus increasing control by the operator. The patient's cooperation is assured if the appliance is either fixed permanently to the teeth, or may be removed by the operator as a fixed/removable component. This is an essential feature of treatment planning when patient motivation does not ensure full-time wear of the appliance.

It has been an objective of the author for many years to design Fixed Twin Blocks, using preformed components as an effective guidance mechanism for mandibular advancement, that may be integrated with conventional fixed appliances, and/or lingual appliances for arch development.

Three distinct phases of treatment may be defined as follows:

- First phase: interceptive treatment and arch development
- Second phase: orthopaedic treatment by a fixed/functional Twin Block system.
- Third phase: detailed orthodontic correction by bonded fixed appliances.

It is recommended that the correct archform is established in both dental arches as a preliminary to fitting fixed Twin Blocks for functional orthopaedic correction. This ensures that the arches will occlude together correctly when the mandible is translated to a forward position.

Occlusal inclined planes

Preformed inclined planes are designed to slide into lingual and buccal horizontal tubes on upper and lower first molar bands, prior to being bonded directly to the occlusal surfaces of the teeth. The method of attachment to the molar bands permits mesio-distal adjustment of the inclined planes to adapt individually in order to achieve a comfortable occlusion. Correct adaptation may be achieved either in the labora-

tory or at the chairside, depending on whether a direct or indirect method is employed. The occlusal inclined planes occlude at a 70° angle to the occlusal plane mesial to the lower molar.

Fitting fixed Twin Blocks

The occlusal components of Twin Blocks are designed to be removable from the tubes on molar bands. This allows the molar bands to be tried in the mouth independently of the Twin Blocks, to check the fit of the bands. The next step is to assemble the Twin Block appliances and molar bands in one piece and to try it in the mouth as a unit. If the appliance is easily inserted in this way it may be cemented as a unit. Alternatively, the bands may be cemented first, before attaching the occlusal and lingual components. As a precaution against occlusal caries it is available to apply fissure sealant prior to fitting the occlusal blocks (Fig 22.12).

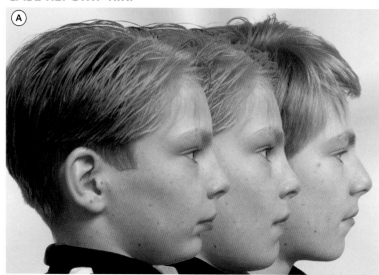

Fig. 22.13 Treatment:
A Profiles at ages 1) 11 years 7 months, 2) first day when fixed Twin Block is fitted, 3) 13 years 6 months.
B Before treatment.
C After fixed Twin Blocks.
D After treatment with fixed appliances.

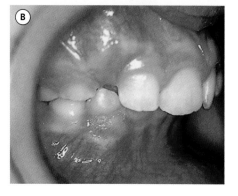

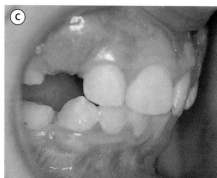

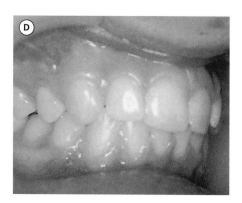

The inclined plane attachments may be fitted directly in the mouth and are bonded directly to the teeth with composite. Light cured composite offers the additional advantage of adequate working time to ensure that the blocks are fully engaged on the occlusal surfaces before the composite is activated to set.

Alternatively the appliance may be constructed by an orthodontic laboratory, with acrylic occlusal blocks. A good adhesive band cement may be used to attach the bands and blocks to the teeth (Figs 22.13, 22.14).

Clinical management

When the appliances are tried in the mouth, it is advisable to check that the blocks occlude correctly and are shaped correctly to allow the objectives of treatment to be achieved. This relates particularly to the patient being able to achieve a comfortable occlusion in a forward mandibular posture. Next, check the effect of the occlusal bite blocks on vertical dental development.

To correct deep overbite vertical development of the lower

molars can normally be delayed until the lower arch has been translated to a forward position. This allows the first permanent molars to be used as a means of fixation for the Twin Block lingual arch component. Vertical elastics to lingual and buccal hooks on opposing molar bands may be used in the support phase to accelerate eruption after the occlusal blocks are removed.

Appliance maintenance

In the early stages of treatment it is necessary to establish that the appliance settles in comfortably and that the patient is consistently occluding the mandible forwards in the desired position. If the correct forward posture is not being achieved consistently, an upper fixed appliance may be fitted, with provision for Class II intermaxillary elastics, to guide the mandible forwards.

When the patient has settled comfortably with fixed Twin Blocks and is posturing forwards correctly, routine maintenance should be at 3- to 4-week intervals. It is advisable to make more frequent checks than with removable appliances,

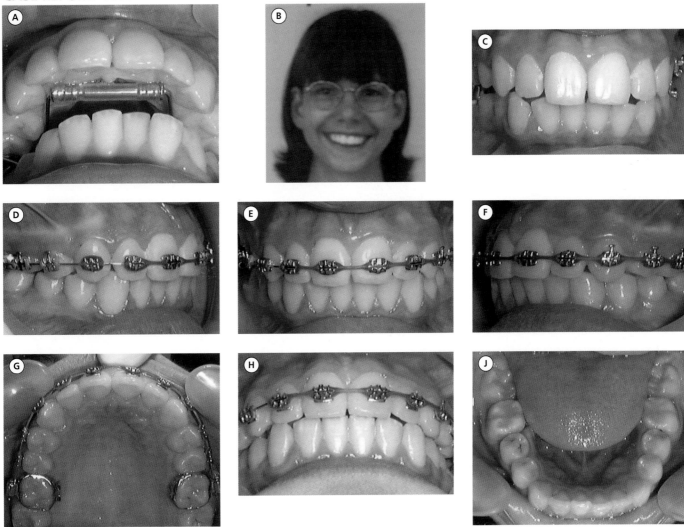

Fig. 22.14 Treatment:
A Overjet = 12 mm before treatment.
B Facial appearance before treatment.
C Occlusion corrected after fixed Twin Blocks.
D–F Upper fixed appliance and lower lingual arch.
G–J Correction after fixed appliances.

and patients should be advised to contact the office immediately if anything breaks or comes loose. If the occlusal blocks become loose they will be retained in position by their attachment to the molar bands. The blocks may be removed and reattached without necessarily removing the molar bands.

Support phase: fixed anterior inclined plane

When the sagittal relationship is fully corrected, usually within 4–6 months, the occlusal blocks are removed and a fixed anterior inclined plane is fitted to support the corrected incisor relationship. The Bite Guide, as described in Chapter 7 (and see Fig. 22.15 overleaf), is an excellent alternative method of providing a fixed inclined plane by bonding lingual attachments on the upper incisors to maintain the correct overjet and overbite. The overjet must first be corrected to 3 mm or less to engage the lower incisors. The molars and premolars are now free to erupt, if necessary with the help of vertical elastics.

Depending on the timing of treatment, if treatment has been initiated in mixed dentition, orthodontic correction may be a separate phase of treatment after the permanent teeth have erupted, or may proceed concurrently with the fixed Twin Blocks. In permanent dentition treatment the support stage is fully integrated with bonded fixed appliances to level the occlusal plane and detail the occlusion.

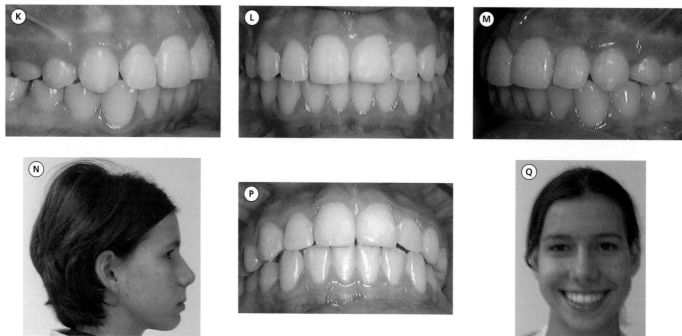

Fig. 22.14 Treatment (cont.):
K–M Occlusion after treatment.
N–Q Facial appearance after treatment.

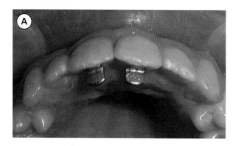
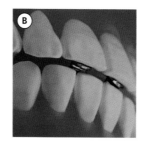
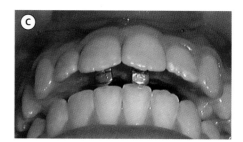

Fig. 22.15 The Bite Guide is an excellent fixed lingual retainer to maintain the correct overjet and overbite (courtesy of Lindsay Brehm, Ortho Organizers).

The bite guides may be used in conjunction with fixed appliances to control the overbite and overjet following the Twin Block phase. If used during retention it is advisable to fit a fixed lower lingual retainer. It should be appreciated that if one of the bite guides is lost this could cause labial displacement of the lower incisor which is in contact with the opposing bite guide. Placement of a lower lingual retainer serves to maintain the alignment of the lower incisors.

REFERENCES

McNamara, J.D. & Brudon, W.L. (1983). Treatment of tooth-size/arch-size discrepancy problems. In *Orthodontic and Orthopedic Treatment in the Mixed Dentition*. Ann Arbor, Needham Press, pp. 67–93.

Melsen, B. (1972). A histological study of the influence of sutural morphology and skeletal maturation on rapid palatal expansion in children. *Trans. Eur. Orthod. Soc.*, 499–507.

Timms, D.J. (1968). An occlusal analysis of lateral maxillary expansion with mid palatal suture opening. *Trans. Eur. Orthod. Soc.*, 73–9.

Timms, D.J. (1976). Long term follow up of cases treated by rapid maxillary expansion. *Trans. Eur. Orthod. Soc.*, 211–15.

CHAPTER 23

The Flat Earth Concept of Facial Growth

Medicine remains too often one-dimensional in its approach
(Charles, Prince of Wales, 1998)

In the Age of Technology statistics speak louder than words. Common sense is not so common!

LIMITATIONS OF CEPHALOMETRIC ANALYSIS

Since the introduction of the cephalostat by Broadbent in 1937, cephalometric analysis has become the most widely used diagnostic aid and research tool in the study of facial growth. The method has proved invaluable in diagnosis as a means of defining and monitoring skeletal and dental relationships. However the technique has limitations as a research tool when used to investigate growth and development and to determine the influence of orthodontic treatment as opposed to normal growth and development.

On cephalometric radiographs, with the teeth in occlusion or in rest position the outline of the condyles and the glenoid fossa is obscured by superimposition of the basal portion of the occipital bone. In addition, the glenoid fossa and the condyle have a cylindrical configuration and are disposed at an angle to the median plane. These bilateral structures may not superimpose exactly on a projected image, thus a number of factors cast doubt on the accuracy of defining the outline of the condyles and glenoid fossae. Ghafari *et al.* (1993) indicate that identification of condylar anatomy affects the evaluation of mandibular growth, and that measurement of mandibular length following orthodontic therapy should be limited to cases where the condyle is clearly identified, not interpreted.

Given these limitations, it is not surprising that attempts to evaluate facial growth from conventional cephalometric studies are inconclusive and open to differing interpretations (De Vincenzo, 1991; Mills, 1991; Nelson *et al.*, 1991; Clark, 1995; Johnston, 1996; Mills & McCulloch, 1998, 2000). All efforts to evaluate growth change from a two-dimensional image are subject to bias due to the inherent inadequacies of the method, and the interpretation placed on results is of equal importance to the recording and measuring of cephalometric data.

RELEVANCE OF STATISTICAL EVIDENCE

In recent years 'evidence based' studies have become the accepted standard of investigation in medical research. Advances in computer technology facilitated statistical analysis, which now forms the basis for most academic studies, to a large extent replacing the philosophical hypotheses of past generations. In a practical subject such as orthodontics many advances in the past were based on clinical experience, usually supported by evidence from clinical records. The basic principles have not changed, although the investigative techniques have become more sophisticated.

Depending on the interpretation of results, several factors serve to limit the usefulness of statistical analysis. Clinical investigation often involves multi-factorial questions, and it is difficult to obtain accurate controls, or to eliminate individual differences in growth and response from small groups used in statistical studies. These are unavoidable limitations of the method of study. Nevertheless it is tempting to accept the results of statistical analysis as the best available method of scientific investigation.

This is in spite of an uncomfortable doubt, expressed so eloquently by Mark Twain, that 'There are three kinds of lies: lies, damned lies and statistics.' The implication is that, given the appropriate sample, we can prove virtually anything by statistics. Thus the endless conflicting results emerging from studies in almost any subject under investigation.

M.L. Moss (1981) observes that 'As statistics developed, the effects of various types of treatment could be statistically analysed, although at times as various observers have pointed out some of the statistical differences have been found to be clinically meaningless.'

The flat earth concept of facial growth

In philosophical terms, the Flat Earth Concept of Facial Growth is an appropriate analogy for the study of facial growth in orthodontics by two-dimensional cephalometric analysis. The concept underlines the inherent disadvantage of attempting to evaluate changes in the form of a three-dimensional structure based on the analysis of a projected two-dimensional image. This deficiency has long been recognized, as observed by Moyers & Bookstein, in their paper 'The inappropriateness of conventional cephalometrics' (1979).

A direct analogy exists between our present state of knowledge of facial growth from cephalometric studies, and early historical misconceptions regarding the shape and form of the earth. Understanding the concept of volumetric growth of the face is as important as realising that the earth is round and not flat.

After a century of investigation, the question is still unresolved as to whether or not we can influence the pattern of facial development by encouraging the mandible to grow. Alternatively we may influence the maxillo-mandibular relationship by bony remodelling in the glenoid fossa, or by a positional change of the mandible relative to the maxilla. Considering the inherent limitations of the method of study it is not surprising that attempts to resolve crucial questions regarding facial growth by statistical analysis have produced inconclusive evidence.

Opinions differ regarding the extent of genetic control versus the influence of environmental factors in the development of the face. At the end of the twentieth century many orthodontists remained philosophically divided between an orthodontic and orthopaedic approach to treatment. Two schools of thought continued to exist regarding the potential to influence facial growth by orthopaedic treatment. Such a fundamental division impacts directly on the organisation of orthodontic practice. It is a significant factor in the timing of treatment, between early or late intervention, or between orthopaedics or surgery to resolve skeletal discrepancies.

Advances in computerized morphometrics may help to resolve questions on craniofacial growth that have persisted throughout the twentieth century, while magnetic resonance imaging is capable of higher resolution than radiographic techniques for the investigation of structural change. Such fundamental technological advances take many years to implement and until we can evaluate three-dimensional images it is possible to arrive at a more meaningful interpretation of the results of cephalometric analysis by adopting a three-dimensional perspective to interpolate volumetric changes from two-dimensional images.

Two-dimensional representation of mandibular length

Present methods of measuring increments in mandibular growth by conventional cephalometric analysis tend to underestimate growth due to the limitations of the two-dimensional method. The cephalometric image represents the reflection of a shadow of a three-dimensional form on a flat surface placed behind the object of study. A typical enlargement of the image on a cephalometric film varies between 6% and 13%, and cephalometric studies commonly make allowance for enlargement of the image on the cephalometric radiograph by introducing an appropriate correction. In addi-

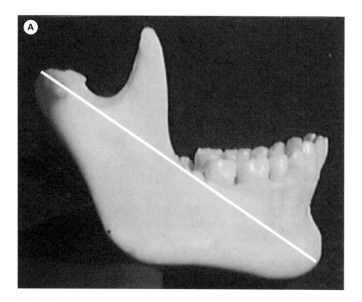
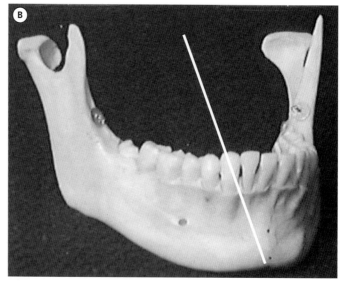

Fig. 23.1
A The mid-sagittal axis is used to measure mandibular growth.
B A simple linear measurement does not represent the complex bi-lateral form of the mandible.

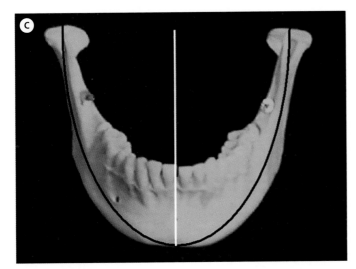

Fig. 23.1 (cont.):
C A line from condylion to pogonion around the exterior surface of the mandible represents the peripheral length of the mandible.

tion, however, the two-dimensional image of the mandible is foreshortened relative to its true shape and it is not customary to make an equivalent allowance for foreshortening of the mandible on the projected image. Similarly conventional analysis makes no allowance for the fallacy of measuring growth increments on the midline projection of a bilateral structure. These fundamental flaws in the method of study have led us to consistently underestimate the effects of treatment on facial growth.

The peripheral length of the mandible

Given the three-dimensional shape of the mandible, and its semi-elliptical morphology, measurement from condyle to condyle is a more meaningful representation of mandibular length than the midline projection of mandibular length from condylion to pogonion. An increase in the peripheral length of the mandible is more significant in the clinical context than a projected midline measurement, which has little direct clinical significance. One of the basic aims of orthodontic treatment is to accommodate the teeth over basal bone in good alignment without crowding. Therefore the peripheral length of the mandible is a more meaningful factor in the clinical equation than the midline projection that is commonly used to evaluate mandibular length.

A line from condylion to pogonion around the exterior surface of the mandible represents the peripheral length of the mandible (Fig. 23.1C). The distance may be measured from the left condylion to the midpoint of the lower border of the mandible. This is repeated on the right side and the sum of the two measurements represents the total length of the mandible from condyle to condyle. Measurement of the peripheral length of the mandible on the dry skull using a

flexible ruler indicates that the peripheral length on each side is 20% greater than the projected cephalometric linear distance from pogonion to condylion. Taking into account the bilateral morphology of the mandible, the following example illustrates how a relative increase in peripheral length would compare to the projected cephalometric image.

Before treatment:
Mid-sagittal measurement Co to Pogonion = 100 mm.
Exterior peripheral measurement Co to Pogonion = 120 mm.
Bilateral peripheral measurement Co to Pogonion = 240 mm.

After treatment:
Mid-sagittal measurement Co to Pogonion = 105 mm.
Exterior peripheral measurement Co to Pogonion = 126 mm.
Bilateral peripheral measurement Co to Pogonion = 252 mm.

An increase of 5 mm in the midline projection of mandibular length is equivalent to an increase in the peripheral length of the mandible of 12 mm. In clinical terms, the difference between the peripheral length and the projected length of the mandible represents a significant factor, which may be important in the resolution of crowding and the space available for eruption of second or third molars.

It is possible that a method could be devised using a panoramic radiograph to measure the peripheral length of the mandible as an alternative to the projected image of the mandible, in order to evaluate more accurately the true length of the mandible (Fig. 23.1).

Comparison of linear and volumetric values

Understanding the concept of volumetric growth of the face is as important as realising that the earth is round and not flat.

In comparing objects of broadly similar shapes, the relationship between linear and volumetric values remains the same. The mathematical formula for the expansion of an object relating to percentage change is expressed as :

$$(1 + r)^3 = 1 + 3r + 3r^2 + r^3$$
$$\text{where } r = \% \text{ change.}$$

In mathematical terms r^2 and r^3 are negligible where the percentage change is small.

Various recognisable three-dimensional forms may be selected to illustrate this principle, and it is immaterial whether the selected form is spherical, cuboid or ellipsoid, as the same principle may be applied using any of these models. For example, a 1% increase in the radius of a sphere increases the volume by 3%. Similarly, a 1% increase in the length of the sides of a cube or cuboid results in a 3% increase in

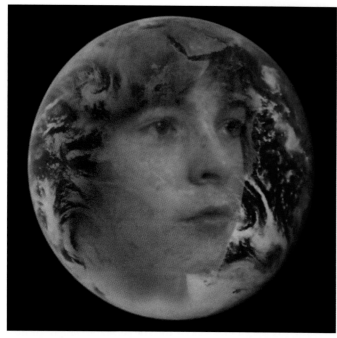

Fig. 23.2 Understanding the concept of volumetric growth of the face is as important as realising that the earth is round and not flat.

volume. The same principle applies to an ellipsoid, where the maximum and minimum radii are expressed in the formula. Thus linear values may be multiplied by three to convert to volumetric values. Irrespective of the shape of the object, the relationship between linear and volumetric values remains the same. This assumption does not rely on hypothesis, but is an established fact based on the mathematical formulae used to calculate volumetric values from the linear dimensions of an object.

The head is more closely related to a sphere or an ellipsoid than the projected two-dimensional image displayed on a cephalometric film. Using mathematical principles it is possible to interpolate volumetric values from linear cephalometric measurements, and to evaluate more meaningful three-dimensional changes occurring in craniofacial growth and development. This principle can be applied with confidence to linear percentage changes of up to 5%, which represents the linear growth increments measured in studies of growth modification in the mandible relative to the maxilla or cranial base during a course of orthodontic or orthopaedic treatment.

It is not suggested that such a mathematical conversion will provide as accurate a result as a sophisticated technological system for three-dimensional measurement. However, until such a system is available this method may serve to provide a more accurate evaluation of the effects of treatment on facial growth by making allowance for the deficiencies of incorrect interpretation of two-dimensional cephalometric techniques. We may be able to interpolate more meaningful

statistics from existing cephalometric records. The method is presented as worthy of further investigation.

Interpolating volumetric changes from cephalometric radiographs

A cephalometric radiograph may be used to interpolate three-dimensional changes in specific areas of the craniofacial complex; the slice of a sphere is an appropriate model to illustrate this mathematical principle.

$$\text{The volume of a slice of a sphere} = \text{Angle}/360° \times 4/3\pi r^3$$

The two variables in the formula which define the slice on a two-dimensional image are the radius and the angle. Accepted linear values from cephalometric analysis may be used to interpolate volumetric changes in the middle third and lower third of the face.

Cranial, maxillary and mandibular base length

The relative length of cranial base, maxilla and mandible is expressed by linear measurements:

Cranial base: Basion – Nasion.
Maxilla: Basion – A-point.
Mandible: Basion – Pogonion.

These linear measurements may be applied in the formula for the slice of a sphere with the appropriate angular measurements to interpolate volumetric changes in the middle and lower thirds of the face. In volumetric terms the face grows radially from basion, and the angle Nasion–Basion–ANS on a cephalometric radiograph may be selected to represent a slice of the middle third of the face, similar to the segment of an orange. Similarly the angle ANS–Basion–Menton represents the lower third of the face. Angular changes are defined in volumetric terms by the formula:

The significance of angular changes may be expressed as follows, assuming the radius were to remain constant:

$$100/\text{Angle} = \%\text{Change in volume per degree}$$

Thus volumetric change in the lower face is relatively greater per degree of change in brachyfacial types relative to dolichofacial types. For example an angle of 20° yields 5% increase in volume, per degree increase in the angle, whereas a 40° angle results in a 2.5% increase in volume.

However changes in the angles defining the middle and lower face in the following studies are not significant. A direct comparison may therefore be made between two-dimensional linear measurements from a cephalometric study and interpolated volumetric measurements by measuring the radius to represent the cranial base, maxillary base or mandibular base, and applying the changes before and after treatment to the appropriate formula.

Linear changes are more significant when converted to three-dimensional values. In mathematical terms linear values should be multiplied by three to convert to volumetric values. Within the parameters of growth studies during a course of orthodontic treatment, a 1% increase in linear values represents a 3% increase in volumetric values in the comparison of objects of broadly similar shapes. As no fundamental change in facial form occurs during treatment, this principle may be applied with confidence. This does not preclude the modification of facial form by subtle changes that may be obvious to the aesthetic senses, without necessarily being statistically significant.

Statistical evaluation of aesthetic factors

As stated above, Moss observes that 'As statistics developed, the effects of various types of treatment could be statistically analysed, although at times as various observers have pointed out some of the statistical differences have been found to be clinically meaningless'.

Statistical methods are limited as a means of measuring aesthetic factors. Clinical examination supported by photographic records may be more effective in interpreting subtle changes in facial form, which may or may not be statistically significant. This does not deny the value of statistical methods, but there is an obvious danger of relegating aesthetic judgement to the level of statistics.

It is therefore important to relate statistically significant changes to the resulting effect on the facial form. For example, an increase in ramus height is a highly significant finding in many statistical studies of functional technique. Vertical changes are extremely important in facial aesthetics. An increase in the height of the ramus has a significant effect on facial appearance. In aesthetic terms it is an important factor in reshaping the contours of the lower third of the face. It is frequently accompanied by an increase in lower facial height, and remodelling of the circum-oral musculature.

The evaluation of growth increments in the mandible by measurement of the mid-sagittal axis falls into the same category. The mandible is an extremely complex three-dimensional structure, and growth of the mandible is by a combination of cartilaginous and subperiosteal apposition. An increase in the mid-sagittal axis is of minor significance in clinical terms. It may have a limited effect on the contour of the chin in profile. However, even a small advancement of the mandible may have a significant effect on the contours of the lower face, in height and width, in addition to changes in the profile. Because the mandible is wedge shaped, the lower

third of the face widens as the mandible is advanced. Therefore volumetric changes in the shape of the face are exponential relative to linear changes.

A change in the mandibular position may be of equal significance compared to an increase in mandibular length in determining the facial contours. This may be related to a small change in the direction of growth at the condyle, or remodelling in the glenoid fossa, or a combination of both of these factors. Measurement of the mid-sagittal axis does not take either of these important factors into account. As a result of these limitations, the evaluation of growth changes in the face from previous cephalometric studies is fundamentally flawed.

While clinical technique must have a sound basis in scientific research, it is equally important to recognise the limitations imposed by inadequate methods of investigation in determining the validity of scientific study. Correct interpretation of results is an important aspect of cephalometric study. This must take into account the limitations of two-dimensional analysis from a projected image. At present we still adhere to a 'flat earth concept of facial growth' and have failed to adjust our vision to accommodate a three dimensional perspective.

The efficacy of functional therapy has been the subject of a great deal of criticism, mostly based on conventional two-dimensional cephalometric studies. However, functional orthopaedics presents a valid alternative to orthognatic surgery that is more acceptable and less costly for the patient in many borderline Class II skeletal cases. In comparison to conventional fixed appliance techniques functional orthopaedics is more effective in the treatment of severe malocclusions resulting from skeletal discrepancies.

Increasing evidence is emerging to support the positive benefits of full-time functional appliances on facial growth. An improved method of interpolating volumetric changes from the study of cephalometric radiographs may help to clarify the changes that result from treatment, until such time as we can evaluate fully the three-dimensional effects of functional orthopaedics by morphometric techniques.

Science is the study of natural processes by observation, hypothesis and experimentation. In an age of rapidly advancing technology, it is inevitable that results that were accepted as correct at the time of investigation, are frequently found subsequently to be incorrect. Methods of investigation tend to compartmentalise knowledge of complex subjects and mechanisms. In our present state of knowledge a doctrinaire approach to the teaching and study of facial growth and the effects of treatment is dangerously misleading. The inherent danger is that undue reliance on the statistical evaluation of past two-dimensional studies from a negative perspective may prejudice students of orthodontics who are at the beginning of their professional career. Such an approach may deny patients the benefits of appropriate treatment for skeletal discrepancies.

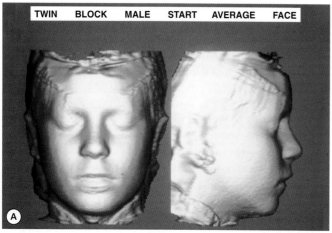

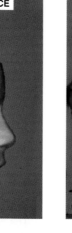

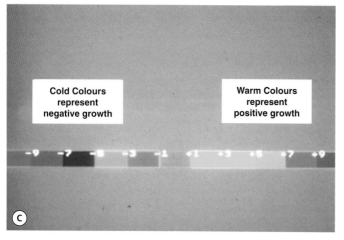

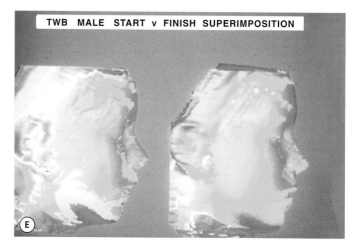

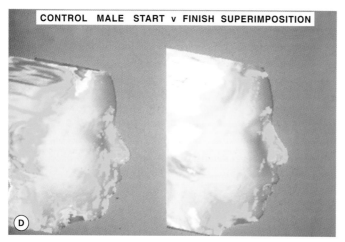

Cold Colours represent negative growth

Warm Colours represent positive growth

Fig. 23.3
A, B Composite facial masks of a group of patients before and after treatment with Twin Blocks.
C Colour coding is used to illustrate areas of positive and negative growth.
D The control group shows no significant growth changes.
E The Twin Block group shows positive three-dimensional changes in the face during treatment over the entire area of the mandible.
By courtesy of Professor J.P. Moss.

The following quotation is relevant to this discussion:

Science has tried to assume a monopoly, even a tyranny, over our understanding (Charles, Prince of Wales, 1998)

To place this quotation in perspective, it is unreasonable to expect that science can resolve all questions at any time, therefore it is dangerous to draw dogmatic conclusions from scientific research in a clinical subject. Results must always be viewed with an open mind, taking into account the limitations of the method of study. It is essential to combine a scientific approach with the pragmatism that is required to resolve clinical problems.

VOLUMETRIC ANALYSIS OF FACIAL GROWTH BY IMAGING TECHNOLOGY

Advances in imaging technology make it possible to examine three-dimensional images. Recent research at University College, London (J.P. Moss and co-workers) employs leading edge technology to investigate three-dimensional growth changes. In a technique for optical surface scanning a laser scanner and a video camera are used to plot accurate facial masks for a group of patients.

The technique of optical surface scanning may be used to illustrate three-dimensional changes in facial form by computer-generated images of facial masks of individual patients, or groups of individuals with or without treatment by creating a composite facial mask to represent the mean facial pattern from a group of patients. At present this technique has been used to show changes in the soft-tissue mask of the face. Colour coding may be used to demonstrate areas of differential growth. Composite masks of a group of untreated patients are used as controls to examine changes in the soft tissues of the face. The masks are colour coded with cold colours representing negative areas of growth, and warm colours showing positive growth. The consistent pattern of colour coding verifies that no significant volumetric changes occur in the three-dimensional masks of the untreated patients before and after observation (Fig. 23.3).

By comparison, the composite masks of Twin Block patients show positive three-dimensional changes in the face during treatment. Significant volumetric changes are registered in the lower third of the face over the entire area of the mandible. Improvement in the profile is expressed in the outline of the lips and chin, with changes in the shape of the mouth affecting the circumoral musculature and the mentalis region. Increased lower facial height is evident in the ascending ramus, extending forward along the lower border of the mandible to the symphyseal region.

The shape of the lower face is equally affected by remodelling in the transverse dimension. Advancing the mandible results in widening of the lower face, affecting both hard and soft tissues, as muscular adaptation occurs to accommodate the underlying bony changes. This accounts for the extensive areas of change registered over the entire mandible, including the ramus and the outline of the masseter muscle.

By contrast, the mid face maintains a similar pattern, indicating no significant changes in the mid-facial profile. There is some evidence that the remodelling over the area of the mandible extends upwards into the maxilla, indicating slight widening of the maxilla as a result of midline expansion.

Morris *et al.* (1998) compared soft-tissue changes in groups of patients treated by three different functional appliances compared to a control group. Normal growth was associated with only minimal changes in the soft-tissue profile and form during the study period of 9 months. Comparison of Bionator, Bass appliance and Twin Blocks with controls showed that each of the functional appliance groups produced further changes in the soft-tissue profile and form than would otherwise have been expected. Greater antero-posterior changes occurred in the male treatment groups. Upper lip landmarks showed no significant changes in any of the appliance groups despite the significant overjet reduction achieved in each appliance group.

The Twin Block appliance group (male and female) achieved greater changes in their facial soft tissues in comparison with the other two functional appliances. The most significant effect found was the advancement and lengthening of the lower lip combined with some forward movement of the chin point and increase in all face height parameters.

The subtlety of these volumetric changes is highly significant in aesthetic terms, and evidently cannot be interpreted from two-dimensional radiographic images. Using similar scanning techniques it will be possible in the future to obtain measurements of volumetric changes in the hard tissues, and therefore to evaluate more accurately changes in facial form resulting from orthodontic and orthopaedic techniques.

MORPHOMETRIC ANALYSIS

by G.D. Singh and W.J.Clark

Kendall's spherical blackboard used the mathematics of spherical space to represent three-dimensional morphology (Kendall, 1989). Finite element analysis uses new mathematical concepts and computerized morphometrics to examine growth changes in greater detail from a three-dimensional perspective.

As cephalometry does not take size variation into consideration, opinion is emerging that it is perhaps a relatively inappropriate method of shape analysis (Bookstein, 1981). Recently, geometric morphometric techniques have become useful to facilitate hypothesis testing (Singh *et al.*, 1997). These methods include superimposition techniques such as Procrustes analysis, Finite-Element Scaling Analysis (FESA), Thin Plate Spline (TPS) analysis and Euclidean Distance Matrix analysis (EDMA) (Singh *et al.*, 1998a,b,c). These techniques are registration-free approaches that rely upon the relative positions of homologous landmarks rather than linear and angular measurements (Bookstein, 1981) (Fig. 23.4).

Whilst the Class II malocclusion is accepted as a classification of the dentition, it does not presuppose a skeletal craniofacial relationship (Coben, 1966). Investigations into linear dimensions and facial proportions conclude that the mandible is of average linear size but proportionally small for the face because the depth of the cranial base is larger than average (Coben, 1960). In the treatment of Class II malocclusion, functional appliances such as the Twin Block train patients in oral and tongue posture; an early phase of

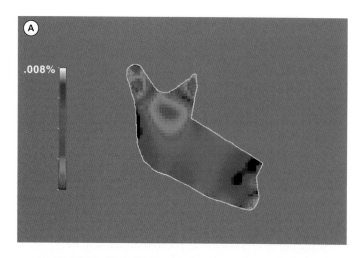

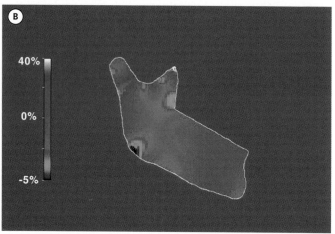

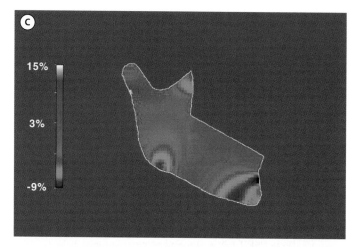

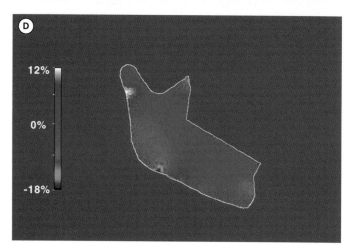

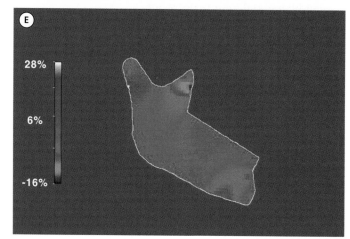

Fig. 23.4
A Postpubertal males – analysis of shape. Shape change is uniform. High isotropy over the entire nodal mesh.
B Prepubertal females – analysis of size. Limited positive differential growth.
C Postpubertal females – analysis of size. Highly significant differential growth.
D Prepubertal males – analysis of size. Highly significant differential growth.
E Postpubertal males – analysis of size. Highly significant differential growth.

functional appliance treatment is commonly used to simplify subsequent therapy, and to optimise the development of the facial skeleton. Unfortunately, this latter expectation enjoys little support in the literature. A prospective trial found no evidence that functional appliances can alter the shape of the mandible. Indeed, a study (Johnston 1996) that examined matched patients from a two-stage bionator/edgewise regimen and a conventional one-stage edgewise treatment found that when the two groups were compared, they underwent essentially indistinguishable skeletal changes; the early phase of functional treatment conferred no obvious measurable benefits. Similarly, another study reported that the length of the mandible did not increase in young adult patients treated with functional regulator therapy.

A morphometric analysis of consecutively treated Twin Block patients

A morphometric analysis was carried out to evaluate the results of treatment of 138 consecutively treated patients in the author's practice (W.J. Clark). The sample was subdivided on the basis of age into four groups of prepubertal and postpubertal males and females. Using finite element scaling analysis it is possible to model regions of proliferative growth and remodelling. It appears that Twin Block (TB) therapy may involve:

- Developmental modulations at the condylar cartilage.
- Epigenetic remodelling of the ramus and corpus.
- Osteogenic deposition that extends from the corpus of the mandible into the dentoalveolar areas.

This latter factor relates to vertical adjustments of the occlusion, in response to the observed increases in ramus height. A slight increase in the length of the body of the mandible was observed following TB treatment. Corpus growth made a significant contribution to mandibular development in both prepubertal males and females. This pattern of development may reflect the natural process of bony remodelling, which occurs in the corpus and dentoalveolar areas during the transition from mixed to permanent dentition.

Localisation of size increase in the condylar neck region appears to relate to chondrocytic proliferation in the growing patient. As might be expected, the contribution of condylar growth and remodelling in the ramus appears to increase during the pubertal stage. The degree of cartilaginous enlargement is greater in the adolescent compared to the prepubertal child.

The study also confirmed that the TB appliance combined with extraoral traction force have a restricting effect on forward maxillary growth, and also restrict forward growth of the maxillary alveolus. This finding is in common with previous studies of the 'headgear effect'.

A morphometric study using both EDMA and TPS analysis

suggested that there was very little change in the length of the body of the mandible either following TB treatment or during untreated growth. By contrast, the height of the ramus was shown by EDMA to increase following TB treatment. Similarly, the oblique length of the mandible was found to have increased slightly.

Thin Plate Spline analysis attempts to show shape changes in the form of deformations of grids such as those associated with D'Arcy Thompson (1917). Examination of mandibular landmarks confirmed that downward and forward rotation of the mandible occurred, and this method of investigation seemed to indicate that correction of the distal relationship of the mandible is achieved predominantly by altered mandibular position, rather than by altering mandibular form.

Affine transformation grids showed downward and forward rotation of the mandibular landmark configuration following TB treatment. Non-affine transformation grids indicated that mandibular form was only slightly altered on completion of treatment. This same pattern of non-affine mandibular transformation was observed in the longitudinal transformation indicating, therefore, that TB treatment had little effect on mandibular form but rather altered mandibular position predominantly.

Similarly, the present study corresponds also with earlier findings using finite element scaling analysis, as positive allometry was noted in the mandibular corpus. Other areas not related to muscle insertions show positive allometry, such as the postero-superior area of the ramus, the mid-region of the corpus, and the dentoalveolar process. Indeed, areas exhibiting isometry and negative allometry may be related to muscle attachment. Specifically, negative allometry at the gonial angle and ante-gonial notch relates to the attachments of the masseter muscle, while isometry extends over its area of insertion on the ascending ramus. Similarly, areas of negative allometry on the coronoid process relate to the insertion of the tendon of the temporalis muscle. The area of the mental protuberance and the symphysis exhibits a negative allometry that may be associated with the insertion of the mentalis muscle. In the pubertal male, however, no negative allometry is observed in the ramus, gonial angle or the symphysis, but these areas appear to be isometric during a period of rapid growth.

By contrast, the distal aspect of the condylar neck consistently showed positive allometry at all stages examined, in line with the lateral pterygoid hypothesis. In normal growth, significant bony remodelling is necessary in this area to maintain the shape of the mandibular ramus to compensate for distal condylar extension, vertical extension of the ramus, and thickening of the posterior border of the ramus. The high degree of isotropy over the entire nodal mesh in the analysis of mandibular shape confirms that a similar remodelling process could occur during functional protraction in order to maintain the shape of the mandible.

In summary, this study attempted to model regions of

proliferative growth and remodelling using FEA. Presumably, localization of size increase in the condylar neck region relates to chondrocytic proliferation in the growing patient and, perhaps not surprisingly, the degree of cartilaginous enlargement was greater in the adolescent compared to the prepubertal child. These geometric changes might reflect increased activity of the lateral pterygoid muscle and subsequent condylar growth that correlates with observed increases in mandibular length in patients treated with TB. The morphology of the glenoid fossa, however, was not assessed in this particular study, and any translatory changes of the mandible require determination by undertaking a similar study of the maxillary and soft-tissue matrices in patients treated with TB.

CONCLUSIONS

- Localization of growth in the condylar neck with concomitant remodelling of the coronoid process may reflect the correction of mandibular form achieved with Twin Blocks.
- TB therapy may involve developmental modulations at the condylar cartilage, remodelling of the ramus and corpus, and osteogenic deposition in dentoalveolar regions.
- Condylar growth is greater in the postpubertal stage.
- Expansion is located in the neck of the condyle.
- Corpus extension is greater in the prepubertal stage.

- Prepubertal changes may relate to dental development.
- Postpubertal changes may relate to cartilaginous proliferation.
- The largest growth increments are localised in postpubertal males.

These results should be interpreted with caution until we fully understand the mechanisms involved in growth modification. Many studies have concentrated on the change in length of the mandible compared to untreated controls. More sophisticated techniques are required to determine the importance of changes in mandibular position in growth modification. In order to resolve questions relating to growth modification by functional mandibular protrusion, three-dimensional analysis is necessary to examine changes in mandibular form and these studies are currently underway.

A similar morphometric study of maxillary growth was carried out on the original series of patients treated by a combination of Twin Blocks with extraoral traction. A configuration of five landmarks encompassing the midfacial region was used to determine whether Twin Blocks with traction restricts growth of the midfacial complex. This study concluded that TBA treatment resulted in a 'normal' Class I occlusion. The improvement in facial balance was shown to be associated with restriction of anterior displacement of the midfacial complex.

REFERENCES

Bookstein, F.L. (1981). *Looking at Mandibular Growth: Some New Geometric Methods*.

Broadbent, H. (1937). The face of the normal child. *Angle Orthod.*, **7**: 183–208.

Clark, W.J. (1995). Growth response to Twin Block treatment. In *Twin Block Functional Therapy, Applications in Dentofacial Orthopaedics*. London, Mosby-Wolfe.

De Vincenzo, J.P. (1991). Changes in mandibular length before, during and after successful orthopedic correction of Class II malocclusions, using a functional appliance. *Am. J. Orthod. Dentofac. Orthop.*, **99**: 241–57.

Ghafari, J., Jacobsson-Hunt, U., Beidman, R.W. & Schofer, F.S. (1993). Identification of condylar anatomy affects the evaluation of mandibular growth. *EJO*, **15**: 445.

Johnston, Jr L.E. (1996). Functional appliances: a mortgage on mandibular position. *Austral. Orthod. J.*, **14**: 154–6.

Kendall, D.G. (1989). A survey of the statistical theory of shape. *Statistical Science*, **4**: 87–120.

Mills, C.M. & McCulloch, K.J. (1998). Treatment effects of the Twin Block appliance: a cephalometric study. *Am. J. Orthod. Dentofac. Orthop.*, **114**: 15–24.

Mills, C.M. & McCulloch, K.J. (2000). Post treatment changes following successful correction of Class II malocclusions with the Twin Block appliance. *Am. J. Orthod. Dentofac. Orthop.*, **118**: 24–33.

Mills, J.R.E. (1991). The effect of functional appliances on the skeletal pattern. *Br. J. Orthod.*, **18**: 267–75.

Morris, D.O., Illing, H.M. & Lee, R.T. (1998) A prospective evaluation of Bass, Bionator, & Twin Block appliances. Part 2 – the soft tissues. *Eur. J. Orthod.*, **20**: 663–84.

Moss, M.L. (1981). Genetics, epigenesis and causation. *Am. J. Orthodont.* **80**: 366–375.

Moyers, R.E. & Bookstein, F.L. (1979). The inappropriateness of conventional cephalometrics. *Am. J. Orthod.*, **75**: 599.

Nelson, C., Harkness, M. & Herbison, P. (1993). Mandibular changes during functional appliance treatment. *Am. J. Orthod. Dentofac. Orthop.*, **104**: 153–61.

Singh, G.D., McNamara, Jr, J.A. & Lozanoff, S. (1997). Morphometry of the cranial base in subjects with Class III malocclusion. *J Dent Res* **76**: 694–703.

Singh, G.D., McNamara, Jr, J.A. & Lozanoff, S. (1998a). Morphometry of the midfacial complex in subjects with Class III malocclusions: Procrustes, Euclidean & cephalometric analyses. *Clin. Anat.*, **11**: 162–70.

Singh, G.D., McNamara, Jr, J.A. & Lozanoff, S. (1998b). Procrustes, Euclidean and cephalometric analyses of the morphology of the mandible in human Class III malocclusions. *Arch. Oral Biol.*, **43**: 535–43.

Singh, G.D., McNamara, Jr, J.A. & Lozanoff, S. (1998c). Craniofacial heterogeneity of prepubertal Korean and European–American subjects with Class III malocclusions: Procrustes, EDMA & cephalometric analyses. *Int. J. Adult Orthodont. Orthognath. Surg.*, **13**: 227–40.

Thompson, D.W. (1917). On the theory of transformations, or the comparison of related forms. In *On Growth & Form*, ed. J.T. Bonner. 1961 reprinted 1988 Cambridge University Press.

Berkowitz, B.K.B, Holland, G.R. & Moxham, B.J. (1992). *A Colour Atlas and Textbook of Oral Anatomy, Histology and Embryology*, 2nd edn. London, Wolfe Publishing.

Bookstein, F.L. (1991). *Morphometric Tools for Landmark Data: Geometry and Biology*. Cambridge,Cambridge University Press.

Bookstein, F.L. (1996). Combining the tools of geometric morphometrics. In *Advances in Morphometrics*, NATO ASI Series A, eds L.F. Marcus, M. Corti, A. Loy, G.J.P. Naylor & D.E. Slice. London, Plenum Press.

Chaplain, M.A.J., Singh G.D., & McLachlan, eds (1999) On growth and form. Spatio-temporal Pattern Formation in Biology. Chichester, John Wiley.

Cole, T.M. (1999). Euclidean Distance Matrix Analysis Computer Program, version 0.1 alpha.

Ferrario, V.F., Sforza, C., Miani, Jr, A. & Serrao, G. (1993). Dental arch asymmetry in young healthy human subjects evaluated by euclidean distance matrix analysis. *Arch. Oral Biol.*, **38:** 189–94.

Illing, H.M., Morris, D.O. & Lee, R.T. (1998). A prospective evaluation of Bass, Bionator & Twin Block appliances. Part 1 – the hard tissues. *Eur. J. Orthod.*, **20:** 501–16.

Lele, S. (1993). Euclidean distance matrix analysis (EDMA): Estimation of mean form AND mean form difference. *Math. Geol.*, **25:** 573–602.

Lele, S. & Richtsmeier, J.T. (1991). Euclidean distance matrix analysis: A co-ordinate free approach for comparing biological shapes. *Am. J. Phys. Anthropol.*, **86:** 415–27.

McDonagh, S., Moss, J.P., Goodwin, P. & Lee, R.T. (2001). A prospective optical surface scanning and cephalometric assessment of the effect of functional appliances on the soft tissues. *Eur. J. Orthod.*, **23:** 115–126.

Moss, J.P., Campos, J.C. & Linney, A.D. (1992). The analysis of profiles using curvature analysis. *Eur. J. Orthod.*, **14:** 457–61.

Nute, S.J. & Moss, J.P. (2000). Three-dimensional facial growth studied by optical surface scanning. *J. Orthod.*, **27:** 31–8.

Rohlf, F.J. (1994). Thin Plate Spline Analysis Computer Program.

Rohlf, F.J. & Slice, D.E. (1991). Generalised Rotational Fit Computer Program, version 1.0

Singh, G.D. & Clark W.J. (2001) Localisation of mandibular changes in patients with Class II Division I malocclusions treated with the Twin-block appliance: finite element scaling analysis. *Am. J. Orthod. Dentofacial Orthop.*, **119 (4)**: 419–425.

Slice, D.E., Bookstein, F.L., Marcus, L.F. & Rohlf, F.J. (1998). A glossary for geometric morphometrics. www.life.bio.sunysb.edu/morph/glossary

Stangl, D.P. (1997). A cephalometric analysis of six Twin Block patients. A study of mandibular (body and ramus) growth and development. *Funct. Orthod.*, **14:** 4–6, 8–14, 17–19.

CHAPTER 24

Growth Response to Twin Block Treatment

INTRODUCTION

by G. David Singh

> *It is the customary fate of new truths to begin as heresies*
> (Thomas Henry Huxley 1825–1895)

After a century of research there is not yet a consensus within the orthodontic specialty regarding the response to functional jaw orthopaedics. Indeed the benefits of functional therapy and the validity of any orthopaedic changes have frequently been questioned in academic circles (Mills, 1991; Johnston, 1996, 1998). One of the objectives of this book is to update information on the effects of Twin Blocks on growth, and to present a summary of studies on this subject. It is imperative that clinical technique has a sound basis in scientific research, rather than relying on the empirical opinions that determined our views in the past. In evaluating the results of treatment it is equally important to take into account limitations imposed by previous methods of investigation and research, and recognise the potential of new technology to improve our understanding, and eventually to resolve philosophical differences, which are often based more on sentiment than on logical analysis.

Throughout the past century orthodontists have expressed different views on the aetiology of malocclusion and this has been reflected in the methods of treatment. A malocclusion is almost always due to some variation in normal growth and development (Proffit, 1985). Class II malocclusion with an increased overjet is unlikely to occur in the absence of skeletal and soft-tissue growth discrepancies. In these Class II cases, the mandible and mandibular dental arch are in a distal relationship to the maxilla; the maxillary incisor teeth are in labioversion (Ast *et al.*, 1968), and the maxilla appears to protrude. In a study of 277 children (8 to 10 year olds) with Class II malocclusions (McNamara, 1981), it was concluded that 50–70% of the Class II population had a skeletal mandibular retrusion. The same study determined that there were more cases of skeletal maxillary retrusion than skeletal

protrusion. This was true regardless of whether the SNA angle or the relationship of point A to the nasion perpendicular to the Frankfort plane was used to assess maxillary position relative to the cranial base.

Treatment philosophy employed in the correction of Class II division 1 malocclusions is governed by the orthodontist's concept of the Class II problem, the possibilities of tooth development and the relationship of growth to treatment (Coben, 1966). To treat this class of malocclusion the molars can be tipped distally to engage the underdeveloped mandible in a normal inclined relationship, thereby attempting to establish functional and muscular stimulation to return the face and occlusion to normal (Coben, 1966), but nevertheless failing to address the fundamental skeletal discrepancy.

During the twentieth century, a common approach to the treatment of a Class II division 1 malocclusion with crowding was to relieve the anterior crowding by extracting premolars and then use the available space to retract and align the maxillary incisors with the mandible. However, this method produces undesired changes in the facial profile in some cases, and orthodontists and patients are becoming more aware of the potential undesirable effects on the facial profile associated with bicuspid extraction. Another approach uses extraoral traction to retract the maxillary dentition into Class I relationship with a distally occluding mandible, thus avoiding premolar extractions. This is often a laboriously slow process which may also produce an unsatisfactory profile, as the nose continues to grow when the dentition is retracted, sometimes resulting in an obtuse naso-labial angle, which is not aesthetically desirable. The other alternative is to use Class II intermaxillary elastics to correct a distal occlusion, but this method produces undesirable anchorage loss in the lower arch, and resulting instability of the lower labial segment. As these disadvantages become more widely realised, many orthodontists prefer a more functional approach (Counihan, 1998).

The purpose of this chapter is to review the status of

current research on growth modification in Twin Block functional appliance therapy. Before considering the results of past and current research the background of development of the technique should be explained.

THE TWIN BLOCK TRACTION TECHNIQUE

The first Twin Block appliances were fitted in 1977 and in the early years of development of the technique the author did not believe it was possible to enhance mandibular growth by functional mandibular advancement, on the basis of the perceived knowledge at that time. Having routinely used extraoral traction for maxillary retraction prior to developing Twin Blocks, the earliest patients were treated by Twin Blocks with the addition of extraoral traction. The Concorde facebow was soon developed to apply functional orthopaedic forces to enhance the action of the inclined planes by a combination of extraoral and intermaxillary traction. The direction of pull could be adapted in vertical growers to intrude the upper posterior teeth. This was an extremely powerful functional orthopaedic mechanism which produced rapid results, and could be used to correct distal occlusion and large overjets, almost irrespective of the mandibular growth response. This mechanism was used in the early patients in the first study. As a result of adding extraoral traction the retraction force on the maxilla was considerably increased. Patients exhibited a characteristic headgear effect with maxillary retraction and autorotation of the mandible in some cases, and potentially undesirable effects on the profile (Clark 1988).

In the first published paper to describe the technique (Clark, 1982), it was observed that the response to treatment varied according to the growth pattern. Patients who were growing strongly exhibited a good mandibular response, while patients who were growing slowly showed more maxillary retraction. The most favourable and sustained mandibular response occurred in boys when treatment coincided with the pubertal growth spurt. In all of the early cases there appeared to be a combination of skeletal and dentoalveolar changes. The dentoalveolar changes appeared to be inversely related to the skeletal adaptation and individual response apparently depended on the growth pattern and the timing of treatment. These early conclusions were reached on the basis of clinical experience, without the benefits of statistical analysis, but subsequent analysis has served to confirm the accuracy of the initial clinical evaluation.

GROWTH RESPONSE TO TWIN BLOCKS WITH TRACTION

The first statistical study was completed in 1985 to investigate the changes occurring in a group of 74 consecutively treated patients with Class II division 1 malocclusion. The sample consisted of 43 girls and 31 boys aged, before treatment, from 9 years 6 months to 14 years. The method of examination was by serial cephalometric analysis before and during treatment, at the end of retention, and on average 18 months out of retention. Where possible patients were followed through to check the long-term results several years out of retention.

Tracings recorded 19 angular and 18 linear measurements to assess a range of craniofacial and dental changes for comparison with control values that relate age to growth changes. Allowance was made for sexual dimorphism in comparison with controls of untreated patients.

Control groups

Two sets of published cephalometric standards were selected as the best available basis for comparison as control values.

Control group 1
An Atlas of Craniofacial Growth
Cephalometric Standards from the University School Growth Study, the University of Michigan: Riolo, M.L., Moyers, R.E., McNamara, J.A. Jr., Stuart Hunter, W. *An Atlas of Craniofacial Growth*. Monograph No. 2. Craniofacial Growth Series, Center for Human Growth and Development, 1979.

This study was based on examination of 83 individuals, 47 males and 36 females, with continuous attendance at the University School from their 6th to 16th birthdays, who were x-rayed on their birthday at yearly intervals.

Magnification
The distance from the x-ray target to the midsagittal plane of the subject was 5 ft (152.25 cm). The distance from the midsagittal plane of the head to the film surface was 7.625 in (17.84 cm). This geometry produces a 12.7% enlargement in all linear measurements reported in this control study.

Control group 2
A Mixed Longitudinal Interdisciplinary Study of Growth and Development
Prahl Anderson, B., Kowalski, C.J., Heydendael, P.H.J.M. *A Mixed Longitudinal Interdisciplinary Study of Growth and Development*. University of Nijmegen, San Francisco Academic Press, 1979.

This control sample examined a group of untreated patients biased towards a Class II dental relationship. This was therefore a more appropriate control sample to use for comparison with a series of patients with Class II malocclusion who received treatment.

Material and method

Cephalometric analysis

Serial cephalometric x-rays were taken at the following intervals:

- Before treatment commenced.
- When the overjet was reduced.
- On completion of stage 1 – the active Twin Block phase.
- On completion of stage 2 – the support phase.
- On completion of stage 3 – retention.
- Post-retention examination, on average 18 months out of retention.

In 57 cases the first x-ray was taken on average 6 weeks before treatment commenced. During that period normal growth occurred. No correction was made for this, and the calculation and summation of growth changes during treatment for statistical analysis includes this short period of normal growth before treatment commenced.

The average time between the first and second x-ray was 7.3 months. That included the 6 weeks pretreatment period in 57 cases. This was equivalent to an average active stage of treatment of 6 months with Twin Blocks in addition to the pretreatment period of 6 weeks.

The control values are based on annual growth increments and in order to allow a direct comparison to be made, radiographs were selected as near as possible to a year after the initial cephalograms. A correction was made to annualise the changes in comparison to the control. On average this includes a period of 7.3 months from the initial cephalogram to the end of the Twin Block phase, followed by 4.7 months of passive support with an anterior inclined plane following the Twin Block stage.

Statistical analysis compared to untreated control samples

The results of analysis were subjected to Students t test, and changes were assessed as follows:
$P < 0.001$ = highly significant (***).
$P < 0.01$ = significant (**).
$P < 0.1$ = significant (*).

Michigan series controls (Group 1)

A comparison with Riolo *et al.*. (1979) control values revealed the following highly significant changes at the level of $P < 0.001$:

1. Reduction of maxillary protrusion by retraction of the A-point.
2. Reduction of anteroposterior skeletal discrepancy by a combination of maxillary retraction and to a lesser degree mandibular advancement.
3. Retraction of the upper incisors.
4. Increase in the interincisal angle.
5. Reduction of convexity by retraction of the A-point relative to the facial plane.

6. Advancement of the lower incisor tip relative to A–Pogonion.
7. Retraction of the upper molars, measured to the pterygoid vertical.
8. Increase in mandibular length, except in the age group 13–13.11.
9. Increase in ramus height, except in ages 11–11.11 and 14–14.11.
10. Increase in facial height, nasion–menton.

Nijmegen series controls (Group 4)

Highly significant changes were noted in the factors compared to controls in the Prahl Anderson series as follows:

1. Reduction of maxillary protrusion by retraction of the A-point.
2. Reduction of anteroposterior skeletal discrepancy by a combination of maxillary retraction and to a lesser degree of mandibular advancement.
3. Retraction of the upper incisors and reduction of the over-jet.
4. Increase in mandibular length in the age group 10–12.5 (articulare–gnathion, Ar–Gn).
5. Increase in facial height (nasion–menton).
6. Increase in the gonial angle, but not throughout the age range. This factor may relate to altered angulation of condylar growth.

Evaluation of mean growth changes

Mandibular growth change in boys

This was assessed by recording the dimension Ar–Gn as follows:

Group 1: Period of treatment
For direct comparison with control values the changes were examined in 31 boys during the first year of treatment (mean age before treatment =11 years 9 months). This represented on average 7.3 months of treatment from the initial cephalogram to the end of the Twin Block stage, followed by 4.76 months of passive support. The mean period examined was 12.06 months, and a slight conversion was made to record the annual change.

Mean before treatment = 109.63 mm.
Mean after treatment = 114.79 mm.
Mean increase in Ar–Gn = 5.16 mm per annum.
Mean annual growth rate of control for this age group = 2.71 mm.
Increased growth compared to control = 2.45 mm.

Group 2: Post-treatment observation period = 27.54 months
Mean at end of treatment = 114.79 mm.

Mean at end of observation = 121.02 mm.

Mean increase in Ar–Gn = 2.71 mm per annum in the period of observation, exactly equivalent to the annual growth rate of the control sample.

Growth in facial height

Period of treatment (boys)

Mean facial height before treatment = 116.90 mm.

Mean facial height after treatment = 123.19 mm.

Increase in facial height during treatment = 6.29 mm.

Mean annual growth rate of control group for this age group = 2.58 mm.

Increased vertical growth in treatment compared to control = 3.71 mm.

Mandibular growth change in girls

A similar calculation was done for 43 girls, mean age before treatment =11.6 years.

Group 1: Period of treatment

Mean before treatment = 106.81 mm.

Mean after treatment = 110.84 mm.

Mean annual increase in Ar–Gn = 4.0 mm.

Mean annual growth rate of control for this age group = 1.83 mm.

Increased growth compared to control = 2.17 mm.

Group 2: Post-treatment observation period = 23.53 months

Mean after treatment =110.84 mm.

Mean after observation = 114.41 mm.

Mean annual increase during observation = 1.89 mm.

Mean annual growth rate for control group for this age group = 1.83 mm.

Growth during the observation period after treatment was exactly equivalent to the mean growth rate of the control sample.

Growth in facial height

Period of treatment (girls)

Mean facial height before treatment = 117.40 mm.

Mean facial height after treatment = 122.33 mm.

Increase in facial height during treatment = 4.93 mm.

Mean increase in control for this age group = 1.16 mm.

Increased vertical growth in treatment compared to control = 3.77 mm.

Evaluation of results

- Small increases (0.7° to 2°) were noted in SNB angle during the Twin Block phase throughout the age range with changes at the level of $P > 0.1$ occurring in the 11 to 13 age group.

- Significant reduction in angle SNA was noted (–0.6° to –3°) in the range of age groups 10–15 years ($P > 0.01$).

- Highly significant reduction in ANB angle (2.3° to 3.2°) in the age range 10–13.5 years ($P > 0.001$) was by a combination of maxillary retraction, and to a lesser degree, mandibular advancement.

- Highly significant vertical changes were recorded in ramus height, and this was reflected in corresponding increases in facial height during treatment.

- Both clinical and statistical evidence indicated that the combined functional orthopaedic approach overcorrected upper incisor angulation and increased the contribution of maxillary retraction in the corrected result. It may be argued that the headgear effect would cause a secondary clockwise rotation of the mandible, thus limiting the increase in the SNB angle.

Discussion

After completing this study the author concluded that the addition of extraoral traction limited mandibular advancement and resulted in overcorrection of upper incisor angulation and maxillary retraction. Subsequently the technique was used without extraoral traction, except in cases with significant maxillary protrusion, where maxillary retraction may be indicated, or in vertical growth where high pull traction may be indicated to intrude upper posterior teeth. Clinical experience subsequently confirmed that in most cases correction of Class II malocclusion could be achieved without extraoral traction.

In addition it was realised that a labial bow is not normally required to retract the upper incisors as the development of a lip seal has the effect of uprighting the incisors. The use of a labial bow was now only indicated to control severely proclined and spaced incisors, and for patients with anterior open bite where incisor retraction was required. More emphasis was now placed on advancing retroclined incisors to enhance the response to functional mandibular protrusion.

It should not be expected that all patients who undergo functional therapy will show increased mandibular growth compared to the norm for their age. Some patients grow at a rate less than the norm while others exceed the normal rate of growth, with or without functional therapy. A lack of growth response may be related to the level of endocrine activity that prevails at the time of treatment. If treatment occurs during a resting phase of growth, the potential for increased mandibular growth is more limited.

As stated in Newton's third law of motion: 'To every action there is an equal and opposite reaction'. Functional appliances, therefore, exert equal and opposite forces in the opposing dental arch and have the reciprocal effect of restricting the forward component of maxillary growth. If a patient grows slowly during treatment, functional mandibular protrusion is more likely to retract the maxilla than advance the mandible.

On the question of the timing of treatment, Enlow (1983) stresses that 'the utilization of the pubertal growth spurt is coming rather late'. This observation applies especially to the treatment of Class II division 1 malocclusion where prominent upper incisors are vulnerable to trauma, and early treatment may be indicated after the eruption of permanent incisors. Class III malocclusion also responds to early intervention in the deciduous or mixed dentition, when the addition of forward pull traction to a facemask may be considered to increase the potential for maxillary advancement.

It is especially important to treat girls early because growth slows considerably after menstruation commences. There is more leeway in boys, who mature later and still show useful growth in their middle and late teens. As a general principle the response to treatment is related directly to the patient's rate of growth. Therefore, after the mid-teenage years, the older the patient the less growth we should expect and we should not presume growth changes in adults. But this does not preclude muscular advancement of retruded mandibles in adults with functional appliances, which may be indicated if

the condyles are displaced posteriorly or superiorly in the glenoid fossae.

The best growth response is to be expected when treatment coincides with the pubertal growth spurt, and a comparison of early and late treatment follows later in this chapter.

A further cephalometric study, completed in 1995, compared a larger group of patients treated with Twin Blocks with a group of patients treated with fixed appliances, in order to compare the growth response.

TWIN BLOCKS VS FIXED APPLIANCES

A statistical comparison was made of two groups of consecutively treated patients, both treated by the author in his orthodontic practice (Clark, 1998). A group of 138 Twin Block patients had an average treatment time of 13 months (Fig. 24.1) followed by 6 months of retention. A group of 30 patients received an average of 27 months of treatment with fixed appliances (Fig. 24.2), followed by 12 months of retention. In order to confirm that the improvements registered in

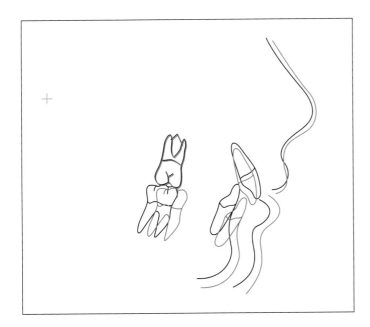

T₁–T₂ = 13 months	T/B n=138	Age 11y 9m	Age 12y 10m	Difference
Cranial Base length Ba–Na		111.9	113.7	1.8
Maxillary length Ba–A		100.7	101.4	0.7
Mandibular length Ba–Pg		108.4	113.4	5.0

Average treatment time: 13 months. Twin Blocks.

Fig. 24.1

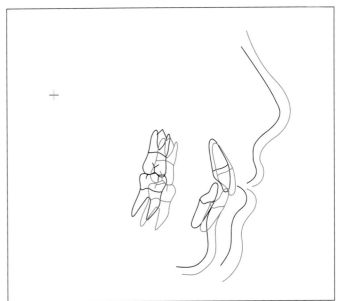

T₁–T₂ = 27 months	Fixed n=30	Age 11y 9m	Age 14y 1m	Difference
Cranial Base length Ba–Na		107.5	111	3.5
Maxillary length Ba–A		96	98.4	2.4
Mandibular length Ba–Pg		107.4	112.9	5.5

Average treatment time: 2 years 3 months. Fixed appliances.

Fig. 24.2

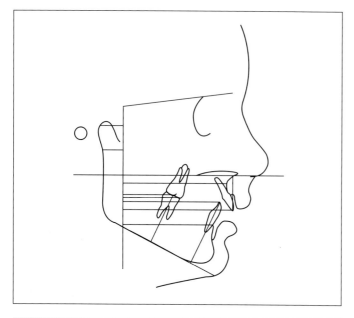

T₁–T₃ = 33 months	T/B n=51	Age 11y 4m	Age 14y 1m	Difference
Cranial Base length	Ba–Na	110.8	114.8	4.0
Maxillary length	Ba–A	100.5	102.9	2.4
Mandibular length	Ba–Pg	107.1	115.4	8.3

Period of treatment and observation: 33 months. Twin Blocks.

Fig. 24.3 Custom analysis used by Mills and McCulloch to measure horizontal distances from skeletal and dental landmarks to a vertical reference plane constructed through sella and perpendicular to the palatal plane.

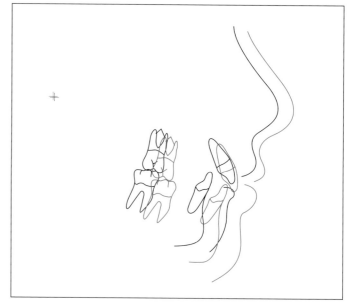

T₁–T₄ = 33 months	T/B n=22	Age 10y 9m	Age 15y 3m	Difference
Cranial Base length	Ba–Na	111.0	116.4	5.4
Maxillary length	Ba–A	100.4	104.4	4.0
Mandibular length	Ba–Pg	105.9	116.7	10.8

Period of treatment and observation: 54 months. Fixed appliances.

Fig. 24.4

mandibular growth were maintained, 51 of the original group of Twin Block patients were reviewed after 33 months (Fig. 24.3), and 22 patients after 54 months (Fig. 24.4).

The Twin Block group was severe Class II with an average convexity of 5.4 mm, an overjet of 10.5 mm and a full unit distal occlusion. The fixed appliance group was mild Class II with a mean convexity of 3.9 mm, an overjet of 6.2 mm and a cusp to cusp molar relationship.

The point basion was selected to measure the comparative lengths of the cranial base (Ba–Na), maxilla (Ba–A) and mandible (Ba–Pg), and to register changes observed. This method of measurement may make allowance for positional change in the mandible, rather than incremental change in the length of the mandible.

Maxillary length, mandibular length and maxillo-mandibular difference were compared before and after treatment. Before treatment maxillary length was slightly less in the fixed appliance group compared to the Twin Block group, while mandibular length was almost identical.

During treatment of the fixed appliance group the mandibular length increased by 3.5 mm, compared to

4.4 mm in the Twin Block group. Significantly, however, the fixed appliance treatment extended over a period of 2 years 3 months, compared to 13 months of Twin Block treatment. During the period of treatment the rate of mandibular growth in Twin Block treatment was double that observed during fixed appliance treatment. This accounts for the faster correction in the Twin Block group of the more severe malocclusions compared to the milder skeletal and occlusal corrections in the fixed appliance group. The more severe malocclusions were corrected more quickly, and the improvement observed in mandibular length was maintained by additional growth increments compared to the maxillary length and cranial base length on further evaluation out of retention at 20 months and 41 months after completion of Twin Block treatment.

As indicated earlier in this chapter a previous study of patients treated with Twin Blocks reinforced by extraoral and intermaxillary traction confirmed that mandibular growth during an observation period of approximately 2 years after completion of the Twin Block phase of treatment was exactly equivalent to the mean growth rate of the control sample.

	Control	Mills	Leishman	Kluzak	Clark
Mx length increase	1.9	1.5	1.2	1.5	1.4
Md length increase	2.3	6.5	7.3	5.6	6.3
Md length gain	0.4	5	6.1	4.1	4.9

Table 24.1 A comparision of cephalometric studies.

In view of the differing opinions expressed in the literature regarding the effectiveness of a functional orthopaedic approach to treatment, it is important to establish the consistency of the growth response achieved by a full-time functional appliance. Data were collected from a number of sources to record the cephalometric changes in patients treated consecutively by the Twin Block technique. The patients were treated by the following practitioners, all of whom are experienced in Twin Block technique, and have contributed examples of clinical technique in previous chapters in this book.

- Mills – Canada.
- Leishman – New Zealand.
- Kluzak – Canada.
- Clark – Scotland.

Table 24.1 illustrates the mean changes in maxillary and mandibular length, and the gain in mandibular length compared to maxillary length during Twin Block treatment.

It is significant that Leishman's group had the largest overjets, and Kluzak's group the smallest overjets. In addition Leishman's appliance design incorporates blocks of 7 mm thickness in the first premolar region. It may therefore be observed that the mandibular growth response is related to the size of the overjet, and to the amount of anterior and vertical activation built into the appliance. To compensate for these factors in the treatment of patients with overjets smaller than 9 mm, overactivation may sometimes be indicated, either by advancing the mandible beyond an edge-to-edge incisor relationship, or by modifying the thickness of the occlusal blocks to increase the vertical activation.

BASS, BIONATOR, TWIN BLOCKS AND CONTROLS

A prospective cephalometric evaluation of Bass, Bionator and Twin Block appliances compared to an untreated control group was carried out at the Royal London Hospital (Illing *et al.*, 1998). The study concluded:

- All the functional appliances produced a measureable change in the skeletal and dentoalveolar tissues, with the untreated sample showing minimal change due to growth alone.
- The appliance groups all demonstrated a forward

movement of pogonion and a more pronounced downward movement of menton in comparison with the control group. The anterior movement of the mandible was greatest in the Twin Block group, followed by the Bass and Bionator groups, respectively.

- Highly statistically significant increases in lower anterior face height ($P < 0.01$) were found between all the appliance groups and the control group. This was the most marked facial change in the study.
- The Twin Block and Bionator groups showed highly significant increases in total face height ($P < 0.01$), suggesting that the Bass appliance, by incorporating headgear, is effective in limiting the vertical development of the maxilla.
- The Twin Block group demonstrated greater restriction of anterior movement of A-point than the Bass group. Highly significant reduction of ANB compared with Bass and controls may be attributed to rotation of the maxillary plane observed in the Twin Block group.

TWIN BLOCKS AND MATCHED NORMATIVE GROWTH DATA

In a comparative study with matched controls Trenouth (2000) found an increase in mandibular length of 7.19 mm (Co–Po) compared to 4.0 mm in controls. This study concluded that the Twin Block appliance not only results in forward positioning of the mandible, but also lengthening as shown by linear measurements. By comparison, restraint of maxillary growth was shown to be purely minimal and not clinically significant. The correction of Class II dental base relationship was greater than that reported for the Andresen and Frankel appliances and comparable to that reported for the Herbst appliance.

TWIN BLOCKS, FR-2 AND CONTROLS

A comparison of the Twin Block appliance and the FR-2 appliance of Frankel (Toth and McNamara, 1999) came to the following conclusions. Statistically significant increases in mandibular length were observed in both treated groups (Table 24.2). The Twin Block appliance achieved an additional 3.0 mm of mandibular length, whereas the Frankel

	Control	Frankel	Twin Block
Md length increase	2.7	4.6	5.7
Md length gain		1.9	3

Table 24.2 Comparision of the Twin Block appliance and the FR-2 appliance of Frankel.

group increased 1.9 mm more than did the controls. No significant restriction in maxillary length was observed in either functional appliance group relative to controls.

A significant increase in lower anterior face height was evident in both treated groups. Vertical increase in the Twin Block patients was significantly greater than in the FR-2 group. In general, more extensive dentoalveolar adaptation was observed with the tooth-borne Twin Block appliance than with the more tissue-borne FR-2. Both samples showed significant retroclination and extrusion (eruption) of the maxillary incisors. The Twin Block patients also exhibited distal movement of the upper molars; however there was no extrusion. Slight lower incisor proclination was noted in both treatment groups, and lower molar extrusion was found to be significantly greater in the Twin Block group compared with the other two samples. No horizontal differences were detected in the lower molars among groups.

It was concluded that Class II correction with the Twin Block appliance is achieved through normal growth in addition to mandibular skeletal and dentoalveolar changes. Class II correction with the FR-2 is more skeletal in nature, with less dentoalveolar change.

TWIN BLOCK APPLIANCE TREATMENT EFFECTS

The following account is based on studies by Mills and McCulloch (1998) to investigate the growth response during Twin Block treatment, with a follow-up to examine post-treatment changes.

A contribution by Christine Mills is the source of a summary of the findings reported here, while the published articles provide a comprehensive account.

Methods and materials

A comparison was made between a sample of 28 consecutively treated patients (11 boys and 17 girls) and matched controls selected from the Burlington study. All of the patients were in the mixed dentition stage of development, had an angle ANB difference of 5° or more, and a full cusp Class II molar relationship on one side and an end-to-end or greater Class II molar relationship on the other side. The mean age and sex distribution of this control group was identical to that of the Twin Block treatment group. In addition, the controls were matched to the treatment group with respect to the vertical facial pattern.

Statistical analysis

Detailed statistical analysis involved the calculation of means and standard deviations for the 31 cephalometric variables.

When the composite tracings of the two groups were superimposed the maxillary structures were almost identical, but due to the difficulty in finding severe skeletal Class II individuals for the control group, the mandibles in the Twin Block treatment group were considerably more retrognathic at the initial observation time (T1) than the mandibles of the control group.

Treatment effects on the maxilla

The Twin Block appliance had an inhibiting effect on the growth of the maxilla as evidenced by a 0.9° decrease in angle SNA as compared to a 0.1° increase in angle SNA in the untreated control group.

Treatment effects on the mandible

The mandibular unit length (as measured from condylion to gnathion) increased nearly three times as much in the Twin Block group as in the controls. Approximately two thirds of the overall increase in mandibular length in the treatment group can be attributed to an increase in mandibular ramus height (Table 24.3).

These mandibular growth changes in turn account for a 1.9° increase in angle SNB in the treatment group as compared to only a 0.3° increase in the untreated control group.

Dentoalveolar changes

In spite of the fact that no labial bows were used on any of the Twin Block appliances in this study, there was nevertheless an uprighting effect on the upper incisors.

The lower incisors proclined 5.2° in the Twin Block group compared to 1.4° in the control group (Table 24.4). Although this labial tipping of the lower incisors contributes somewhat

	Control	Twin Block	Twin Block gain
Md length increase	2.3	6.5	4
Ramus height	1.2	4.1	2.9
Md Corpus (Go-Gn)	1.7	3	1.3
SNB Angle	0.3°	1.9°	1.6°

Table 24.3 Treatment effects on the mandible.

	Controls	Twin Block
Upper incisors	+0.2°	-2.5°
Lower incisors	+1.4°	+5.2°
Overjet	+0.3 mm	-5.6 mm

Table 24.4 Dentoalveolar changes.

to the 5.6 mm of overjet correction that occurred in the Twin Block group, nearly two thirds of the overjet correction was accounted for by forward growth of the mandible (Fig. 24.5A). The overjet change in the control group was minimal.

In the Twin Block treatment group the net reduction in the Class II molar relationship was 6.2 mm compared to a reduction of only 0.4 mm in the control group. Approximately 50% of the molar correction was accomplished by skeletal improvement in the lower jaw and 50% by dentoalveolar change in the upper and lower molars (Fig. 24.5B).

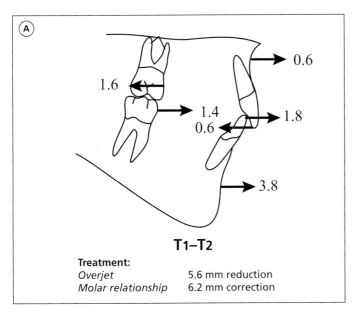

T1–T2

Treatment:
Overjet — 5.6 mm reduction
Molar relationship — 6.2 mm correction

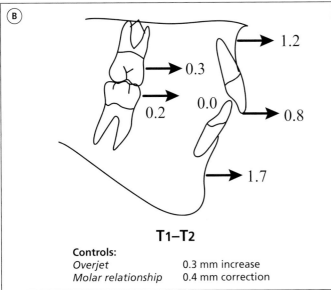

T1–T2

Controls:
Overjet — 0.3 mm increase
Molar relationship — 0.4 mm correction

Fig. 24.5 A, B Skeletal and dental changes in the (**A**) Twin Block treatment group between T1 and T2 and (**B**) in the control group between T1 and T2

POST-TREATMENT STABILITY

To better understand the impact of this appliance on growth and development over the long term, the patients from the Twin Block study outlined above were followed for approximately 3 years post-treatment (Mills & McCulloch, 2000).

Methods and materials

Of the original sample of 28 consecutively treated severe skeletal Class II patients (mean age at start of treatment 9 years 1 month), a total of 26 individuals were available for follow-up cephalometric tracings at a mean age of 13 years 1 month (T3). Of these 26 patients, 11 were males and 15 were females.

A comparison group of 24 Class II individuals (11 males, 13 females) obtained from the Burlington group provided data for the control group. This control group had a mean age of 9 years 1 month at the time of the initial observation (T1) and 12 years 11 months at the time of the final follow-up cephalometric tracing (T3).

Results

A study was completed of 31 cephalometric variables to assess post-treatment changes in the Twin Block group compared to untreated Class II controls. Only five of the 31 variables showed statistically significant differences between the two groups when Student's t-tests were used to compare rates of change.

Of the five variables showing statistically significant differences, four were dental measurements. The only skeletal variable that showed a statistically significant difference in growth rate during the post-treatment follow-up was the ramus height as measured from condylion to gonion (Co–Go).

Maxillary changes post-treatment
None of the three cephalometric variables used to assess maxillary growth showed any statistically significant differences in the post-treatment phase. However, there was a trend toward reduced forward growth of the maxilla in the Twin Block group from T2 to T3. The measurements for angle SNA, maxillary unit length (Co–SubANS) and the horizontal distance from point A to the vertical reference plane, all suggest that slightly less forward maxillary growth was taking place in the Twin Block group than in the untreated controls at the same age.

	Control	Twin Block		
Md length increase	6.7	6	0.7	Control gain
Ramus height	4.3	2.7	1.6	Control gain
Md Corpus (Go-Gn)	4.5	5.2	0.7	Twin Block gain
SNB Angle	0.6°	0.3°	0.3°	Control gain

Table 24.5 Mandibular changes post-treatment.

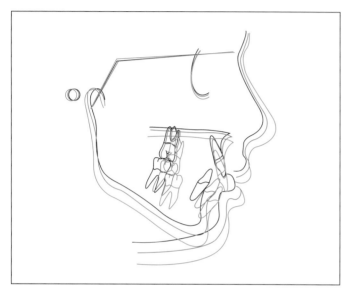 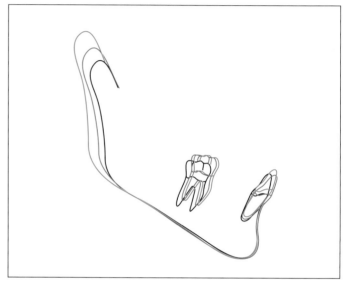

Fig. 24.6 Twin Block Treatment: T1 – 9 years, 1 month; T2 – 10 years 3 months; T3 – 13 years, 1 month. Controls: T1 – 9 years, 1 month; T2 – 10 years 2 months; T3 – 12 years, 11 months.

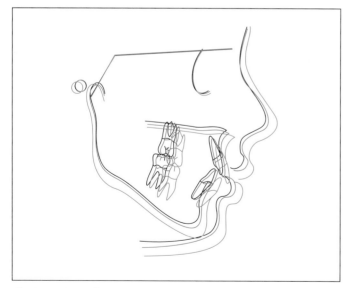 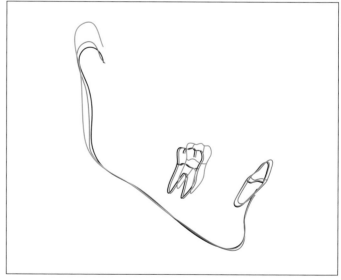

Fig. 24.7 Controls: T1 – 9 years, 1 month; T2 – 10 years 2 months; T3 – 12 years, 11 months. Treatment: T1 – 9 years, 1 month; T2 – 10 years 2 months; T3 – 13 years, 1 month.

Mandibular changes post-treatment (Table 24.5)

Most of the mandibular changes in the Twin Block group during the post-treatment phase indicate a tendency toward reduction of the growth rate compared to the controls. However, only one of the variables used to assess mandibular growth changes in this study showed a significant difference between the two groups. This variable was the ramus height as measured from condylion to gonion (Co–Go). In the 3 years post-treatment, this measurement increased 2.7 mm on average in the Twin Block group and 4.3 mm on average in the control group. The net 1.6 mm difference was statistically significant at the $P < 0.05$ level.

A decline in growth rate in the mandibular unit length of 0.7 mm in the Twin Block group compared to the controls is compensated by a corresponding increase in corpus length of the same amount. Although this difference was not statistically significant, it may have the effect of offsetting some of the rebound seen elsewhere in the mandible so that the net change in Angle SNB is not much different in the two groups (0.3°).

Dental changes post-treatment

The greatest differences between the Twin Block and control groups in the T2–T3 phase were seen in the molar and incisor measurements. In particular, there was an uprighting tendency for the lower incisors in the Twin Block group.

The net residual proclination of the lower incisors in the Twin Block group compared to the control group was thus only 1.7°.

The upper incisors showed some tendency to rebound as well but this difference in response was not statistically significant.

These changes in incisor angulations contributed an increase in overjet of 1.0 mm on average in the Twin Block group compared to a slight decrease (–0.1 mm) in the controls. This difference was statistically significant at the $P < 0.01$ level of confidence.

The molar relationship as measured in the sagittal plane showed a mean relapse of 1.2 mm in the Twin Block group as compared to almost no change (0.1 mm) in the control group ($P < 0.05$).

- The Twin Block appliance as used in this study provided mandibular growth increments greater in magnitude than those obtained with other removable functional appliances described in the literature. In addition, the direction of the mandibular growth was favourable and thus contributed substantially to the anteroposterior skeletal correction.
- Johnston (1996, 1998) has suggested that functional appliances work temporarily by using up the mandibular growth potential in advance. In fact, he proposes that there is a limited or preordained amount of mandibular growth that can occur in any particular patient.
- By contrast, the present study indicates that much of the gain in mandibular length achieved during the active treatment with the Twin Block appliance was maintained 3 years later (Fig. 24.6). When compared post-treatment, the Twin Block and control group experienced similar growth characteristics in the mandible (Figs 24.7–24.9).

Conclusions

This study has shown that the Twin Block appliance can achieve substantial skeletal improvement in young growing Class II individuals. Much of this skeletal improvement is related to increases in mandibular length and these changes are, for the most part, stable 3 years post-treatment.

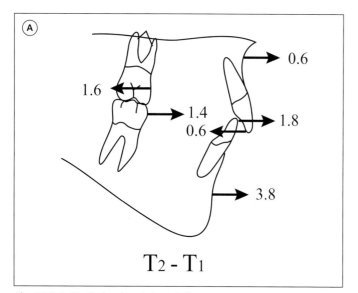

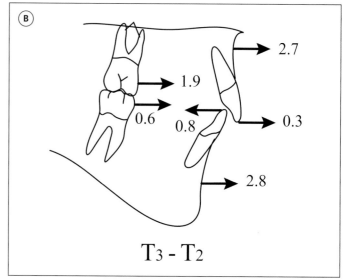

Fig. 24.8 A, B Skeletal and dental changes in the Twin Block treatment group during active treatment (T1–T2) and following treatment (T2–T3).

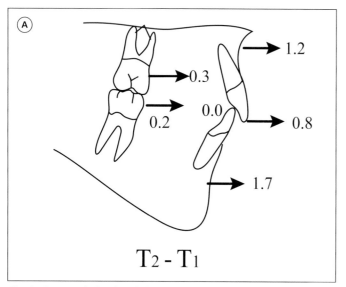

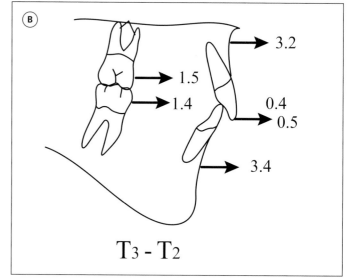

Fig. 24.9 A, B Skeletal and dental changes in the untreated Class II control group from ages 9 years 1 month to 10 years 2 months (T1–T2) and from age 10 years 2 months to 12 years 11 months (T2–T3).

TWIN BLOCK THERAPY TREATMENT TIMING

The following report is based on a published paper by Franchi *et al.* (2000a) on the subject of treatment timing in Twin Block therapy.

This cephalometric study evaluated skeletal and dentoalveolar changes induced by the Twin Block appliance in two groups of subjects with Class II malocclusion treated at different skeletal maturation stages (before and during the pubertal peak in mandibular growth) in order to define the optimal timing for this type of therapy. Skeletal maturity in individual patients was assessed on the basis of the stages of cervical vertebrae maturation. The method of determining skeletal maturity is described in detail in a published article referring to this study.

The findings of this short-term cephalometric study indicate that optimal timing for Twin Block therapy of Class II disharmony is during or slightly after the onset of the pubertal peak in growth velocity. When compared with treatment performed before the peak, late Twin Block treatment produces more favourable effects that include:

- Greater skeletal contribution to molar correction.
- Larger increments in total mandibular length and in ramus height.
- More posterior direction of condylar growth, leading to enhanced mandibular lengthening and to reduced forward displacement of the condyle in favor of effective skeletal changes.
- The importance of the biological evaluation of skeletal maturity in individual patients with Class II disharmony to be treated with functional appliances is emphasized.

Late treatment with the Twin Block starting during or slightly after the onset of the peak in mandibular growth appears to be more effective than early treatment, as it induces more favourable mandibular skeletal modifications.

Supplementary elongation of the mandible compared to controls (Table 24.6)

The amount of supplementary elongation of the mandible in the late-treated group was more than twice that of the early-treated group.

The greater additional growth of the mandible in the

late-treated group was concomitant with significant changes in the direction of condylar growth. Late-treated individuals showed significantly more backward direction of growth in the mandibular condyle, as revealed by the significant opening of the angle formed by the condylar line in relation to the mandibular line (cl–ml, 2.8°/year). This growth modification has been described previously as 'posterior mandibular morphogenetic rotation' (Lavergne & Gasson, 1977), a biological mechanism leading to greater increments in total mandibular length and, thus, efficiently improving the skeletal sagittal relationships in Class II malocclusion.

Further investigation, however, is needed in order to clarify the role of glenoid fossa modifications following protrusive mandibular function in groups treated at different stages of skeletal maturation.

Comparison of Herbst and Twin Block (Table 24.7)

Due to the similarity in skeletal maturation at the start of treatment and in the nature of control groups, the results of the present study with regard to the late-treated group can be contrasted with the effects induced by the acrylic splint Herbst appliance as analysed in a previous investigation by the authors of this study. Twin Block therapy is able to produce greater increments in mandibular length and in the height of the mandibular ramus (Franchi *et al.*, 2000b).

Comparison of Frankel and Twin Block (Table 24.8)

Of some interest also is the comparison of the Twin Block treatment results with those produced by the Fränkel appliance by McNamara (1981).

Although the significance of a direct comparison among different appliances in separated investigations is limited by a series of factors, two major considerations may still be deducted:

- The assessment of the growth potential and of the stage of skeletal maturation in individual patients definitely is important for treatment effectiveness, regardless of the

Increase (mm/year)	Herbst	Twin Block
Mandibular length	2.7	8
Ramus height	1.2	2.7

Table 24.7 Comparison of Herbst and Twin Block

Gain vs controls mm/year	Early treatment	Late treatment
Mandibular length (Co–Pg)	1.88	4.75
Ramus height (Co–Go)	N.S.	2.73
Corpus height (Co–Pg)	N.S.	1.66

Table 24.6 Supplementary elongation of the mandible compared to controls

Supplementary Bi-annual increments of growth with Twin Blocks vs Frankel	
Mandibular length	3.6 mm/2 years
Ramus height	3.1 mm/2 years

Table 24.8 Comparison of Frankel and Twin Block

functional/orthopaedic appliance that is used to correct the skeletal disharmony.

- Both the Twin Block and the FR-2 appear to be more effective in inducing supplementary mandibular lengthening than the acrylic splint Herbst appliance.

Summary

Optimum treatment timing for Twin Block therapy of Class II disharmony appears to be during or slightly after the onset of the pubertal peak in growth velocity. Major favourable effects induced by functional therapy at this time in comparison with earlier phases are:

- Greater skeletal contribution to the correction of the molar relation.
- Larger and clinically significant increments in total mandibular length and in ramus height.
- More posterior direction of condylar growth, a biological mechanism enhancing supplementary mandibular lengthening and reducing the amount of forward condylar displacement in favour of effective mandibular growth and reshaping.

Conclusion

As stated in the Preface, the purpose of this book is to advance the recognition of dentofacial orthopaedics as the treatment of choice for correction of malocclusion that results from abnormal skeletal developments. As new information becomes available from research, philosophical differences expressed in the past will surely be resolved in the application of dentofacial orthopaedics.

Time's Glory is to calm contending kings
to unmask falsehood and bring truth to light
The Rape of Lucretia
(William Shakespeare 1564–1616)

In the pursuit of ideals in orthodontics, facial balance and harmony are of equal importance to dental and occlusal perfection. We cannot afford to ignore the importance of orthopaedic techniques in achieving these goals by growth guidance during the formative years of facial and dental development.

At the dawn of a new century, the integration of orthodontic and orthopaedic techniques offers a new challenge in restoring facial balance for patients who present skeletal growth discrepancies.

To catch dame Fortune's golden smile
Assiduous wait upon her,
And gather gear for ev'ry wile,
That's justified by honour.
Epistle to a young friend
(Robert Burns 1759–1796)

REFERENCES

Ast D.B., Carlos J.P., Cons N.C. (1965). The prevalence and characteristics of malocclusion among senior high school students in upstate New York. *Am. J. Orthod.*, **51**: 437–445.

Clark, W.J. (1982). The Twin Block Traction Technique. *Eur. J. Orthod.*, **4**: 129–38.

Clark, W.J. (1998). The Twin Block Technique: a functional orthodontic appliance system. *Am. J. Orthod. Dentofac. Orthop.*, **93**: 1–18.

Coben, E.S. (1966). Growth and Class II treatment. *Am. J. Orthod.* **52**: 5–26.

Enlow, D.H. (1983). Enlow on craniofacial growth. ICO interviews. *ICO*, **17**: 669–79.

Franchi, L., Baccetti, T., & McNamara, J.A., Jr. (2000a). Treatment timing for Twin-block therapy. *Am. J. Orthod. Dentofac. Orthop.*, **118**: 159–70.

Franchi, L., Baccetti, T. & McNamara, J.A., Jr (2000b). Mandibular growth and cervical vertebrae maturation and body height. *Am. J. Orthod. Dentofac. Orthop.*, **118**: 335–40.

Illing, H.M., Morris, D.O. & Lee, R.T. (1998). A prospective evaluation of Bass, Bionator and Twin Block appliances. Part 1 – the hard tissues. *Eur. J. Orthod.*, **20**: 501–24.

Johnston, L.E., Jr (1996). Functional appliances: a mortgage on mandibular position. *Austral. Orthod. J.*, **14**: 154–6.

Johnston, L.E., Jr (1998). Early and often: growing jaws for fun and profit. In: *Salzmann Lecture, 98th Annual Session of the American Association of Orthodontists, San Diego.*

Lavergne, J. & Gasson, N. (1977). Operational definitions of mandibular morphogenetic and positional rotations. *Scand. J. Dent. Res.*, **85**: 185–92.

Lund, D.I. & Sandler, P.J. (1998). The effects of Twin Blocks: a prospective controlled study. *Am. J. Orthod. Dentofac. Orthop.*, **113**: 104–10.

McNamara, J.A. Jr. (1981). Components of Class II malocclusion in children 8–10 years of age. *Angle Orthod.*, **51**: 177–202.

Mills, C.M. & McCulloch, K.J. (1998). Treatment effects of the Twin Block appliance: a cephalometric study. *Am. J. Orthod. Dentofac. Orthop.*, **114**: 15–24.

Mills, C.M. & McCulloch, K.J. (2000). Post treatment changes following successful correction of Class II malocclusions with the Twin Block appliance. *Am. J. Orthod. Dentofac. Orthop.*, **118**: 24–33.

Mills, J.R.E. (1991). The effect of functional appliances on the skeletal pattern. *Br. J. Orthod.*, **18**: 267–75.

Prahl Anderson, B. Kowalski, C.J. & Heydendael, P.H.J.M. (1979). A mixed longitudinal interdisciplinary study of growth and development. University of Nijmegen, San Francisco Academic Press.

Proffit W.R. (1986). On the aetiology of malocclusion. *Br. J. Orthod.* **13 (1):** 1–11.

Riolo, M.L., Moyers, R.E., McNamara, J.A., Jr. & Stuart Hunter, W. (1979). An atlas of cranofacial growth. Monograph No. 2. Craniofacial Growth Series. University of Michigan, Center for Human Growth and Development.

Toth, L.R. & McNamara, J.A., Jr. (1999). Treatment effects produced by the Twin-block appliance and the Fr-2 appliance of Frankel compared with an untreated Class II sample. *Am. J. Orthod. Dentofac. Orthop.*, **116:** 597–609.

Trenouth, M.J. (2000). Cephalometric evaluation of the Twin-block appliance in the treatment of Class II division 1 malocclusion with matched normative growth data. *Am. J. Orthod. Dentofac. Orthop.*, **117:** 54–9.

FURTHER READING

Carmichael, G.J., Banks, P.A. & Chadwick, S.M. (1999). A modification to enable progressive advancement of the Twin Block appliance. *Br. J. Orthod.*, **26:** 9–13.

Chadwick, S.M., Banks, P. & Wright, J.L. (1998). The use of myofunctional appliances in the UK: a survey of British orthodontists. *Dent. Update* **25:** 302–8.

Lund, D.I. & Sandler, P.J. (1998). The effects of Twin Blocks: a prospective controlled study. *Am. J. Orthod. Dentofac. Orthop.*, **113:** 104–10.

Petrovic, A, Stutzmann, J. & Lavergne, J. (1990). Mechanism of craniofacial growth and modus operandi of functional appliances: a cell-level and cybernetic approach to orthodontic decision making. In *Craniofacial Growth Theory and Orthodontic Treatment*, ed. D.S. Carlson. Craniofacial Growth Monograph series, Vol. 23. Ann Arbor, Center for Human Growth and Development, The University of Michigan.

Turner, M. & Guiltan, A.S. (1999). Comparison of the effects of monobloc and twin-block appliances on the skeletal and dentoalveolar structures. *Am. J. Orthod. Dentofac. Orthop.*, **116:** 460–8.

List of recommended Orthodontic Laboratories

Laboratory Construction is a very important factor in the successful application of Twin Block therapy. For many years the author has made a point of working with the best orthodontic laboratories wherever possible in order to ensure that their technicians are correctly trained in the design and construction of Twin Block appliances. The following licensed laboratories are recommended to construct Twin Blocks.

USA

Allesee Orthodontic Appliances Inc.
13931 Spring Street
PO Box 725
Sturtevant, WI 53177
Tel: ++1 414 886 1050

Dental Services Group
5775 Wayzata Blvd., Suite 670
Minneapolis, MN 55416

Dockstader Ortho Lab, Inc.
340 West Cromwell, Suite 102
Fresno, CA 93711
Tel: ++1 559 439 5160

Dynaflex
PO Box 142399
St Louis, MO 63114-0399
Tel: ++1 314 426 4020; Fax: ++1 314 429 7575

E.M. Ortho Lab, Inc.
6 Lafayette Place,
Waldwick NJ 07463
Tel: ++1 201 652 4411

Great Lakes Orhodontics Ltd
200 Cooper Avenue
Tonawanda, NY 14150
Tel: ++1 800 828 7626

John's Dental Laboratories
423 South 13th Street
PO Box 606
Terre Haute, IN 47808
Tel: ++1 812 232 6026; Fax: ++1 812 234 4464

North Star
Industrial Park
PO Box 146
Park Rapids, MN 56470
Tel: ++1 218 732 9503 or 880 346 0011; Fax: ++1 218 732 1372

Ohlendorf Company
2840 Clark Avenue
PO Box 7212
St Louis, MO 63103
Tel ++1 314 533 3440; Fax: ++1 314 533 7331

Ortho Technology Inc.
PO Box 4871
Houston, TX 77210 9649
Or 5524 Cornish
Houston, TX 77007 4304
Tel : ++1 713 861 0033

Space Maintainers
PO Box 4184
9129 Lurline Av.
Chatsworth, CA 91311
Tel: ++1 818 998 7460; Fax: ++1 818 341 4684

Specialty Appliances
PO Box 105224
1670 Oakbrook Dr., Suite 390,
Norcross, Atlanta GA 30348
Tel: ++1 770 416 1822; Fax: ++1 770 446 6958

AUSTRALIA

Ortholab
50 Garden Street
South Yarra
Victoria 3141
Tel: ++61 3 9826 0088; Fax: ++61 3 9826 9661

BELGIUM

Cordie Orthodontie CV
Holstraat 70 8790 Waregem
Tel: ++32 (0) 56 60 66 46; Fax: ++32 (0) 56 61 52 64

THE NETHERLANDS

Laboratorium Bosboom
Herenstraat 99
3431 CB Neuwegein
Tel: ++31 30 603 3645; Fax; ++31 30 605 2295

Ortholab. B.V.
Dorpsplein 8
Postbus 65
3940 A B Dourn
Tel: ++31 343 415441; Fax: ++31 343
416403

ITALY

Napoli Ortodonzia,
80128 Napoli
Via Mariano D'Amelio 80
Tel/Fax: ++39 081 241 1966

Sergio Postir
Laboratorio Ortodonzia
34133 Trieste
Via C Beccana 7
Tel: ++39 040 362830; Fax: ++39 040
369147

Gruppo Europeo di Ortodonzia
Via Gasperina 217/219/221
00173 Roma
Tel: ++39 06 72671754; Fax: ++39 06
72675490

Or T. Italia
Via F. Illi Saugo
2 – 36016 Thiene (VI)
Tel: ++39 0443 380523; Fax: ++39 0443
376161

MEXICO

Labok – Dental Kawasaki Dental
Martires Iriandeses #120
Col. Parques San Andres
CP 04040
Mexico City
Tel: ++52 55 5689 4982; Fax: ++52 55
5336 0317

SPAIN

Ortobao – C/. Hurtado de Amezaga
no. 27
48008 Bilbao
Tel: ++34 94 421 80 19; Fax: ++34 94
421 73 90

LICENSE PENDING

GERMANY

TB Alink
Sieringhoeker Weg 17
48450 Bad Bentheim
And Postfach 1164
48442 Bad Bentheim
Tel: ++49 5924 785900; Fax: ++49 5924
7859090

Dr Hinz Dental – Vertriebages
Mbh & Co. Kg
Friedrich der Grope 64
44628 Herne

International Straightwire
BahnofStrase 40,
48599 Gronau,
Tel: ++49 5924 785920

Further licenses are pending for laboratories in Portugal.

Index